SPORT AND EXERCISE PSYCHOLOGY RESEARCH ADVANCES

SPORT AND EXERCISE PSYCHOLOGY RESEARCH ADVANCES

MARTIN P. SIMMONS AND LIMAN A. FOSTER
EDITORS

Nova Biomedical Books
New York

NOTICE TO THE READER

The Publisher has taken reasonable care in the preparation of this book, but makes no expressed or implied warranty of any kind and assumes no responsibility for any errors or omissions. No liability is assumed for incidental or consequential damages in connection with or arising out of information contained in this book. The Publisher shall not be liable for any special, consequential, or exemplary damages resulting, in whole or in part, from the readers' use of, or reliance upon, this material.

Independent verification should be sought for any data, advice or recommendations contained in this book. In addition, no responsibility is assumed by the publisher for any injury and/or damage to persons or property arising from any methods, products, instructions, ideas or otherwise contained in this publication.

This publication is designed to provide accurate and authoritative information with regard to the subject matter covered herein. It is sold with the clear understanding that the Publisher is not engaged in rendering legal or any other professional services. If legal or any other expert assistance is required, the services of a competent person should be sought. FROM A DECLARATION OF PARTICIPANTS JOINTLY ADOPTED BY A COMMITTEE OF THE AMERICAN BAR ASSOCIATION AND A COMMITTEE OF PUBLISHERS.

Library of Congress Cataloging-in-Publication Data

Sport and exercise psychology research advances / Martin P. Simmons and Liman A. Foster, editors.
    p. cm.
  ISBN 978-1-60456-157-9 (hardcover)
 1. Sports--Psychological aspects. 2. Exercise--Psychological aspects. I. Simmons, Martin P. II. Foster, Liman A.
  GV706.4.S65 2008
  796.01--dc22
                        2007051477

Published by Nova Science Publishers, Inc. ≃ New York

Contents

Preface

The application of psychology to sport and exercise settings is a relatively new field which is rapidly developing and expanding. This branch of psychology is concerned with understanding the behaviour, mental processes, and well-being of people who are involved in sport and exercise. Practitioners typically specialise in either the sport or exercise branches, though some work equally in both fields. This new book presents invigorating recent research in the field.

Short Communication A - The aim of the study was to examine the relationship between body esteem, objectively measured physical activity and anthropometry and in British school children. Two hundred and twenty four children aged 8-14years (114 boys and 110 girls) took part in the study. Body esteem was measured using the Body Esteem Scale for children and physical activity was assessed by pedometer worn over 4 consecutive days (2 weekday, 2 weekend). Additionally, body mass index (BMI), waist to hip ratio and waist circumference was assessed. Percent body fat was also determined by skinfold measures. Results indicate that body esteem was significantly and negatively related to BMI, waist circumference and percent body fat. No significant differences in body esteem according to gender were evident. In regard to physical activity, no significant difference according to gender was evident although weekday physical activity was significantly greater than weekend physical activity. The results of the present study appear to indicate that body image is related to body fatness and waist circumference but not physical activity. Therefore, when examining children's body image it may also be prudent to consider body fatness and/or waist circumference.

Short Communication B - The purpose of the study was to assess the effectiveness of self-modeling videotapes as a tool for improving self-efficacy and the performance of shooting skills in ice hockey. Self-modeling tapes consisted of previous performances edited to include only the correct elements of performance, which result in positive outcomes. Participants consisted of 22 members of a NCAA Division I ice hockey team. A pretest-posttest, control group design with repeated measures was used, such that half of the athletes viewed self-modeling tapes for 10 weeks, and the other half acted as controls. Measurements took place prior to the intervention, after 5 weeks and after 10 weeks of intervention. Results indicated that the experimental group showed greater shooting accuracy and reported higher shooting efficacy than the control group, with the largest difference occurring after 5 weeks. No interactions occurred with time.

Chapter I - In order to explain and predict health behaviors like physical exercise, it is essential to have good theoretical backdrops. In recent years, a number of models were designed to map proximal determinants of physical activity. These models can be categorized into continuum models and stage models.

Continuum models try to identify variables that determine behavior change. A linear prediction equation combines the different variables. Based on this assumption, interventions to promote physical exercise focus on increasing all associated variables in all individuals. On the contrary, stage theories model health behavior change as discrete stages along the way to the goal behavior. Depending on the stage that a person is in, specific social-cognitive variables are important. Every stage has its own equation that predicts the progression to the next stage. Stage-based interventions propose intervention packages matched to the stage a person is in, i.e., to the prevalent needs.

The chapter goes into more detail for stage models. An overview of stage theories such as the Transtheoretical Model (TTM) by Prochaska and DiClemente (1983) and the Health Action Process Approach (HAPA) by Schwarzer (1992) is given. Measurements for exercise stages are discussed and state-of-the art examples are presented. Research strategies, empirical evidence and criticism on stage theories are outlined. The chapter identifies stage-specific mechanisms and provides guidance to design theory-based expert systems and physical exercise promotion programs.

Chapter II - Despite the wealth of productive research examining the concept of competitive anxiety, the notion of 'facilitating' or 'positive anxiety' has recently stimulated an exciting conceptual debate amongst researchers. One perspective postulates that high levels of cognitive anxiety can be perceived as facilitating to performance. The opposing view maintains that, such cognitive symptoms are purported to reflect positive expectations of coping and goal achievement and lead to positive emotions including 'challenge' or 'excitement'. The purpose of the study therefore was to examine the suggestion that facilitating interpretations of symptoms associated with the competitive stress response may be representative of some other positive affective state other than anxiety. 322 competitive athletes, sampled from a range of team and individual sports aged 18-29 years ($M = 24.8$, $SD = 3.1$) completed the modified Competitive Trait Anxiety Inventory-2 (CTAI-2; Martens, Burton, Vealey, Bump, and Smith, 1990), the Positive and Negative Affect Schedule, and adapted from the work of Jones and Hanton (1996, 2001) a measure of feeling states, the Pre-Performance Feelings Scale (PPFS; Mellalieu, 2000). Three separate one-way MANOVA's were conducted with groups (debilitated versus facilitated) as the independent variable and performers' PPFS, PANAS and CTAI-2 subscales as the dependent variables respectively. All three MANOVA's were found to be significant with follow-up univariate analyses revealing differences between debilitators and facilitators of competitive trait anxiety for mental readiness, confidence and perception of physical state subscales of the PPFS and the positive and negative affect subscales of the PANAS. Correlation analyses revealed negative affect as more important in mediating competitive trait anxiety intensity, while positive affect was found to be more important in mediating competitive trait anxiety direction. Strong relationships were also found between the direction of competitive trait anxiety and positive and negative subscales of the PPFS. The findings indicate that sports performers' facilitative interpretations of symptoms associated with competitive anxiety responses may indeed be representative of some other positive affective state. Further, this positive affective state experienced in the precompetition period may therefore be more influential in determining successful sports performance than the existing belief that suggests competitive anxiety *per se* is the key factor in accounting for performance. Finally, the oxymoron of 'positive anxiety' is discussed in light of the study findings regarding the difference between true feelings of anxiety resulting in performance benefits versus the interpretation of associated symptoms having a similar positive influence. Practical implications and significant future recommendations for the practitioner are also offered.

Chapter III - The study of motivation has a long history in sport and exercise psychology research. Almost as long is the inclusion of social goals in relation to motivation. Despite this inclusion of social goals, they have not received the same attention as other ability focused goals. In this article the 'past' and 'present' research that has included social goals in sport and exercise is reviewed. Drawing on this research, as well as related research from education and social psychology, a discussion of the possibilities to further develop this area of motivation research is presented. Review of the social goal research revealed the lack of a sustained systematic examination of social aspects of motivation, and specifically social goals. Furthermore, that this maybe due to a narrow focus of on just one social goal, social approval. The social approval goal was conceptualised within achievement motivation theory as a universal view of success and was defined as aiming to maximize the probability of gaining others' approval. Despite attempts to operationalize and assess this social approval goal orientation questions remain regarding the measurement, consequences of holding a social approval orientation and its utility in furthering the authors understanding of motivation. Recently, however, a number of researchers in sport, education, and social psychology have begun to explore multiple social goals. An examination of this literature revealed a variety of conceptualizations of social goal constructs including what individuals are striving for and why individuals are striving. Therefore, despite this advance in social goal research, how social goals are conceptualised, assessed, and related to motivation remains unclear. Based on this review of past and present social goal research, possibilities for future development of social goal research are discussed. The focus of this discussion is on developing conceptual clarity with regard to how many, what content, and what level of goals are necessary to adequately capture socially focused motivation, as well as the meaning of social goal pursuit.

Chapter IV - There has been an ongoing debate in the motor learning literature regarding the role of performance error. Some practices assume that errors promote learning (i.e., learning from mistakes; Schmidt, 1975) whereas others consider the elimination of error as necessary because repeated errors may interfere with correct performance. A second debate has revolved around considerations of the extent to which individuals' motor learning should be reliant upon processes that are explicit/declarative (readily verbalisable and attention demanding) or implicit/procedural (difficult to verbalise and minimally attention demanding; e.g., Masters and Maxwell, 2004; Willingham, 1998). In this chapter the authors review recent research, which suggests that errors in performance have important implications for the involvement of implicit and explicit processes in movement control, and discuss the implications for sports performance and rehabilitation.

Chapter V - The present report overviews the on- and off-ice challenges of elite junior (major junior) hockey players located in one remote region of Canada. The data was gathered with a purposive sample of 10 athletes through semi-structured interviews, with the guidance of an advisory panel. There were three stages of data collection and content analysis, with 3-4 respondents elicited during each stage. Based on guidelines espoused by Côté, Salmela, Baria, and Russell (1993) and Schinke and da Costa (2000), the data were segmented into meaning units, coded into a hierarchy of themes, and verified with each respondent. From the data, there is indication that elite junior athletes from ice-hockey can adjust to and benefit from placements within remote locations. Peers, team-mates, coaching staff, billets, and community resources within the remote region offered the aspiring major junior athletes assistance with their adaptation. Implications are provided for applied sport psychology researchers and practitioners interested in placements within remote regions.

Chapter VI - In this study the authors examined the perceptions of a group of adolescents representing a variety of sport experiences regarding the motivational impact of what Bronfenbrenner (1979) called "second party" or "third order" effects, in allusion to the influence of other members of the social group on the interactions between two people. Qualitative analyses of semi-structured interview data highlighted several circumstances where participants took an active role in negotiating multiple interpersonal influences in the context of their sport participation. Specifically, exercising personal judgment and choice when faced with conflicting information and seeking to compensate the motivational deficits associated with particular relational contexts were two ways through which participants negotiated multiple influences and became active agents of their socialization and development in sport. The authors situate the findings and suggest avenues for future research in the context of a systems-style approach for the study of socialization processes in youth sport.

Chapter VII - Interest in the area of sport career termination has grown considerably in recent years among sport psychology researchers. Over 270 references could be identified on the topic of career transitions in sport during the last three decades. The present chapter aims to review and update existing research and to present some future theoretical and methodological issues emerging from recent advances in this field. Existing research have been guided by three main interests. The first is related to the identification of the nature of retirement from elite sport. Second, a descriptive view has been adopted by researchers to identify athletes' reactions to sport career termination. A third main question in the area of sport career termination concerns the mechanisms and variables playing a role in athletes' reactions and adaptation. The number of explanatory variables identified has grown during the last years, and hypothesized risk or facilitating factors span an enormous range, from individual characteristics to cultural determinants, taking also into account several transition-related variables. The present chapter proposes a reorganisation of the many explanatory variables in two interrelated categories, pre-conditions and transitional factors, which determine the quality of adaptation to retirement. Its appears that transition out of elite sport is a dynamic, complex, and multidimensional phenomenon, given the crucial importance of time in its definition, and the number of variables playing a role in the adaptation process of former athletes.

Chapter VIII - Despite the highly recognized benefits of exercise, 51% of Canadian adults do not achieve a level of physical activity equivalent to walking 30 minutes per day. These low activity rates have prompted the development of strategies to increase physical activity. One strategy has been to enhance perceptions of cohesion among group exercisers. Cohesion has been shown to be positively related to adherence and negatively related to dropout behavior. Carron and Spink (1993) suggested that one method to increase perceptions of cohesion is to provide greater opportunities for social interaction. The *quantity* of social contacts represents a construct termed structural social support and has been theorized to be linked to relational outcomes such as cohesion. Consequently, the primary purpose of the present study was to examine the relationship between perceptions of cohesion and the percentage of social contacts that exercisers (a) knew, and (b) interacted with in a group exercise context. Importantly, the percentage of social contacts does not necessarily provide an indication of the *quality* of those relationships. Therefore, a secondary purpose of the study was to examine perceived social support as a potential mediator of the social contacts-cohesion relationship. Adult exercisers ($N = 87$; $M_{age} = 34.47 \pm 13.23$) completed measures of cohesion, perceived social support and a sociogram of their exercise class used to indicate the percentage of other group members whom they knew and interacted with. Results demonstrated that the percentage of group members *known* to the participants was positively related to the cohesion dimensions of Attractions to the Group-Social and Group Integration-Social. The percentage of other group members with whom the participants *interacted with* was negatively related to the cohesion dimension Attractions to the Group-Task. Furthermore, the social support function Opportunity for Nurturance was found to be a mediator of the social contacts-cohesion relationship. Specifically, the percentage of group members known to participants was positively related to perceptions of being relied upon by others which, in turn, was positively related to the Attractions to the Group-Social dimension of cohesion. Results are discussed in relation to group dynamics theory and applied relevance.

Chapter IX - This is the second section of a broader study focusing on athletes' retirement decision process. A preliminary study dealt with the reasons which lead athletes to end their career and provided a new tool for assessing the pattern of these reasons, namely a self-report questionnaire called the Athletes' Retirement Decision Inventory based on the Push Pull Anti-push Anti-pull theoretical framework. This questionnaire provides a comprehensive view of how athletes fluctuate between Push, Pull, Anti-push and Anti-pull factors when they decide to end their career. The first objective of the present study was to extend this earlier work by examining the relationship between a number of personal characteristics (chronological age, gender, marital status, family status and subjective health) and the four ARDI subscales. The second goal was to identify the relative contribution of the four factors (Push, Pull, Anti-push and Anti-pull) in athletes' intention to retire. About 190 competitive athletes participated in this study. The results of standard multiple-regression analyses revealed first that the personal characteristic variables had no effect on the pattern of reasons for retirement measured by the ARDI. Secondly, the results of a sequential regression analysis indicated a relationship between the ARDI and the athletes' intention to retire; the four subscales of the ARDI predicted the athletes' intention to retire more accurately than the socio-demographic variables typically studied in the literature, with the Pull subscale emerging as the most predictive. The present study highlights the importance of how the future is perceived in the retirement decision process. This finding should allow the development of specific career transition programs for athletes in which career counsellors do not confine their interview to exploring the present situation, but systematically enlarge it to analysing how the future is perceived.

It can be hoped that future studies will continue to investigate the possibilities offered by this tool for a better understanding of the athletes' retirement process.

Chapter X - Two studies were conducted pertaining to gender differences in perceived physical effort. In the first study male (n = 7) and female (n = 8) volunteer participants (M age = 24.33, SD = 3.30) rated nine perceived effort sensations, arranged into three sensation clusters (sensory-discriminative, motivational-affective and cognitive-evaluative sensations), at regular intervals during a sustained handgrip-squeezing task. Female participants were found to report significantly higher ratings of physical and affective sensations, but significantly lower ratings of motivational sensations, than males. Females in this study were also found to report significantly lower perceived self-efficacy during the handgrip task than males. Several theories have attempted to explain gender differences in the perception of physical effort. Psychosocial theories consider socialization factors that encourage physical robustness among men, and the expression of distress among women, as important contributors to gender differences in effort perception. An alternative to this assumption is the suggestion that gender differences in athletic experience may account for observed gender differences in perceived effort and self-efficacy.

A follow-up study examined gender differences in perceived effort in male and female participants with similar athletic experience and current physical activity participation. Participants completed two exertive tasks: a sustained handgrip-squeezing task (n = 35) and a sustained cycle task (n = 13). As in the previous study three dimensions of physical effort (sensory-discriminative, motivational-affective and cognitive-evaluative sensations) were measured at regular intervals during the two tasks. Results of this study indicated no significant differences between male and female participants on any of the sensation dimensions. Additionally, males and female participants did not differ significantly on either physical or task-specific measures of self-efficacy. Based upon these findings it is concluded that previously observed gender differences in effort perception are likely due to pre-existing gender differences in athletic experience, rather than socialization factors.

Chapter XI - The purposes of the study in this chapter were to evaluate the use of salivary cortisol to measure stress experienced by athletes and to study the relationship between pre-competitions stress and personality of athletes. Sixteen swimmers representing Hong Kong in regional and international competition were recruited for the study. In the laboratory, swimmers were instructed to perform a mental arithmetic test and its purpose is to arouse the participant's stress level. They were then being led through the diaphragmatic breathing technique to help them relax. The stress levels of the swimmers at pre-arousal, post-arousal, and post-relaxation were monitored by salivary cortisol, skin conductance, respiratory rate, shortened State Trait Anxiety Inventory (STAI-6), and self-reported subjective score. Changes in salivary cortisol agreed with changes in all other stress measurements (skin conductance, respiratory rate, STAI and subjective stress score). Salivary cortisol is a possible parameter to be used for monitoring stress level of athletes. The pre-competition stress experienced by the swimmers was also measured at a local competition. Athletes were instructed to provide a saliva sample for cortisol measurement, to complete the Competitive State Anxiety Inventory-2 (CSAI-2) and a subjective stress scale 30-60 minutes prior to their respective competition event. The average of saliva cortisol levels as obtained on three rest days were used as baseline for comparison. Salivary cortisol as obtained prior to competition although was higher than that obtained on the rest days, the difference was not statistically significant. It seems that the competition under study was not stressful enough to the swimmers. Attempt was also made to study whether pre-competitive stress correlated to individual's personality (sensation seeking and coping skill). No significant correlation between pre-competition stress and personality was identified in the study.

Chapter XII - Muscle injuries are one of the most common traumas in sports and can be produced by intense or even moderate physical activity, especially eccentric exercise. It has been suggested that the immediate effects associated with muscle injury are mechanical, largely caused by the excessive tension to which muscle sarcomeres are subjected. Intense physical exercise induces muscle fiber lesions, whose severity depends on the duration and characteristics of the exercise, the training stage at which the sportsperson is found, and the presence of dietary or muscular (agonist/antagonist) imbalance. Although eccentric exercise has undoubted biomechanical and bioenergetic benefits, its intense or only occasional practice can produce structural and functional alterations of the muscles involved.

Immunoassay is the most widely used approach in clinical biochemistry to identify and quantify molecules and offers high sensitivity and specificity. Although some debate remains, it is generally considered that the detection of proteins bound to intracellular structures (mitochondria, nucleus, etc.), even in small amounts, usually indicates necrosis.

The molecular diagnosis of muscle damage is largely based on measurement of the plasma activity of different sarcoplasmatic enzymes (creatine kinase [CK] and lactate dehydrogenase [LDH]). These enzymes are normally strictly intracellular, and their increased activity in plasma reflects their escape via membrane structures.

Although the direct demonstration of muscle damage is histological, in practice the diagnosis is largely based on the measurement of plasma enzyme concentrations. Thus, the diagnosis can be supported by the combined measurement of biological and clinical parameters, e.g., plasma LDH activity, myoglobin, malondialdehyde (MDA), leukocyte count and changes in muscle parameters.

The diagnosis of exercise-induced muscle lesions by the measurement of markers remains controversial. Thus, the presence in plasma of increased CK activity and MDA levels reflects only muscle overload and offers low specificity and sensitivity as a muscle damage marker.

Increasing attention has been focused on the clinical relevance of the detection in plasma of cellular proteins released after tissue injury, commonly referred to as biochemical markers. The detection of α-actin and myosin molecules, closely related to muscle contraction, is of special interest and requires a reliable technique that offers high sensitivity and specificity. The aim is to be able to detect biochemical markers quickly and with high accuracy, especially when clinical and analytical findings fail to deliver an unequivocal diagnosis. The sensitivity of Western blot and the biological material used (serum obtained by a simple extraction of blood without need for biopsy) offer two major advantages for the study of skeletal muscle damage.

Chapter XIII - The ways in which people deal with the stresses of sports competition are called coping strategies. Recently Gaudreau and Blondin (2002) developed the multidimensional Coping Inventory for Competitive Sports (CICS) and provided strong evidence using confirmatory factor analysis for the existence of ten coping strategies used in sporting competition (thought control, mental imagery, relaxation, effort expenditure, logical analysis, seeking support, venting of unpleasant emotion, mental distraction, disengagement and social withdrawal). The aims of this study were to extend the findings of Gaudreau and Blondin (2002) to test the higher-order factor structure of the CICS, and examine the structural and differential stability of the CICS over four time points. Results suggested that a two-factor higher order model of task oriented and emotional oriented coping best fitted the data. Measurement invariance was observed for all subscales. Latent growth curve models suggested subscale scores decreased over time. At the second order factor level the use of task oriented coping decreased over the 10-week season, whereas the use of emotional oriented coping remained stable.

Chapter XIV - The aim of this study was to investigate the immunological (lymphocytes and lymphocytes subset), the hypothalamus pituitary adrenocortical (cortisol) and the hypothalamus pituitary (growth hormone GH) responses to an immersion with self-contained underwater breathing apparatus (SCUBA) in an unexplored siphon, placed in a cave about 700 m under the surface. The combination of heavy and long duration exercise before (5 hours of descending) and after (13 hours of ascending) the immersion in a demanding environment, the siphon altitude (quota: 1200 m), the exercise effort during diving in cold water (cave temperature: 2°C; water temperature: 2°C), the absolute darkness, the confinement, the restrictions with the associated risk of getting stuck and the emotion for the exploration as well as the awareness that if an accident happened the situation became drastically very critical represent a unique multiple stress model that may be helpful in understanding the immune and endocrine expression of acute physiological and psychological stress. Owing to the high skill of the performance and to the enormous difficulties for carrying all the technical equipment on the bottom of this cave, only one cave-diver was tested; however this subject repeated the same immersion in two different days following the same schedule. Five blood drawings were performed. 1. at 7:30 am, at the hospital (sea level), 2. 7:30 pm on the bottom of the cave (quota: 1230 m), before the siphon immersion, 3. after the immersion, 4. at the exit of the cave (quota: 1930m), 5. 24 hours after resting and the authors focused their attention on the pre-post immersion time interval. Moreover, blood drawings, as controls, were performed at the same resting time envisaged for the day of the experiment to minimize the specimen processing time influences and any circadian fluctuation. A marked increase in GH and cortisol hormone was measured while a dramatic decrease in the total absolute number of lymphocytes and all studied lymphocytes subpopulations (CD3+ T cells, CD4+ T helper cells, CD8+ T cytotoxic cells, CD19+ B cells and CD16+CD3- natural killer cells was found. The authors data confirm that extreme physiological/psychological conditions of cave diving are stressors that are able to alter both the immune and hormonal response. In particular the marked rise of GH values during diving underlines the great intensity of cave diving effort due to the difficult route that the cave diver covered and the bulky technical equipment dressed while the rise of cortisol is likely due to the combination of emotional stress and exercise. Moreover, cold temperature, darkness and sleep deprivation could also enhance cortisol secretion. The unusual and marked drop of total absolute number of lymphocytes as well as all the lymphocytes subpopulations, just during the exercise appear dependant at least in part, to the very long duration characteristic of all the performance (spelunking and diving) and the associated effects induced by the augmented cortisol levels with respect to basal condition, in particular during the immersion. Finally it should be noted that also sleep deprivation could negatively influenced the immune response to physical exercise.

Chapter XV – Despite the benefits of participation in sport and physical activity, there is a clear prevalence of sport dropout behavior beginning in early adolescence. A potential influence on youth sport and physical activity participation is sport status. The purpose of the present investigation was to examine levels of sport and physical activity participation for youth of various sport status (i.e., high status/starting athlete, low status/non-starting athlete, non-athlete) prior to the academic transition from elementary school (Grade Eight) to high school (Grade Nine) and examine this situation within the Theory of Planned Behavior (i.e., attitudes towards physical activity, perceived behavioral control, subjective norms, intentions to be physically active). Grade Eight students (n = 79) were administered a set of questionnaires to assess physical activity participation, sport participation (including starting status), and perceptions of physical activity (i.e., TPB variables). Multivariate analyses of variance revealed significant differences between sport status levels in perceptions of attitudes towards physical activity, $F(2,76)$ = 8.98, p < .001, η^2 = .19, intentions to be physically active, $F(2,76)$ = 3.64, p < .05, η^2 = .09, perceived behavioral control, $F(2,76)$ = 3.46, p < .05, η^2 = .08, and vigorous physical activity levels, $F(2,76)$ = 5.14, p < .01, η^2 = .12. Specifically, post-hoc tests indicated significant differences (p < .05) between starting athletes and non-athletes with regard to attitudes, intentions, and vigorous physical activity levels. However, youth athletes with lower sport status held similar perceptions of physical activity (i.e., attitudes and intentions) and engaged in similar levels of vigorous physical activity as both higher status athletes and non-athletes.

Chapter XVI – It is generally accepted emotional stress may increase the risk of several diseases such as arrhythmia, myocardial ischemia, cancer, chronic inflammatory diseases, immunodeficiency, etc.. However the mechanisms regarding how emotional stress causes disruption of homeostasis are complex and remain unclear.

Recent studies have reported it may be explained, at least in part, since psychological stress may change the balance between pro-oxidant and antioxidant factors, inducing oxidative damage. Further, "unhealthy" lifestyle factors such as smoking, sedentary, low-fruit consumption, among others, may be pointed out as potential targets by health care professionals since it was reported a significant synergistic influence on the decrease in the antioxidant capacity when combined to emotional stress.

On the contrary, physical activity is recognized as an important component of a healthy life style and consequently is highly recommended by scientists and clinicians. This finding may be explained at least in part, since regular exercise may improve redox metabolism by increasing significantly antioxidant defense system. At the present moment, this field is at an exciting stage. And fortunately, ample evidence of this progress can be found in the literature.

In this line, several studies focused on the management of emotionally stressed animals concluded regular exercise improved their redox metabolism. In humans, long-term aerobic training program at low-moderate intensity increased significantly both enzymatic and non-enzymatic antioxidant systems. Conversely, short-term supramaximal anaerobic exercise increased significantly lipid, protein and DNA oxidation whose evaluation may provide a significant clue to the magnitude of oxidative damage.

To explain the double role of physical activity, existing data indicated on one hand that, moderate long-term exercise may cause adaptation of the antioxidant and repair systems, which could result in a decreased base level of oxidative damage and increased resistance to oxidative stress. On the other hand, a single bout of vigorous exercise result in oxidative damage as a sign of incomplete adaptation.

Consequently, in order to be effective and healthy, these intervention programs based on physical activity should be adequately designed and supervised during their application by a multidisciplinary team of healthcare professionals, psychologist, bachelor's degree on exercise science, etc.

Chapter XVII - Background: Perceived competence, relatedness, and autonomy embody the basic psychological needs subtheory housed within Self-Determination Theory (SDT). Fulfillment of these basic psychological needs represents an important avenue for the promotion of well-being and the optimization of motivation for health behaviors including exercise. Few attempts, however, have been made to systematically measure the fulfillment of basic psychological needs in exercise contexts using a construct validation approach.

Purpose: The main purpose of this article is to review the available evidence attesting to the measurement of psychological need satisfaction in exercise contexts using SDT as a guiding framework. The subpurposes of this review were to identify key issues associated with the current measurement of psychological need satisfaction in exercise using a construct validation framework and illustrate salient issues pertinent to the selection and development of instruments designed to measure perceived competence, autonomy, and relatedness specific to exercise contexts for future research.

Summary: Early work in this area relied on instruments that had not been developed specifically for measuring perceived psychological need satisfaction in exercise contexts. A number of psychometric concerns were evident in the data reported in these studies including reliability issues and a lack of convincing evidence for convergent and nomological validity. More recent construct validation work has produced the Psychological Need Satisfaction in Exercise Scale and the Basic Psychological Needs in Exercise Scale. Both instruments appear to hold promise for furthering the authors understanding of the influential role afforded competence, autonomy, and relatedness perceptions in the context of exercise.

"We must believe that even in prehistoric times Og, the cave man, made rudimentary appraisals of his fellows. He saw Zog go by, made some such judgment as "Big, strong, keep out of way," and acted upon it; or he came upon the campfire of Wog, observed "Small, weak, take dinner," and did so forthwith. But for much of recorded history, the appraisals that man has made of his fellows have been of this crude and subjective type.".

In: Sport and Exercise Psychology Research Advances   ISBN: 978-1-60456-157-9
Editors: M. P. Simmons, L. A. Foster, pp. 1-8   © 2008 Nova Science Publishers, Inc.

Short Communication A

Relationships between Body Esteem, Objectively Measured Physical Activity and Anthropometry in Children

Michael J. Duncan[1], Yahya Al-Nakeeb and Lorayne Woodfield
Newman University College, UK

Abstract

The aim of the study was to examine the relationship between body esteem, objectively measured physical activity and anthropometry and in British school children. Two hundred and twenty four children aged 8-14years (114 boys and 110 girls) took part in the study. Body esteem was measured using the Body Esteem Scale for children and physical activity was assessed by pedometer worn over 4 consecutive days (2 weekday, 2 weekend). Additionally, body mass index (BMI), waist to hip ratio and waist circumference was assessed. Percent body fat was also determined by skinfold measures. Results indicate that body esteem was significantly and negatively related to BMI, waist circumference and percent body fat. No significant differences in body esteem according to gender were evident. In regard to physical activity, no significant difference according to gender was evident although weekday physical activity was significantly greater than weekend physical activity. The results of the present study appear to indicate that body image is related to body fatness and waist circumference but not physical activity. Therefore, when examining children's body image it may also be prudent to consider body fatness and/or waist circumference.

Keywords: *Pedometer, Body Esteem, Waist Circumference, Body Fat.*

1 Please address correspondence and requests for reprints to Michael J. Duncan, Department of Physical Education and Sports Studies, Newman College of Higher Education, Birmingham, England, B32 3NT or e mail m.j.duncan@newman.ac.uk.

Body image is a multidimensional phenomenon that has been variously defined and is a construct that has received substantial research attention (Grogan, 1999). Previous research has found that a positive body image is significantly related to greater self esteem (Mendelsen et al., 2002), lower incidence of depression (Ackard, Croll, and Kearney-Cooke, 2002) and lower levels of body fatness (Duncan, Al-Nakeeb, Jones, and Nevill, 2006a).

Children have reported considerable body esteem concerns (Thompson and Smolak, 2001). This is of concern as body image disturbance among children might be a risk factor for the later development of eating disorders (Stice, 2002). This issue is doubly important given rising levels of overweight and obesity in the U.K. and internationally. Moreover, overweight and obesity have additionally been identified as a risk factor in the development of body image problems in children (Duncan et al., 2006a). Coupled with increasing rates of overweight and obesity worldwide, the study of physical activity, obesity and body esteem merits further study. This may be particularly so in childhood as obese children are more likely to become obese adults (Thompson and Smolak, 2001) and an investigation of factors that may impact on overweight and obesity in children could be useful for targeting intervention strategies aimed at obesity reduction.

Body image may also be influential in terms of an individual's physical activity behaviour (Williams and Cash, 2001). Previous adult based studies have examined related issues including the impact of excessive exercise or specific training programmes on body dissatisfaction (Williams and Cash, 2001; Davis, 2004) and body dissatisfaction differences between exercisers and non-exercisers (Furnham, Titman, and Sleeman, 1994). More recently research has focused on the relationship between physical activity and body image/esteem in pediatric populations. However, the relationship between body image and physical activity in children is unclear as some studies report no significant relationship (Duncan, Al-Nakeeb, Jones, and Nevill, 2004) and others have reported a positive association between body dissatisfaction and physical activity (Duncan et al., 2006a). Furthermore, results of a recent intervention study suggested that 6 weeks of aerobic dance significantly reduced body image dissatisfaction in adolescent girls (Burgess, Grogan, and Burwitz, 2006). The lack of agreement across studies examining body image and physical activity may be due to a number of reasons. Firstly, body image is comprised of cognitive, affective and behavioural components (Grogan, 1999). Previous studies may have therefore focused on the relationship between physical activity and different components of body image. Secondly, previous studies examining this issue have tended to rely on self-report methods to assess physical activity (Duncan et al., 2004; Duncan et al., 2006a). The use of self-report methods to assess physical activity has been criticised and there have been recommendations for researchers to use objective measures when assessing children's physical activity (Trost, 2001). One such measure, the pedometer, has recently shown promise as an objective tool for assessing children's physical activity as they are relatively inexpensive compared to accelerometry and heart rate monitoring, unobtrusive and demonstrate good reliability and validity (Tudor-Locke, Williams, Reiss, and Pluto, 2004a).

Despite the lack of clarity in prior studies, physical activity may have a beneficial impact on body dissatisfaction (Grogan, 1999) and obesity (Ackard et al., 2002). Therefore, the aim of this study was to examine the relationships between body image, multiple measures of weight status and physical activity using objective measures in a group of British children.

Method

Participants Two hundred and twenty four children (114 boys and 110 girls) from 10 schools in Central England volunteered and returned signed parental informed consent forms to participate in the study. Children were from school years 4-8 (aged 8-14years) and were from white (n = 154), black (n = 12) and Asian (n = 58) ethnic groups as classified by the Department for Education and Skills (2002). The mean age (± *SD*) of the children was 10.8 ± 1.8 years. All schools were located in the same geographical area of central England and the study was approved by institutional ethics committee.

Procedures

Body Image

The Body Esteem Scale for children (Mendelsen, and White, 1982) was used to assess body image. This scale was specifically developed to assess body image in children from 7 to 17 years of age and has been identified as suitable to measure attitudinal body image in children (Smolak, and Levine, 2001) and the psychometric properties of this scale have previously been established (Mendelsen, and White, 1982). The body esteem scale for children assesses how a child values his or her appearance based on yes or no responses to 24 items such as 'I wish I were thinner' and 'I worry about the way I look'. Unlike other measures of body image that have been used with child and adolescent populations the body esteem scale for children avoids problems associated with using likert scales with children and does not ask questions that other body image measures include relating to sex organs or sexual activities which may be considered inappropriate. The body esteem scale for children was administered to participants on an individual basis prior to collection of physical activity or anthropometric data.

Physical Activity

Physical activity was assessed using a sealed, piezo-electric pedometer (New Lifestyles, NL2000, Montana, USA) worn over four days (2 X weekdays and 2 X weekend days). Four days of monitoring is a sufficient length of time to determine habitual physical activity levels in children (Trost , Pate, Freedson, Sallis, and Taylor, 2000). Prior to the monitoring period children were familiarized with the pedometers (all children had prior experience wearing pedometers as part of school science classes) and were briefed as to the nature of their involvement in the study. On the first day of monitoring, the children were instructed on pedometer attachment (at the waist), its removal (only during showering/bathing, swimming or sleeping), and reattachment before going to school each morning. The children were also asked not to tamper with the pedometer and to go about their normal activities during the monitoring period. The research staff attached the pedometers on the each day of monitoring and collected them at the end of the four days of monitoring. Daily step counts were stored in the internal memory of each pedometer enabling recall of each day's step count on collection of each pedometer. Across the period of measurement, the children were asked to complete a brief survey to verify that the pedometers were worn for the entire time of the study. Survey results were used to identify those participants who reported removing the pedometer for ≥ 1 h. Their data was subsequently deleted before analysis in accordance with other studies investigating pedometer determined physical activity in children (Tudor Locke et al., 2004b). This resulted in twenty two exclusions of physical activity data from the data set.

Anthropometry

Body mass (kg) and height (m) were directly measured using a Stadiometer and weighing scales (Seca Instruments, Germany, Ltd) prior to the monitoring period. Body mass index was determined as kg/m^2. Overweight/obesity status was determined using child-specific, International Obesity task force cut-off points (Cole, Bellizi, Flegal, and Dietz, 2000). Waist circumference was assessed midway between the rib cage and the superior border of the iliac crest using an anthropometric tape measure with participants in a standing and at the end of gentle expiration. Hip circumference was measured at the maximum circumference over the buttocks. Both measurements were assessed in duplicate and rounded to the nearest 0.5 centimetre and were used to determine waist to hip ratio. In addition, Percent body fat was determined using skinfold measures at two sites (tricep and medial calf) employing the child specific Slaughter, Lohman, Boileau, Horswill, Stillman, Van Loan and Bemben (1988) skinfold equation.

Analysis

Data was analysed in a number of ways. The relationship between body esteem, physical activity, BMI and WHR was determined using Pearsons' product moment correlations. Gender differences in body esteem, BMI, percent body fatness and waist circumference were examined using independent t-tests. Differences in physical activity according to gender were examined using a 2 (gender) by 2 (mean weekday steps vs mean weekend steps) repeated measures analysis of variance (ANOVA). SPSS version 13 (SPSS inc, Chicago, USA) was used for all analysis.

Results

Results from Pearson's correlations revealed significant relationships between body esteem and BMI ($r = -.350$, $p = .001$), body esteem and waist circumference ($r = -.360$, $p = .001$) and body esteem and percent body fat ($r = -.355$, $p = .001$). No significant relationships were evident between body esteem and physical activity or body esteem and waist to hip ratio (all $p > .05$).

Table 1. Mean ± *SD* for weekend and weekday steps/day, body esteem scores and anthropometric data according to gender group

	Body Esteem		BMI (kg/m^2)		% Fat		Waist Circumference (cm)		Waist to Hip Ratio		Average Weekday Steps		Average Weekend Steps	
	M	SD	M	SD	M	SD	M	SD	M	SD	M	SD	M	SD
Boys (n = 114)	15.5	5.6	18.5	3.6	20.5	7.6	70.3	9.9	0.84	0.05	19485	6359	16386	8197
Girls (n = 110)	14.9	5.7	19.2	4.2	27.8	9.1	69.7	9.9	0.76	0.04	18429	5846	14849	5201

Independent t-tests indicated significant gender differences in waist circumference (t (222) = 1.980, p = 0.045) and percent body fat (t (222) = -3.849, p = 0.01). In both cases boys had lower waist circumference and percent body fat compared to girls. In regard to BMI, no significant gender difference was evident (t (222) = -.566, p > .05). Furthermore, there was no significant difference in body esteem scores between boys and girls (t (222) = -.542, p > .05). Mean ± S.D. for body esteem was 15.5 ± 5.6 for boys and 14.9 ± 5.7 for girls. Mean ± S.D. for body esteem scores and anthropometric data according to gender groups are shown in Table 1.

In regard to physical activity values, repeated measures analysis of variance indicated significant differences in mean step/day between weekdays and weekends (F (1, 174) = 27.5, p = .0001). Bonferroni multiple comparisons indicated that physical activity was significantly greater during weekdays compared to weekends (*Mean Diff* = 4608, p = .0001). Mean ± *SD* of steps/day was 19260 ± 6249 and 15618 ± 6682 for weekdays and weekends respectively. No significant difference was evident between gender groups (F (1, 174) = 0.29, p > .05). Mean ± S.D. for steps/day was 17935 ± 3509 for boys and 16942 ± 4071 for girls. Mean ± S.D. for weekend and weekday steps/day according to gender groups are shown in Table 1.

Discussion

Results of this study support previous work conducted by Duncan et al. (2004) that reported significant negative relationships between body fatness and body esteem in a sample of British children. However, in the case of the current study, multiple measures of children's weight status (BMI, Waist circumference and % body fat) were all significantly and negatively related to body esteem. Furthermore, the results of this study indicated that no gender difference was evident in body esteem scores. These results refute previous studies which have indicated that males have more positive body image than females (McCabe, Ricciardelli, and Finemore, 2002; Smolak and Levine, 2001) but support previous studies that have controlled for weight status and have also found no difference in body image between boys and girls (Duncan et al., 2004).

Results from physical activity data support a range of prior studies that have documented increased physical activity during weekdays compared to weekends (Duncan et al., 2006b;

Oliver, Schofield, and McEvoy, 2006). No gender difference was evident in terms of ambulatory physical activity. This is somewhat surprising as it contradicts a number of previous research studies (Oliver et al., 2006; Loucaides, Chedzoy, and Bennet, 2003). However, these findings do agree with heart rate monitor based data taken from a similar sample of British primary school children (Al-Nakeeb, Duncan, Lyons, and Woodfield, 2007).

Although previous research has suggested that there may be a relationship between physical activity and body image (Williams and Cash, 2001) and that participation in physical activity may have an impact on an individual's body image (Burgess et al., 2006; Krane, Stiles-Shipley, Waldron, and Michalenok, 2001) the results of the current study indicated no significant relationship between objectively measured physical activity and body esteem. Although physical activity was assessed using objective measures in the current study, the results agree with previous research that has relied on self-reported estimates of activity in children (Duncan et al., 2004). This is an interesting finding as it clearly contradicts research from exercise intervention studies that have documented improvements in body image following a structured exercise programme. When considered alongside the significant relationships found between body esteem and multiple measures of weight status in the present study, perhaps it is the change (or perceived change) in weight status variables that leads to improvements in body image rather than the physical activity/exercise itself. Future research is needed to fully elucidate whether this is the case.

The results of the present study appear to indicate that body image, body fatness and waist circumference are related. When examining children's body image it may also be prudent to consider body fatness and/or waist circumference. Furthermore, results of the present study may seem to indicate that health professionals aiming to implement interventions or educational programmes aimed at enhancing children's body image need to also focus on children's levels of body fatness. Additional examination of the role that physical activity and exercise may play in children's body image is warranted given the conflicting evidence between physical activity intervention studies and studies of free living physical activity and body image.

References

Ackard D. M., Croll J. K., and Kearney-Cooke, A. (2002) Dieting frequency among college females: Association with disordered eating, body image, and related psychological problems. *Journal of Psychosomatic Research,* 52, 129-136.

Al-Nakeeb, Y., Duncan, M. J., Lyons, M., and Woodfield, L. (2007) Body fatness and physical activity levels of young children. *Annals of Human Biology,* 34, 1-12.

Burgess, G., Grogan, S., and Burwirz, L., (2006) Effects of a 6-week aerobic dance intervention on body image and physical self perception in adolescent girls. *Body Image,* 3, 57-66.

Cole, T. J., Bellizzi, M. C., Flegal, K. M., and Dietz, W. H. (2000) Establishing a standard definition for child overweight and obesity worldwide: International Survey. *British Medical Journal,* 320, 1240-1243.

Davis, C. (2004) Body image and athleticism. In: T. Cash and T. Pruzinsky (Eds), *Body Image* (pp219-225). New York: Guildford Press.

Department for Education and Skills (2002) *Guidance for local education authorities on schools' collection and recording data on pupils' ethnic background.* DFES Circular DfES/0002/2002.

Duncan, M., Al-Nakeeb, Y., Jones, M., and Nevill, A. (2004) Body image and physical activity in British school children. *European Physical Education Review*, 10, 243-260.

Duncan, M., Al-Nakeeb, Y., Jones, M., and Nevill, A. (2006a) Body Dissatisfaction, Body Fat and Physical Activity in British Children. *International Journal of Pediatric Obesity,* 1, 89-95.

Duncan, J. S., Schofield, G., and Duncan, E. K. (2006b) Pedometer-determined physical activity and body composition in New Zealand children. *Medicine and Science in Sports and Exercise,* 38, 1402-1409.

Furnham, A., Titman, P., and Sleeman, E. (1994) Perception of female body shapes as a function of exercise. *Journal of Social Beahvior and Personality,* 9, 335-352.

Grogan, S. (1999) *Body Image: Understanding body dissatisfaction in men, women and children.* London, Routledge.

Krane, V., Stiles-Shipley, J. A., Waldron, J., and Michalenok, J. (2001) Relationships among body satisfaction, social physique anxiety, and eating behaviours in female athletes and exercisers. *Journal of Sport Behavior*, 24, 247-264.

Loucaides, C. A., Chedzoy, S. M., and Bennett, N. (2003) Pedometer-assessed physical (ambulatory) activity in Cypriot children. *European Physical Education Review,* 9, 43-55.

McCabe, M. P., Ricciardelli, L. A., and Finemore, J. (2002) The role of puberty, media and popularity with peers to increase weight, decrease weight and increase muscle tone among adolescent boys and girls. *Journal of Psychosomatic Research.* 52, 145-153.

Mendelson, B. K., McLaren, L., Gauvin, L. and , Steiger, H. (2002) The relationship of self-esteem and body esteem in women with and without eating disorders. *International Journal of Eating Disorders*, 31, 318-323.

Mendelson, B. K., and White, D. R. (1982) Relation between body-esteem and self-esteem of obese and normal children. *Perceptual and Motor Skills.* 54, 899-905.

Oliver, M., Schofield, G., and McEvoy, E. (2006) An integrated curriculum approach to increasing habitual physical activity in children: A feasibility study. *Journal of School Health,* 76, 74-79.

Slaughter, M. H., Lohman, T. G., Boileau, R. A., Horswill, C. A., Stillman, R. J., Van Loan, M. D., and Bemben, D. A. (1988) Skinfold equations for estimation of body fatness in children and youth. *Human Biology*, 60, 709-723.

Smolak, L., and Levine, M. P. (2001) Body Image in Children. In J. K. Thompson and L. Smolak (Eds.). *Body Image, Eating Disorders and Obesity in Youth* (pp 41-66). Washington DC: American Psychological Association.

Thompson, J. K., and Smolak, L. (2001) Body image, eating disorders and obesity in youth. The future is now. In: J. K. Thompson and L. Smolak (Eds.), *Body Image, Eating Disorders and Obesity in Youth* (pp. 1-19). Washington, DC : American Psychological Association.

Trost, S.G., (2001) 'Objective measurement of physical activity in youth: Current issues, future directions', *Exercise and Sports Science Reviews*, 29, 32-36.

Trost, S.G., Pate, R.R., Freedson, P.S., Sallis, J.F., and Taylor, W.C. (2000) 'Using objective physical activity measures with youth: How many days of monitoring are needed', *Medicine and Science in Sports and Exercise*, 32, 426-431.

Tudor-Locke, C., Williams, J.E., Reis, J.P., and Pluto, D. (2004a) 'Utility of pedometers for assessing physical activity – Construct validity', *Sports Medicine*, 34, 281-291.

Tudor-Locke, C., Pangrazi, R.P., Corbin, C.B., Rutherford, W. J., Vincent, S.J., et al. (2004b) BMI-referenced standards for recommended pedometer-determined steps/day in children. *Preventive Medicine*, 38, 857-864.

Williams, P. A., and Cash, T. (2001) Effects of a circuit weight training program on the body images of college students. *International Journal of Eating Disorders*, 30, 75-82.

In: Sport and Exercise Psychology Research Advances   ISBN: 978-1-60456-157-9
Editors: M. P. Simmons, L. A. Foster, pp. 9-18   © 2008 Nova Science Publishers, Inc.

Short Communication B

The Effect of Self-Modeling on Shooting Performance and Self-Efficacy with Intercollegiate Hockey Players

Deborah L. Feltz[2], Sandra E. Short and Daniel A. Singleton
Michigan State University, USA
University of North Dakota, USA
National Hockey League, Columbus Blue Jackets, USA

Abstract

The purpose of the study was to assess the effectiveness of self-modeling videotapes as a tool for improving self-efficacy and the performance of shooting skills in ice hockey. Self-modeling tapes consisted of previous performances edited to include only the correct elements of performance, which result in positive outcomes. Participants consisted of 22 members of a NCAA Division I ice hockey team. A pretest-posttest, control group design with repeated measures was used, such that half of the athletes viewed self-modeling tapes for 10 weeks, and the other half acted as controls. Measurements took place prior to the intervention, after 5 weeks and after 10 weeks of intervention. Results indicated that the experimental group showed greater shooting accuracy and reported higher shooting efficacy than the control group, with the largest difference occurring after 5 weeks. No interactions occurred with time.

Keywords: *Athletes, Ice hockey, Self-efficacy, Video feedback*

In today's world, athletes have the ability to watch their sport experiences through digital or video recordings (e.g., television productions, coach's film, "family" movies, etc.). These

2 Correspondence concerning this article should be addressed to Deborah L. Feltz, Kinesiology, Michigan State University, I.M. Sports-Circle, East Lansing, Michigan, 48824. Phone # (517) 355-4732. Fax # (517) 353-2944. Electronic mail may be sent via Internet to Dfeltz@Msu.Edu.

recordings can help athletes relive positive moments when specific skills were performed flawlessly, strategies were executed perfectly, championships were won or personal bests were obtained. Using personal recordings can be considered as a form of self-modeling (or observational learning; Feltz, Short, and Sullivan, 2008).

Modeling, in general, is one of the most powerful means of transmitting values, attitudes and patterns of thoughts and behaviors (Bandura, 1997). Within sport psychology, models are a stimulus for affecting some type of psychological or behavioral change, and in that way, the use of models is considered an intervention technique (Feltz et al., 2007). Recently, Clark, Ste-Marie, and Martini (2006) used the label "self-as-a-model" for interventions when athletes view themselves performing sport skills on video as a means of performance improvement.

Self-modeling is one of two types of self-as-a-model interventions (self-observation is the other). Self-modeling involves an individual repeatedly observing an edited recording of the correct or best parts of his or her own past performance, and using that as a model for future performance (Dowrick, 1999; Dowrick and Dove, 1980). Self-observation is the process of viewing oneself performing a skill at one's current skill level. The primary difference between self-observation and self-modeling is that in self-modeling any errors in the performance are eliminated from the recording so that the individuals are shown performing more skillfully than normally (McCullagh, 1993). Self-modeling is preferred over self-observation because it is assumed that eliminating errors will enhance self-efficacy and lead to enhanced performance (McCullagh and Weiss, 2001). Recent research by Clark and Ste-Marie (2007) comparing self-modeling and self-observation interventions on children's self-regulation of learning and swimming performance showed that the self-modeling group demonstrated superior swimming performance and increased self-regulatory processing compared to the self-observation and the control groups during both acquisition and retention phases.

The theoretical basis for the effectiveness of self-modeling is grounded in efficacy theory. That is, self-modeling affects performance through its impact on self-efficacy beliefs (Bandura, 1997). Feltz et al. (2008) define self-efficacy is a situationally specific self-confidence. It refers to the belief in one's capability to produce given levels of performance (Bandura, 1986, 1997). According to self-efficacy theory, people's self-efficacy beliefs influence their thought patterns, emotional reactions, motivation, and performance. One's self-efficacy beliefs rely on the cognitive processing of diverse sources of information, including past performance accomplishments, vicarious experiences (e.g., modeling), verbal persuasion, emotional arousal, and physiological states. Self-modeling is a source of self-efficacy information based on the vicarious experiences of one's own performance. Bandura (1986, 1997) contends that the more similarity between the model and the observer, the greater the influence on the self-efficacy of the observer. The model –observer similarity is maximized when the individual serves as his or her own model (Bandura, 1986, 1997). Model similarity studies in the area of motor performance have typically shown that observers of similar models outperform and have higher efficacy levels than observers of dissimilar models (e.g., George, Feltz, and Chase, 1992; Gould and Weiss, 1981; Landers and Landers, 1973; Lirgg and Feltz, 1991; McCullagh, 1987).

Several researchers have studied the effectiveness of self-modeling on sport skill performance and self-efficacy (see Table 1 for a review).

In their study, Winfrey and Weeks (1993), assigned female intermediate-level gymnasts ($N = 11$) to view a 60-90 s. videotape of themselves three times a week for 6 weeks prior to practice or to a control group who just participated in their normal practice program. The authors found that self-modeling had no effect on self-efficacy or balance-beam performance, but their study was limited by their small sample size. In addition, they did not use Bandura's (1986) recommended procedures for assessing self-efficacy beliefs (Feltz and Chase, 1998).

Table 1. Literature review of self-modeling studies that investigated both performance and self-efficacy in sport

Authors	Task	Sample	Experimental groups and sample size	Dependent Variables	Statistical Analysis	Results
Clark and Ste-Marie (2007)	Swimming skills	Semi-experienced children (Aquaquest 3 level)	Self-model group: (n=11) 60 second video watched during 6 consecutive swimming lessons Self-observation group (n=11) Control group (n=11)	Swimming performance Task-specific self-efficacy	3 (group) by 3 (session) repeated measures ANOVA	Self-modeling group improved more than self-observation and control groups (acquisition and retention). Self-modeling group higher self-efficacy scores compared to other groups, but not significant.
Law and Ste-Marie (2005)	Figure skating jumping	Intermediate level figure skaters	Self-model group (n=12) Watched 30 second video 2/week for 3 weeks Control group (n=7)	Jump performance (outcome and form) Task-specific self-efficacy (single item)	2 Condition (self-modeling, control) x 3 Time (pre-, mid-, final intervention session) analysis of variance (ANOVA) with repeated measures for both factors	No significant differences between the two conditions for the self-modeling group on any of the dependent variables (although scores for each of the variables showed a slight change in the desired direction, the changes were evident for both conditions).
Ram and McCullagh (2003)	Volleyball serve	Intermediate level volleyball players	Self-model group: (n=5) Watched 50 second videos (over possible 8 test days)	Volleyball serve performance Self-efficacy	Multiple baseline single-participant design	Self-modeling contributed to increases in serving accuracy. Performance form and self-efficacy results were inconclusive.

Table 1. (Continued)

Authors	Task	Sample	Experimental groups and sample size	Dependent Variables	Statistical Analysis	Results
Starek and McCullagh (1999)	Swimming skills	Beginner swimmers (adult)	Self-model group: (n=5) Watched 3 minute long videotape in 2 sessions Other-model group: (n=5) Watched 3 minute long videotape in 2 sessions	Swimming performance Task-specific self-efficacy measure	2 (group) by 2 (time) repeated measures ANOVA	Self-modeling group had better swim performance by fourth session compared to other-model group. No significant differences between modeling conditions on self-efficacy.
Winfrey and Weeks (1993)	Balance beam performance	Intermediate level gymnasts (8-13 yrs).	Self-model group: (n=5) Watched video 3 times/week for 6 weeks Control group (n=6)	Balance beam performance State Sport Confidence Inventory	Group by time ANOVA	Confidence scores increased over time Skill test scores increased over time No group differences

Another published study that assessed the effect of self-modeling on self-efficacy and skill performance was completed by Starek and McCullagh (1999). The authors compared self- and other-modeling on the learning of beginning swimming skills and self-efficacy beliefs across two instructional sessions. Although they used Bandura's (1986) recommended procedure for assessing self-efficacy, they only found performance differences between modeling groups, with self-modeling producing greater improvements. Both groups improved in their swimming efficacy from baseline, but not significantly so. This study was also limited by the small sample size ($N = 10$) and low number of training sessions.

The effectiveness of a self-modeling intervention on performance and self-efficacy was also tested by Ram and McCullagh (2003). Using a multiple-baseline single-subject design, five participants (intermediate volleyball players) were differentially exposed to a self-modeling video over a possible 8 intervention sessions. Results from a visual analysis of the data showed that self-modeling contributed to increases in serving accuracy. Performance form scores and self-efficacy results were inconclusive (likely due to the variability in the baseline measures).

More recently, Clark and Ste-Marie (2007) examined whether children ($n = 33$) randomly assigned to a self-modeling group would demonstrate superior swimming performance and increased self-regulatory processing compared to self-observation and control groups. Results showed that the self-modeling group demonstrated superior swimming performance, greater self-satisfaction, was more intrinsically motivated, and, although not significant, displayed a tendency towards higher self-efficacy beliefs as compared to both the self-observation and the control groups.

Similar to our current study, Law and Ste-Marie (2005) examined whether self-modeling plus physical practice would improve intermediate level figure skaters' jump performance, as well as their self-efficacy, motivation, and state anxiety, when compared to physical practice alone. Twelve female figure skaters who received a self-modeling intervention were compared to a separate control group of seven skaters. Their results showed no differences between the two groups on any of the dependent variables although there were slight changes favoring the self-modeling group. Law and Ste. Marie stated that a limitation of their study was the potential for ceiling effects. The skaters' initial mean self-efficacy score was 7.2 out of a maximum of 10 for jumps in the self-modeling condition and 6.7 out of 10 for jumps in the control condition, which, in their opinion, left little room for improvement. For elite competitors, even a small improvement in performance may produce a large improvement in results. They also speculated that self-modeling interventions may be more successful for continuous skills as compared to discrete skills. They encouraged further research in these areas.

Thus, the purpose of our study was to examine the effectiveness of a self-modeling intervention on shooting performance and self-efficacy beliefs with intercollegiate ice hockey players. If self-modeling is an effective tool for improving self-efficacy and elite performance in complex open skills, it could be of great value to many athletic programs. Not only would performance be enhanced, but resources and time would be spent more efficiently. We hypothesized that regular viewing of self-modeling videotapes by elite intercollegiate ice hockey players would produce improvements in self-efficacy beliefs and shooting performance, compared with players who did not view self-modeling tapes.

Method

Participants

The participants consisted of 22 hockey players on one varsity intercollegiate NCAA Division I team. They were all Caucasian, male, undergraduates aged 18-23 years. Participants were divided by class (i.e., 6 freshman, 8 sophomore, 5 junior, 4 senior), then assigned randomly to either the experimental ($n = 11$) or control group ($n = 11$). Each athlete provided informed consent to participate in the study.

Research Design

A pretest-posttest, control group design with repeated measures was used. The experimental group participated in a treatment session that consisted of 10 weeks of viewing self-modeling tapes, once per week. The control group did not receive treatment. Skill specific self-efficacy questionnaires and a shooting test performance were administered to all participants at the start of the study, which took place 3 weeks into the hockey season, and twice more at 5 week intervals. Multiple testing allowed differences in the rate of improvement to be observed.

Instrumentation

A Shooter Tutor[TM] was used to test shooting accuracy. The Shooter Tutor consists of a sheet of thick industrial grade plastic that attaches to the net posts to cover the net opening. There are four holes in the sheet, one in each corner. The holes are the shape of a quarter circle, 1 ft (0.3048 m) in radius, with the center of the circle located at the corner on the net. The four holes were the targets. An illustration of the target is presented in Figure 1. A preliminary open ended questionnaire, consisting of one item, identified the backhand as the shot which the majority of players were least confident in performing. Thus, backhand shots were used for all shooting tests.

Participants stood directly in front of the target and fired five consecutive shots, from a distance of 20 ft. (6.10 m), at each of the four targets, for a total of 20 shots. The first five shots were directed to the lower left target, followed by lower right, upper left, and upper right. The five consecutive shots were taken in less than 20 s. The time between each of the four series of shots did not exceed 1 min. The total number of shots that hit the targets was used as the measure of shooting accuracy. All testing was done on fresh ice.

A skill specific self-efficacy questionnaire was constructed, in accordance with Bandura's (1986) recommendations, to measure the participants' confidence in their ability to perform certain shooting skills correctly 100% of the time. The questionnaire was designed to assess beliefs about performing in competition rather than on the Shooter Tutor because of its more practical benefit. Confidence in performing well on the Shooter Tutor does not necessarily mean that one is confident in performing shots in a game. Thus, we were interested in the generalizability of self-modeling effects on the Shooter tutor to self-efficacy beliefs for shots within game situations. The questionnaire comprised five items based on a conceptual analysis of the shots used in collegiate hockey. Players were asked, "How confident are you in your ability to perform the following skills correctly 100% of the time in the next game," for the wrist shot, snap shot, slap shot, backhand shot, and one-timer shot. Each efficacy rating was made on a 10-point probability scale, ranging from 1 (*not at all confident*) to 10 (*extremely confident*). The efficacy scores were computed by summing the five questions, which resulted in a possible scale range of 5 to 50. An internal consistency analysis of the pretest scores revealed a Cronbach alpha of .80 on the five items.

Procedure

Prior to the collection of data, approval was obtained from the Institutional Review Board and the participating team. Each player was tested individually.

The efficacy questionnaire was administered just prior to the shooting test and took place prior to regular practice, on a non-game day. The first measurement time occurred one week prior to the intervention. On the second and third administrations of the instruments, the player was given the questionnaire and the shooting test immediately after viewing his individualized video.

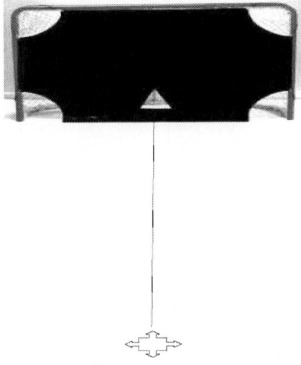

Target 20 ft. from goal

Figure 1. Shooting accuracy task.

Each participant in the experimental group viewed a 90 s self-modeling video tape once, in its entirety, once a week. The tape was constructed by a video technician with 3 years experience as video coordinator for hockey and 2 years of hockey coaching experience. The video consisted of multiple repetitions (range = 40 - 50) of successful shooting test trials of the backhand shot from two different camera angles. The technician assembled the clips without respect to the order in which they were performed or the angle from which they were shot. The self-modeling videotapes were viewed privately, either in the video room or in a vacant room or office on a large RCA 52 in. (132.08 cm) television screen.

Results

Because of the exploratory nature of this study, the rejection region for finding significance was set at $p < .10$ (same as Winfrey and Weeks, 1993), with effect sizes reported. Raising the rejection region to $p < .10$ increases the probability of accepting the research hypothesis when it may be false (Type I error). However, because of the exploratory nature of the study, leniency toward Type I errors may be warranted (Keppel, 1991).

Means and standard deviations for shooting performance and self-efficacy are presented in Table 1. The results of the shooting accuracy test and the self-efficacy questionnaire were analyzed using two separate 2 X 3 (Group by Time) ANOVAs with repeated measures.

A significant main effect was found between the experimental and control groups on the shooting accuracy test, $F(1, 20) = 3.90$, $p < .10$. The experimental group showed greater shooting accuracy ($M = 5.86$, $SD = 1.83$) than the control group ($M = 4.69$, $SD = 2.14$). The effect size, using the Control Group SD was .55. A two tailed t test showed that there was no significant difference between the groups in pretrial test scores, $t(20) = 1.53$, $p > .10$.

The ANOVA on shooting self-efficacy also showed differences between the groups, $F(1, 20) = 5.12$, $p < .10$. The experimental group scored higher on the shooting self-efficacy questionnaire ($M = 37.91$, $SD = 6.41$) than the control group ($M = 33.41$, $SD = 6.81$). The effect size, using the Control Group SD was .66. There was no difference between the groups in pretrial scores, $t(20) = 1.10$, $p > .10$.

Discussion

Regular viewing of self-modeling videotapes by elite intercollegiate ice hockey players produced a moderate, short term improvement in shooting performance, compared with players who did not view self-modeling tapes. The largest difference between the two groups occurred at the Week 5. This result was similar to Franks and Maile (1991), who used self-modeling to train a competitive power lifter. Viewing the tapes produced the greatest gains for the power lifter early in the intervention such that no additional gains were made in the next 4-6 weeks. At the elite level of Division I collegiate hockey, it may be difficult to continue to make substantial improvements in shooting beyond the gains initially made. The self-modeling group's efficacy scores did not fall correspondingly, but rather continued to increase for the intervention group.

In comparison to the other researchers who have not found significant self-modeling effects on performance or self-efficacy, our study used a very difficult shooting task allowing for a greater margin of improvement. In addition, we had a larger sample size and used a skill-specific self-efficacy measure. As a comparison, Winfrey and Weeks (1993) used a modified version of the State Sport Confidence Inventory (Vealey, 1986). As Feltz and Chase (1998) have noted, it is important to have a high correspondence between performance tasks and self-efficacy measures, if one is to have any chance of finding self-efficacy effects with motor performance tasks. Even though our self-efficacy measure was skill specific, it was not context specific to the performance task. Thus, we still found self-efficacy effects in a competitive context based on performance in a practice context.

Our results imply that with a larger sample size and a specific self-efficacy measure self-modeling can influence self-efficacy beliefs as well as performance. In terms of practical implications from our study, self-modeling in sport may be used in two ways. It can be used as a short term aid to performance. For example, footage collected during the previous playing season could be used to create self-modeling tapes to prepare for the upcoming season. Self-modeling may also be of value in ending a slump, an extended period of poor performance. A short-term improvement in performance combined with a long term increase in self-efficacy should help the athlete to recover, and avoid relapse. Post intervention follow-up tests are recommended for future studies to determine the length of self-modeling benefits to self-efficacy. Research that investigates the effects of self-modeling on performance in competition, though difficult to carry out, would also be of benefit to test the generality of effects.

**Table 2. Means and Standard Deviations by
Group for Shooting Performance and Self-Efficacy**

Group		Time 1	2	3
		Shooting Performance		
Self-Model	M	5.18	6.55	5.86
	SD	1.66	1.13	2.59
Control	M	4.18	4.56	5.36
	SD	1.40	2.62	2.11
		Self-Efficacy Scores		
Self-Model	M	36.82	36.91	39.56
	SD	7.80	6.20	13.53
Control	M	33.67	33.82	32.40
	SD	5.33	11.85	14.79

References

Bandura, A. (1986). *Social foundations of thought and action*. Englewood Cliffs, NJ: Prentice-Hall.

Bandura, A. (1997). *Self-efficacy: The exercise of control*. New York: Freeman.

Clark, S.E., and Ste-Marie, D.M. (2007). Investigating the impact of self-as-a-model interventions on children's self-regulation of learning and swimming performance. *Journal of Sport Sciences, 25*, 577-586.

Clark, S.E., Ste-Marie, D.M., and Martini, R. (2006). The thought processes underlying self-as-a-model interventions: An exploratory study. *Psychology of Sport and Exercise, 7*, 381-386.

Dowrick, P. W. (1999). A review of self-modeling and related interventions. *Applied and Preventive Psychology, 8*, 23–39.

Dowrick, P. W., and Dove, C. (1980). The use of modeling to improve the swimming performance of spina bifida children. *Journal of Applied Behavior Analysis, 13*, 51-56.

Feltz, D. L., and Chase, M. A. (1998). The measurement of self-efficacy and confidence in sport. In J. Duda (Ed.), *Advancements in sport and exercise psychology measurement* (pp.63-78). Morgantown, WV: Fitness Information Technology.

Feltz, D.L., Short, S.E., and Sullivan, P.J. (2008). *Self-efficacy in sport*. Champaign, IL: Human Kinetics.

Franks, I. M. and Maile, L. J. (1991). The use of video in sport skill acquisition. In P. W. Dowrick (Ed.), *Practical guide to using video in the behavioral sciences* (pp. 231-243). New York: John Wiley and Sons.

George, T. R., Feltz, D. L., and Chase, M. A. (1992). Effects of model similarity on self-efficacy and muscular endurance: A second look. *Journal of Sport and Exercise Psychology, 14*, 237-248.

Gould, D., and Weiss, M.R. (1981). The effects of model similarity and model talk on self-efficacy and muscular endurance. *Journal of Sport Psychology, 3*, 17-29.

Keppel, G. (1991). *Design and analysis: A researcher's handbook (3rd ed.)*. Englewood Cliffs, NJ: Prentice-Hall.

Landers, D.M., and Landers, D.M. (1973). Teacher versus peer models: Effects of model's presence and performance level on motor behavior. *Journal of Motor Behavior, 5*, 129-139.

Lirgg, C.D., and Feltz, D.L. (1991). Teacher versus peer models revisited: Effects on motor performance and self-efficacy. *Research Quarterly for Exercise and Sport, 62*, 217-224.

Law, B., and Ste-Marie, D.M. (2005). Self-modeling and figure skating performance. *European Journal of Sport Sciences, 5*, 143-153.

McCullagh, P. (1987). Model status as a determinant of observational learning and performance. *Journal of Sport Psychology, 8,* 319-331.

McCullagh, P. (1993). Modeling: Learning, developmental, and social psychological considerations. In R. N. Singer, M. Murphey, and L. K. Tennant (Eds.), *Handbook of research on sport psychology* (pp. 106-126). New York: Macmillan.

McCullagh, P. and Weiss, M.R. (2001). Modeling: Considerations for motor skill performance and psychological responses. In R.N. Singer, H.A. Hausenblas, C.M. Janelle (eds.), *Handbook of sport psychology* (2nd ed., pp.205-238). Toronto, Canada: Wiley and Sons.

Ram, N., and McCullagh, P. (2003). Self-modeling: Influence on psychological responses and physical performance. *The Sport Psychologist, 17*, 220-241.

Starek, J., and McCullagh, P. (1999). The effect of self-modeling on the performance of beginning swimmers. *The Sport Psychologist, 13*, 269-287.

Vealey, R. (1986). Conceptualization of sport-confidence and competitive orientation: Preliminary investigation and instrument development. *Journal of Sport Psychology, 8*, 221-246.

Winfrey, M. L. and Weeks, D. L. (1993). Effects of self-modeling on self-efficacy and balance beam performance. *Perceptual and Motor Skills, 77*, 907-913.

In: Sport and Exercise Psychology Research Advances
Editors: M. P. Simmons, L. A. Foster, pp. 19-51

ISBN: 978-1-60456-157-9
© 2008 Nova Science Publishers, Inc.

Chapter I

Psychological Stage Models of Physical Exercise – Research Advances

Lisa Marie Warner and Sonia Lippke
Freie Universitaet Berlin, Germany

Abstract

In order to explain and predict health behaviors like physical exercise, it is essential to have good theoretical backdrops. In recent years, a number of models were designed to map proximal determinants of physical activity. These models can be categorized into continuum models and stage models.

Continuum models try to identify variables that determine behavior change. A linear prediction equation combines the different variables. Based on this assumption, interventions to promote physical exercise focus on increasing all associated variables in all individuals. On the contrary, stage theories model health behavior change as discrete stages along the way to the goal behavior. Depending on the stage that a person is in, specific social-cognitive variables are important. Every stage has its own equation that predicts the progression to the next stage. Stage-based interventions propose intervention packages matched to the stage a person is in, i.e., to the prevalent needs.

The chapter goes into more detail for stage models. An overview of stage theories such as the Transtheoretical Model (TTM) by Prochaska and DiClemente (1983) and the Health Action Process Approach (HAPA) by Schwarzer (1992) is given. Measurements for exercise stages are discussed and state-of-the art examples are presented. Research strategies, empirical evidence and criticism on stage theories are outlined. The chapter identifies stage-specific mechanisms and provides guidance to design theory-based expert systems and physical exercise promotion programs.

Keywords: *stages of change, stage-matched intervention, theories of health behavior change, tailoring*

1. Introduction

Explaining and predicting health behaviors like physical exercise requires good theoretical grounding. In past decades, numerous models have been designed to map proximal determinants of physical activity. These models can be broadly grouped into continuum models and stage models.

Continuum models of physical exercise try to identify predictors (such as goals or risk-perception) for behavior or behavior change. These different variables are typically combined into a linear prediction equation. By enhancing the determinants, the equation predicts an increase in the probability of behavior or behavior change. Thus, all persons are placed along a continuum of behavior likelihood depending on their level of considered variables. This assumption implies that interventions to promote physical exercise based on continuum models focus on increasing all associated variables in all individuals. Along this line, interventions are designed as "one-size-fits-all"-programs (for a recent overview on continuum models see Richert and Lippke, 2007). However, many studies have shown that one size does not fit all individuals (Kreuter, Strecher, and Glassman, 1999).

On the contrary, stage models assume that health behavior change takes place in several discrete stages, steps or mindsets. Depending on the stage a person belongs to, specific social-cognitive variables are more important than others. According to stage models, every stage has its own equation that predicts the progression to the next stage up to the final stage, where the recommended level of physical exercise is maintained. If interventions are based on stage models, they provide different intervention packages for people in different stages. Hence, these programs are, according to researchers in favor of stage models, matched to the stage-specific needs of each participant.

Why are Stage Models so Attractive?

To illustrate the purpose of stage theories, imagine a group of three individuals who should be motivated to exercise regularly. One of them has never been physically active in his life and is not thinking of being active one day. The second person is not active either but is thinking about starting a fitness center course next week. The third one has been active for three years but has recently moved to a new town and has suddenly stopped exercising. Would it be appropriate to try to persuade these three persons with the same arguments to become more active?

It is known from continuum models that an increase in some social-cognitive variables like self-efficacy, risk-perception or goals might raise the probability of becoming more active. However, which of these determinants will have the best effect in which state of mind? Do certain topics (like the communication of the risks of a physically inactive lifestyle) need to be addressed before others (like how to maintain regular exercise)?

Stage theories would categorize our participants into discrete stages and apply matched intervention programs for each stage. Stage-matched interventions provide tailored treatments for the needs of every participant and omit those issues that are not relevant for the focused stage. Thus, if health behavior change really takes place through qualitatively distinct stages, these intervention packages should be more efficient than "one-size-fits-all"-approaches, as they address nothing but relevant issues in every stage. At the same time, stage-matched interventions should be less time consuming and less cost intensive than "one-size-fits-all"-interventions.

How people are categorized into the different stages and whether the theoretically-driven advantages of stage models can be supported empirically will be discussed after a short description of stage models in general and some current stage models in particular.

The Basic Concept of Stage Models

There are different stage theories. Many theories have unique stages and corresponding staging algorithms (the rules according to which people are classified into the stages). However, according to Weinstein, Rothman and Sutton (1998) all stage models of health behavior change are based on the same basic concepts; they share four defining properties:

(a) Persons can be clearly categorized into different stages.
(b) There is a clear order of stages and it is specified to which stage people progress when leaving a particular stage. People in the highest stages have reached the goal of being physically active.
(c) There are relatively small differences among people in the same stage; e.g., they have to overcome similar barriers to progress to the next stage.
(d) There are relatively large differences among people in different stages; e.g., they face different barriers to progress to the next stage.

Besides these general properties, every stage model has its specific character but also overlapping elements with other stage models. In the following section, the distinctive features of different stage models will be described.

2. Current Stage Models

The idea of mapping the process of health behavior change reaches back to the early 1980s when Prochaska and DiClemente observed that changes in behavior might be illustrated in different stages. In 1982, the first stage theory was published – the *Transtheoretical Model* (*TTM*) by Prochaska and DiClemente. Since then, the TTM is the best known and most prevalent of all stage models.

Other stage models followed throughout the last decades, such as the *Precaution Adoption Process Model* (*PAPM*) by Weinstein and Sandmann (1992), the *Health Action Process Approach* (*HAPA*) by Schwarzer (1992), the *Berlin Stage Model (BSM)* by Fuchs (1999) or the *Multi Stage Model (MSM)* by Lippke and Ziegelmann (2006).

The Transtheoretical Model (TTM)

The *Transtheoretical Model (TTM)* by Jim Prochaska and Carlo DiClemente has initially been developed by Jim Prochaska in the clinical context of smoking cessation, using both therapy literature on quitting smoking and data from self-changers (Prochaska and DiClemente, 1982). The aggregation of constructs drawn from different theories is captured by the term "transtheoretical".

In their original works, Prochaska and DiClemente (1982) identified five stages. However, in the following years, they consistently found only four groups (*precontemplation, contemplation, action and maintenance*) and worked with these four stages the following seven years (McConnaughy, Prochaska, and Velicer, 1983; McConnaughy, DiClemente, Prochaska, and Velicer, 1989; Prochaska and DiClemente, 1983, 1985, 1986). In 1992, Prochaska and DiClemente realized that the same studies analyzed with cluster analyses instead of principal component analyses, identified groups of individuals who were in a stage between *contemplation* and *action*, namely in the *preparation stage*. These studies supported the importance of assessing *preparation* as a fifth stage of change (DiClemente, Prochaska, Fairhurst, Velicer, Velasquez, and Rossi, 1991; Prochaska and DiClemente, 1992). Hence, in 1992, Prochaska and DiClemente finally established their model as today's most widely used version with five-stages (Prochaska, DiClemente and Norcross, 1992) as illustrated in Table 1:

Table 1. The TTM stages of change and their characteristics; staging algorithm applied to exercise by Marcus, Selby, Niaura and Rossi (1992)

Stage	Characteristic	Staging algorithm
Precontemplation	Having no intention to change the behavior in the near future.	"I do not participate in physical activity and I don't think that I will begin to do so in the next 6 months."
Contemplation	Being aware that a problem exists and seriously thinking about overcoming it but having not yet made a commitment to take action.	"I do not participate in physical activity but I will start exercising in the next 6 months."
Preparation	Intending to take action in the very near future. Having done some changes in the right direction (preparatory behavior).	"I exercise somewhat but not on a regular basis."
Action	Adopted the goal behavior since less than 6 months.	"I exercise regularly but have only begun to do so during the last 6 months."
Maintenance	Maintaining the goal behavior for more than 6 months.	"I exercise regularly and have begun to do so more than 6 months ago."

People are assumed to progress through the stages in order, but they may fall back from the *action* and *maintenance stage* to earlier stages as well and they may cycle through the stages several times before reaching the *maintenance stage* (Prochaska and Norcross, 2003). Further developments within the framework of the TTM assume a sixth stage in which the temptation of falling back to previous health-compromising routines is no longer experienced. This stage is called *termination* and may be reached after a long period of time (e.g., five years of successful behavior change) resulting in a temptationless state of regular exercise (Prochaska and Norcross, 2003). However, it is not clear whether in health behavior domains as physical activity a *termination* it possible at all (Marcus and Forsynth, 2003). Therefore, and for the reason that its investigation requires large longitudinal studies with extensive time-frames, nearly no publication in the exercise domain includes the *termination stage* and in the following, this sixth stage will not be included.

In 1992, the first group of researches applied the TTM to physical exercise. The results according to the stages were consistent with applications of the model to smoking cessation and other areas of behavior change (Marcus, Rakowski, and Rossi, 1992). An exemplary staging algorithm developed by the same group of researchers can be found in Table 1 (Marcus, Selby, Niaura, and Rossi, 1992).

The stages provide the basic organizing principle of the TTM and explain *when* changes occur. However, the postulated *social-cognitive variables* and *processes of change* are important contributors to the model as well. The social-cognitive variables are indicators of belonging to a stage and at the same time indicators of stage-progression. One of these social-cognitive variables is the concept of *decisional balance* that contains the reflection of *pros* and *cons*.

From the contemplation stage on, persons begin to weigh up the pros and cons of a change in behavior (Prochaska and DiClemente, 1992). Cons are decreasing with a progression in stage whereas pros increase (DiClemente et al., 1991).

Two additional social-cognitive variables that are often measured within the context of the TTM are *self-efficacy* – the belief in one's competence to overcome potential barriers and *temptation* – the feeling of being tempted to relapse to the problematic behavior in difficult situations (DiClemente et al., 1991; Prochaska, Velicer, Rossi, Goldstein, Marcus, Rakowski, Fiore, Harlow, Redding, Rosenbloom, and Rossi, 1994). Similar to the development of pros and cons, self-efficacy increases throughout the stages whereas temptation decreases (DiClemente et al., 1991).

Within the framework of the TTM, the cognitive-affective and the behavioral processes of change act as predictors and activators for stage-progression and explain how these shifts occur. Prochaska and DiClemente (1998, p. 6) comment: "the most interesting and useful research advances for the TTM are the continued reliable relationships between the stages and processes of change". Table 2 illustrates that cognitive-affective processes are assumed to be used most frequently during the first three stages and the behavioral processes during the last two stages (Prochaska et al., 1992). The processes are postulated as being uniquely effective for the progression from a specific stage to the next stage but not for the progression into others stages. However, Sutton (2005) criticizes that the relation between the processes of change and the social-cognitive variables are not specified in the TTM.

Table 2. Theoretical effects of the processes of change on stage-progression

Processes of change	PC	C	P	A	M
A) COGNITIVE-AFFECTIVE PROCESSES					
Consciousness raising	Pr/K/B	Pr/K/B			
Social liberation	K	K	Pr	Pr	
Dramatic relief, emotional arousal	Pr/B	Pr/K/B	K		
Self-reevaluation		Pr/K/B	Pr/K/B		
Environmental reevaluation	B	K/B	K		
B) BEHAVIORAL PROCESSES					
Self-liberation, commitment			Pr/K/B	Pr/K/B	
Helping relationships			K	Pr/K/B	P/B
Reinforcement management, reward				Pr/K/B	Pr/K/B
Counterconditioning				Pr/K/B	Pr/K/B
Stimulus control				Pr/K/B	Pr/K/B

Note.   PC = Precontemplation; C = Contemplation; P = Preparation; A = Action; M = Maintenance; Pr/K/B = indicates that these strategies theoretically promote progression to the next stage (but not to other stages); Pr = according to Prochaska et al., 1992; K = according to Keller, Velicer and Prochaska, 1999; B = according to Biddle and Mutrie, 2001. The inconsistency reflects today's theoretical disaccord and lack of empirical evidence. (Table based on Lippke & Renneberg, 2006).

Hence, it would be possible that the processes lead to a change in social-cognitive variables, which in turn promote stage-progressions. However, the reverse pattern could also be true. Therefore, Sutton claims that Prochaska and his team should specify any "causal model for each of the four forward stage transitions" (Sutton, 2005, p. 227).

There has been a number of studies that compared the social-cognitive variables, processes and exercise level of persons in different stages on a cross-sectional basis (e.g., Lippke, and Plotnikoff, 2006), in longitudinal programs (e.g., Plotnikoff, Hotz, Birkett, and Courneya, 2001) and intervention studies (e.g., Napolitano, Fotheringham, Tate, Sciamanna, Leslie, Owen, Bauman, and Marcus, 2003) all theoretically framed by the TTM. Keeping in mind that stage theories assume the occurrence of discontinuity patterns (non-linear developments of indicative variables across the stages) both in processes and in social-cognitive variables across the stages, the results of two meta-analyses on the TTM will be summarized in section 3.2.

The Precaution Adoption Process Model (PAPM)

In 1988, Neil Weinstein developed the *Precaution Adoption Process Model* (*PAPM*; Weinstein, 1988; Weinstein and Sandmann, 1992) in the context of home radon (a naturally occurring carcinogenic gas) testing. In 1992, Weinstein and Sandman published a revised version, which will be described in this section. The model contains seven stages as illustrated in Figure 1.

Stages	Characteristics
1. Unaware of issue	1) People are unaware of the health issue
2. Unengaged by issue	2) People are aware of the health issue but they have never thought of adopting the precaution
3. Deciding about acting	3) People are undecided whether or not to adopt the precaution, depending on their decision they move to stage 4 or stage 5.
5. Decided to act 4. Decided not to act	4 & 5) If they decide not to act, they may still return to stage 3 at any time, if they decide to act they may move to further stages
6. Acting	6) People act according to their goals
7. Maintenance	7) People maintain the new behavior

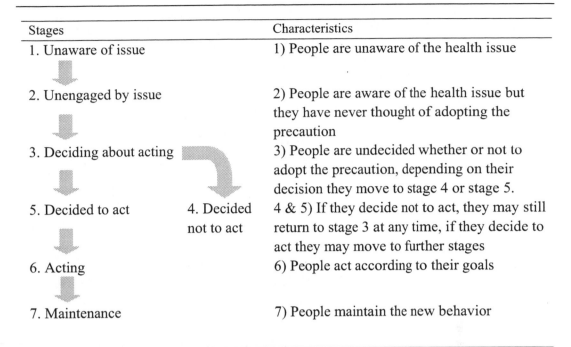

Figure 1. The PAPM adapted from Weinstein and Sandmann (1992).

According to Weinstein and Sandmann (1992), the PAPM has some similarities to the TTM, but it differs in several ways, too. Firstly, it contains seven instead of five stages. Additionally to the TTM stages, there is a stage that contains people who are completely unaware of a health threat (*unaware of issues*). Another additional stage is the *decided not to act* stage.

The *precontemplation stage* of the TTM contains both, individuals that know about the health issue, but who have never thought of changing their behavior and individuals who have decided not to act. The PAPM provides two distinct stages for these different sets of mind, the *unengaged by issue* and the *decided not to act stage*. A detailed analysis of these groups of people may be reasonable in terms of the resistance to treatment as it might make a difference if individuals have never thought of changing their behavior (*unengaged by issue*) and individuals that are already determined not to act (*decided not to act*). Weinstein and Sandman (1992, p. 171) state: "Certainly people who have come to a definite position on an issue - especially an issue regarding their own behavior - will be more resistant to persuasion than people who have never formed an opinion (Frey, 1986; Janis and Mann, 1977; Nisbett and Ross, 1980)".

Even if the *contemplation stage* of the TTM and the *deciding about acting stage* of the PAPM seem to be identical, they differ substantially. The *contemplation stage* in the TTM is usually defined as a serious contemplation of change in behavior within the next six months. This is not the matter in the *deciding about acting stage* in the PAPM, as seriously thinking about doing something in the foreseeable future is not like being undecided whether or not to act.

Table 3. Issues likely to determine progress between the PAPM stages, adapted from Weinstein and Sandman (2002b)

Stage transition	*Important issues*
Stage 1 to stage 2	Media messages about the hazard and precaution
Stage 2 to stage 3	Communications from significant others
	Personal experience with hazard
Stage 3 to stage 4 or stage 5	Beliefs about hazard likelihood and severity
	Beliefs about personal susceptibility
	Beliefs about precaution effectiveness and difficulty
	Behaviors and recommendations of others
	Perceived social norms
	Fear and worry
Stage 5 to stage 6	Time, effort and resources needed to act
	Detailed "how-to" information
	Reminders and other cues to action
	Assistance in carrying out action

The *decided to act stage* of the PAPM and the *preparation stage* in the TTM are similar, if the *preparation stage* is defined in terms of intending and planning a behavior (however, the *preparation stage* sometimes also requires past behavior per definition).

The *maintenance stage* was directly inspired by the TTM, as for home radon testing there is no need for such a stage, because the best precaution would be the elimination of any dangers at home or a lifetime vaccination. Hence, in the context of home radon testing, there is no need for the *maintenance stage*, but Weinstein and Sandmann (1992) integrated it for other health behaviors. Theoretically, individuals progress through the stages in order (1-2-3-5-6-7), some stages may also be skipped, but there is no minimum period of time that has to be spent in any of them. Movements backwards may occur as well, even if not every regression is allowed in the PAPM (e.g., one can not fall back into the first stage after reaching the third or higher stages; Weinstein and Sandman, 2002). Hence, unlikely to the TTM, there are no time criteria for the stages.

The PAPM further postulates several factors that may ease stage-progressions. Up to now, there is little empirical evidence for these factors and whether they have the same effects in different behavioral domains. However, they are listed in Table 3 to cover all aspects of the PAPM.

To date, the PAPM has been applied in studies on physical exercise only in combination with other behaviors in the context of osteoporosis intervention (such as calcium intake; Blalock, DeVellis, Giorgino, DeVellis, Gold, Dooley, Anderson and Smith, 1996; Blalock, DeVellis, Patterson, Campbell, Orenstein and Dooley, 2002; Sharp and Thombs, 2003). Blalock and colleagues conducted a first study on osteoporosis precautions in 1996. They found some evidence for the PAPM stages as women differed in 2/3 of tested knowledge and attitudinal variables like self-efficacy, subjective norms or perceived barriers. However, the effects were better for calcium intake (Blalock et al., 1996). Another study on women's osteoprotective behavior examined the effects of an intervention program that integrated some stage assumptions of the PAPM and compared it to a non-tailored intervention (Blalock et al., 2002). Both programs did not integrate the factors that Weinstein and Sandman postulate to influence stage-progressions (see Table 3), but were based on different communication strategies for three of the PAPM stages (*unengaged, engaged* and *action*). Individuals in the tailored group showed more stage-progressions in calcium intake than in the non-tailored group. However, there were no such effects for exercise behavior.

In 2003, Sharp and Thombs analyzed college students according to their osteoprotective behavior with cluster analyses. They found only two stages, which were referred to as *less engaged* and *engaged*. These stages differed in terms of health motivation, sex, perceived barriers to exercise, and exercise self-efficacy. Sharp and Thombs concluded that the PAPM is not perfect to explain the adoption of osteoprotective precautions. These contrary findings should stimulate further research on the PAPM in the context of physical exercise (Sharp and Thombs, 2003).

Health Action Process Approach (HAPA)

In 1992, Ralf Schwarzer proposed his *Health Action Process Approach (HAPA)*. Instead of further differentiations into more stages, the HAPA (Schwarzer, 1992, 2008) tries to get by with the least possible number of stages. It summarizes the sub-stages of other models under broader categories (see Figure 6). Originally, the HAPA was developed containing only two stages: the *non-intentional/pre-decisional motivational* and the *intentional/post-decisional volitional phase*. The *motivational phase* is assumed to frame all processes that result in the setting of the *goal* to change a behavior. Hence, it comprises individuals that have not yet formulated an intention to act, so the related stage is called the *non-intentional stage*. In the *volitional phase*, planning and realization of the behavior are supposed to be dominant.

In recent publications on the HAPA, the *volitional stage* is further split up into (a) *continuous inactivity* although the individual is decided to be active, also referred to as the *intentional stage*, (b) *adoption* of the new behavior, also referred to as the *action stage* (c) and *maintenance* of behavior (Schwarzer and Lippke, 2005). However, previous studies have only tested the first three stage of the model: The *non-intentional stage* (motivational), the *intentional stage* (volitional-inactive) and the *action stage* (volitional-active). In addition to the specification of stages, the HAPA postulates several social-cognitive variables as affecting a change in behavior like continuum models would. Hence, the HAPA explicitly combines continuous assumptions and phases and is therefore often referred to as a *hybrid model* (Biddle, Hagger, Chatzisarantis, and Lippke, 2007; Schwarzer, 2008). Linear assumptions of the HAPA are for example that the probability of the adoption of regular exercise increases with an increase in levels of self-efficacy and exact *plans* when, where and how the exercise will be adopted (also known as *implementation intentions* see Gollwitzer, 1999). However, planning is only efficient if a person has previously formulated the goal to exercise regularly. That means, that the social-cognitive variables are not overall predictive for changes, but they depend on the stage a persons belongs to. In other words, according to the HAPA, the social-cognitive variables influence goal setting, the planning process and the implementation of behavior in a stage-specific way. See Figure 2 for an overview of the HAPA variables and stages.

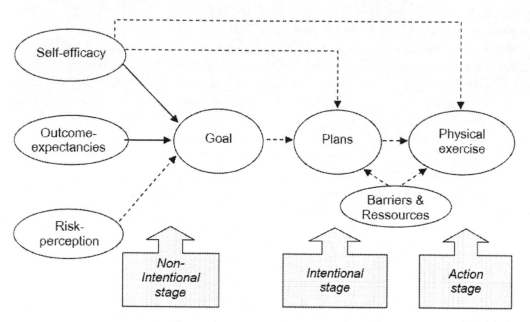

Figure 2. The Health Action Process Approach (HAPA; Schwarzer, 1992) adapted from Schwarzer and Lippke (2005).

As long as individuals have not formulated a goal to change their behavior, they are classified as *non-intentional*. In this phase an increase in *risk-perception* is important as well as the elaboration of *outcome-expectancies* (also known as pros and cons). Another prerequisite of goal setting is self-efficacy, as individuals that are not confident in being able to perform physical exercise on a regular basis are not supposed to formulate the goal to do so. By setting the goal to exercise regularly, a person moves from the *non-intentional* to the *intentional stage*. The *intentional stage* starts with detailed action planning on how, when and where the exercise will be performed. Cognitive links between the concrete opportunities and the intended behavior are built, so that physical exercise is tied to situational cues (Lippke, Ziegelmann, and Schwarzer, 2004). Individuals that specify when, where and how plans are more likely to recognize opportunities for physical exercise; they adopt physical exercise more automatically, and take the opportunity earlier than individuals without action plans. Furthermore, intentions are not forget easily, when specified in a when, where, and how manner (for an overview and meta-analysis, see Gollwitzer and Sheeran, 2006).

Self-efficacy is again an important contributor to the formulation of plans. Outcome-expectancies remain important whilst risk-perception is no longer influential in the *intentional stage*.

By implementing the new behavior, the *action stage* is reached. During the *action stage*, the behavior as well as the goal have to be shielded from distractions and hence constant self-regulatory processes are required (Schwarzer, 2004). Self-regulatory skills and strategies make sure that the goal is not abandoned, the behavior is not given up and the attention is not drawn-off by other goals (Schwarzer, 2008). Barriers that emerge initially and later on in the *maintenance process* have to be coped with, and personal and social resources have to be applied in a way that the behavior can be performed regularly. Even in the *action stage*, self-efficacy and coping planning have a huge impact, as they operate relapse-preventive (c.f. relapse model by Marlatt and Gordon, 1985; for the concept of coping planning in contrast to action planning see Ziegelmann, Luszcysnka, Lippke, and Schwarzer 2007; Ziegelmann and Lippke, 2007). There is a large amount of research that analyzed the continuous assumptions of the HAPA (for an overview see Schwarzer, 2004; Sutton, 2005). However, studies that analyze the stage assumptions have been rare (Lippke et al., 2004; Lippke, Ziegelmann, and Schwarzer, 2005; Warner, Lippke, Wiedemann, Reuter, and Ziegelmann, 2007). The studies that dealt with the HAPA stages supported numerous assumptions. Such studies will be resumed in section 3.2.

Berlin Stage Model (BSM)

A stage model that was mainly designed for exercise is the *Berlin Stage Model* (*BSM* Fuchs, 1999, 2003). Some stages are similar to stages of the TTM (*precontemplation*, *contemplation*). However, the BSM offers a more precise differentiation in the post-decisional phase than the TTM.

The BSM comprises eight stages. The process of behavioral change begins with the stage of *precontemplation*, where engaging in physical activity on a regular basis is not even considered. In the *contemplation stage* people play with the idea of becoming physically active some day. They are beginning to balance the pros and cons of a change in behavior. Consequently, persons in the *contemplation stage* are relatively susceptible for information concerning the pros and cons of physical exercise (Fuchs, 2005). *Precontemplation* and *contemplation* correspond to the first two TTM stages but the BSM abandons the time criteria of the TTM stages.

Once a person decides to engage in regular exercise, the *disposition stage* is entered and a goal is set. With that, the person moves into the post-decisional phase. Details of implementing this goal into action are not yet formulated. The question is no longer if a behavior change is intended but how it can be carried out. Once this *how* is settled a person is allocated to the *preaction stage*. According to Gollwitzer (1999), the details on how to implement a certain goal are called implementation intentions. These implementation intentions contain information such as the type of exercise a person chooses, how to assign for it and when and were to perform it.

If these when, where and how plans lead to the performance of exercise, the *implementation stage* is reached. The challenge in this stage is to integrate the physical exercise into the daily routine and to shield it against competing goals and wishes. To reach stability of regular exercise, persons profit from meta-cognitive strategies such as self-regulatory skills that protect the intended behavior from distractions. If the new behavior becomes such a routine that it does no longer require volitional control to perform it on a regular basis, the *habituation stage* is reached. Hence, in the BSM the *habituation stage* is not defined by a certain period of time, but by the strong anchorage of exercise in the daily routine. A person in the *habituation stage* no longer questions whether to exercise on a special day or not, the cycle of exercise is constant and the person is able to cope with sudden distractions (Fuchs, 2005).

If a person is not able to integrate exercise into his or her lifestyle and exercises on an irregular basis only, he or she is assigned to the *fluctuation stage*. In contrast to the *implementation stage*, where people do also exercise irregularly, the *fluctuation stage* follows a period of regular implementation, hence it follows on the *habituation stage* if the regularity is neglected. Fuchs assumes that persons in the *fluctuation stage* are especially vulnerable to distractions like stress, lack of time, holidays or other incidences that disturb the daily routine. These difficulties cannot be coped within the *fluctuation stage* and therefore provoke a complete drop of exercise. A fluctuating exercise pattern may stabilize after a while but it can also regress to inactivity. A complete abort of exercise is in most cases neither intended nor planned, but rather a quietly sneaking process of disengagement.

People that fell back into an inactive lifestyle may return to the first stages of the BSM, but more often their goals remain and they stay in the post-decisional phase. For previously active people who still intend to resume their engagement some day, Fuchs (1999) created the *resumption stage*. The mindsets of people in this stage resemble the cognitions in the *disposition stage*, with the difference that people in the *resumption stage* know about the barriers that occur whilst integrating regular exercise into the daily routine. However, individuals in the *resumption stage* also know how to overcome these barriers as they experienced it in the *habituation stage* for a while. The incorporation of a *resumption stage* might invalidate the criticism the TTM had to face for grouping individuals who have cycled through the stages and those individuals who have not had any experience of passing through the behavior change process together in the *precontemplation stage* (Kraft, Sutton, and McCreath-Reynolds, 1999). The BSM stages have to be assessed with the Questionnaire for the Diagnosis of Exercise Stage developed by Fuchs in 2001.

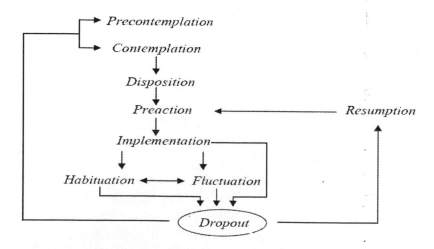

Figure 3. The Berlin Stage Model (Fuchs, 1999).

Some evidence for the existence of the BSM stages could be confirmed in a cross-sectional study, which is discussed in section 3.2 (Fuchs, 2001). Up to now, there are no longitudinal or experimental studies on the BSM.

Multi-Stage Model (MSM)

The *Multi-Stage Model* (*MSM*; Lippke, Sniehotta, and Luszczynska, 2005; Lippke and Ziegelmann, 2006) has been developed to expand the range of the BSM. It models comparable stages of health behavior change as the BSM (see Figure 4). However, it extends the BSM in several ways: Firstly, it was developed to model different behaviors, not merely physical activity. Secondly, it is more flexible, as the initially proposed eight stages may be merged (as in Lippke, Sniehotta, and Luszczynska, 2005) or subdivided (see Lippke, 2004) depending on the research question. Thirdly, the stages can be assessed more flexible, as with the algorithm shown in recent publications (Lippke, Sniehotta, and Luszczynska, 2005; Lippke and Ziegelmann, 2006).

The stage assessments refrain from applying time criteria (except for the differentiation between the *implementation* and the *fluctuation/habituation stage*); instead, they only consider psychological variables, like planning, easiness or habit to diagnose stages. Fourthly, the MSM postulates that persons in all *actional stages* are performing the goal behavior with some frequency. Hence, in contrary to the BSM, the MSM diagnoses the *implementation stage* only if the goal behavior is met (e.g., performing activities at least 5 days per week 30 minutes or more).

Consequently, individuals in the *fluctuation stage* have to perform the goal behavior repeatedly (Lippke, 2004). In contrast, the BSM assesses the *fluctuation stage* in case of sporadic occurring exercise behavior ranging from several times during the week to not even a single time in four weeks (Fuchs, 1999).

Lippke and Ziegelmann (2006) applied a staging algorithm to assess the MSM stages in a study on rehabilitation patients. This staging algorithm is illustrated in Figure 4.

If participants answered "no", they were instructed to choose from one of the possibilities on the left side of Figure 4, if they answered "yes" they should fill in all items on the right side. The *precontemplation stage* was diagnosed if an individual ticked "I am not thinking about exercise", the *contemplation stage* if an individual ticked "I was thinking about exercising (again) but I have not decided yet".

The *disposition stage* was diagnosed if an individual ticked "I have made the decision to start soon a new activity" and the *resumption stage* if an individual ticked "I have made the decision to soon restart exercising an old activity". Those indicating on an additional planning question that they were absolute sure when, where and how they would perform their intended physical activity were re-categorized into the *preaction stage* (out of *disposition* and *resumption stage*). All others explicating to be decided to start a physical activity were categorized into the *disposition stage* (those intending to start a new activity) or into the *resumption stage* (those intending to start an old behavior).

On the right side of Figure 4, individuals were assigned to the *implementation stage*, if they were exercising for at least six months. The *habituation stage* was diagnosed if an individual indicated that performing the physical activity was "very easy" and became "absolutely" a habit; otherwise, the *fluctuation stage* was categorized.

What was a typical week like for you (before the rehab started): Have you engaged in physical exercises for 20 minutes or longer, in such a way that you were at least moderately exhausted?

No ❑ → please choose one of the following four statements that applies to you most	Yes ❑ → please answer the following three questions
❑ I am **not thinking** about exercise.	1) **Since when** have you been exercising with this frequency? For the past ____ weeks/ ____ months/ ____ years
❑ I was **thinking about** exercising (again) but I have **not decided** yet.	
❑ I have made **the decision to start** soon a new activity.	2) **How easy** is it for you to exercise **regularly**, even if your week is busy? ❑ ❑ ❑ ❑ very hard little hard little easy very easy
❑ I have made **the decision to soon restart** exercising an old activity.	3) How much has it become your **habit** to exercise regularly? ❑ ❑ ❑ ❑ not at all not very much a little absolutely

Figure 4. The Multi-Stage Model (Lippke, Sniehotta, & Luszczynska, 2005; Lippke & Ziegelmann, 2006).

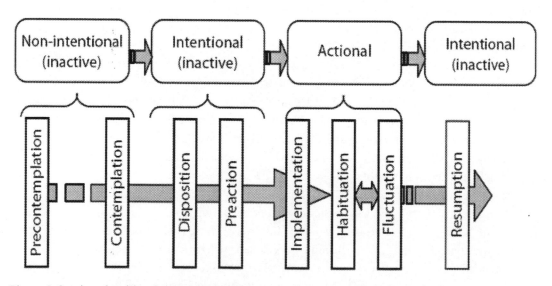

Figure 5. Staging algorithm for the MSM (Lippke and Ziegelmann, 2006).

Until now, there has only been the study by Lippke and Ziegelmann (2006) that analyzed the MSM with regard to exercise behavior: Its results concerning discontinuity patterns will be described in section 3.2.

Summary

To conclude, there are a number of differences between current stage models. They differ in the postulated number of stages and in the way, these stages are characterized and operationalized, respectively. Furthermore, stage models vary in their degree of precision with regard to stage transitions and in their assumptions of how these transitions are carried out. Although theory-guided studies on stage-matched interventions and discontinuity patterns have been conducted, none of the presented models has been tested to the extent, that all of its assumptions could be confirmed. Figure 6 illustrates the stage assumptions of the presented models and gives an overview of similarities and differences in the number and notation of stages.

There are some general questions that remain to be answered: Are stages actually distinct categories and not just subdivisions of a homogenous group of individuals more or less active? How many stages are best and can this number be empirically supported? (c.f. Lippke, Sniehotta, and Luszczynska, 2005; Schwarzer, 2008)?

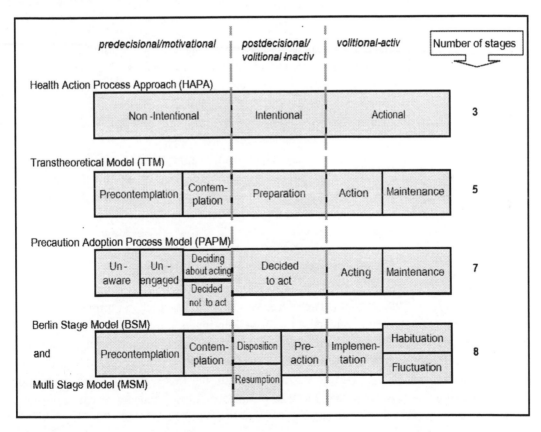

Figure 6. Synopsis of the current stage models: Notation of the general phase; notation of the model; notation of the models stages and number of stages (Lippke, 2004).

3. Theoretical and Empirical Criticism on Stage Models and How to Deal with it

Stage models enjoy great popularity, especially in health and exercise promotion. However, the critique on stage models increased in recent years (Adams and White, 2005; West, 2005; Brug, Conner, Harré, Kremers, McKellar, and Whitelaw, 2005). Already in 1997, Albert Bandura reproached stage models of not being able to capture the complexity of human behavior and of dividing the underlying continuous process into arbitrary parts that are then labeled stages (Bandura, 1997). The main critique on stage models face time spans (because they appear arbitrary), measurement inconsistencies (different stage algorithms used and very less investigated measurement qualities) and categorizing into groups that represent rather pseudo-stages than qualitative different stages.

In 1998, Weinstein, Rothmann and Sutton summarized criticism on stage models in their review article and upgraded it with possible solutions for current problems and ways to test stage assumptions. The research designs Weinstein, Rothmann and Sutton (1998) suggested were:

- Cross-sectional comparisons of persons in different stages (see section 3.2).
- Longitudinal observation studies that observe stage-progressions. These could reveal (a) whether persons are progressing according to the predicted stage transitions (i.e. whether stage B always follows on stage A etc.) and (b) whether stage transitions may be predicted by the assumed social-cognitive variables and processes (see Table 2).
- Randomized controlled trials, to test whether the manipulation of those factors that are assumed to be important, lead to stage-progressions or an increase in other outcome variables (i.e. more exercise) and whether the manipulations of factors that are not assumed to be important have no such effects (see section 3.3).

In the following, criticism on stage models and specific problems that derive by applying stage models will be pointed out. Thereby, it should be considered that some stage models (especially the TTM) meet criticism that does not concern the theoretical conception, but the operationalizations of the model. Therefore, it should be kept in mind, that the operationalizations are often not conducted by those who invent a model, but rather by those who apply a model. The problems with stage models are often methodological ones and evoked by those practitioners and researchers, that have not yet incorporated the idea of stages to the degree that proper operationalizations result. For this reason, it is necessary not only to know the assumptions of stage models, but also to know adequate research designs, which will be illustrated in the following (c.f. Weinstein et al., 1998; Sutton, 2005).

How to Operationalize Stages

Stage models were repeatedly accused of insufficiently operationalizating their stages (Bandura, 1997; Littell and Grivin, 2002; Sutton, 2005; Weinstein et al., 1998; West, 2005).

Stage classification may either be operationalized with multi-dimensional questionnaires like the University of Rhode Island Change Assessment for the TTM (URICA; McConnaughy, DiClemente, Prochaska and Velicer, 1989; McConnaughy, Prochaska, and Velicer, 1983) or with staging algorithms. Multi-dimensional questionnaires assess stages with a set of items for each stage. The derived scores represent an individual's position on each dimension. This approach is quite problematic, as it allows individuals to score high on more than one stage. This phenomenon could often be observed in studies using multi-dimensional questionnaires and contradicts the idea of distinct stages in stage models (for an overview see Littell and Girvin, 2002; Sutton, 2001). The use of staging algorithms prevent the occurrence of double classifications as staging algorithms focus on a few questions that are mutually exclusive.

Hence, many studies on the TTM applied staging algorithms to allocate persons into different stages. In general, these algorithms were at least partly based on time criteria (see Table 1). The problems of using time criteria are apparent: Why should this periods of time (i.e. 6 months) exclusively be crucial and not any other period of time? However, the allocation to the *maintenance stage* of the TTM is still mostly operationalized over the requirement of at least 6 months of regular exercise (see Table 1). Knowing that the TTM goes back to smoking cessation, these time criteria might be appropriate. For other health behaviors like physical exercise, such time criteria seem to be arbitrary and lack any empirical evidence (Sutton, 2005). In other words, their practical usefulness is questionable. This problem contains two implications for further research:

- Aspects of time should be analyzed in more detail in the context of physical exercise as well as for other behaviors, as their usefulness lacks evidence and
- the problems with time criteria may be avoided, if psychologically grounded concepts like habituation ("I am exercising without inner temptations not to do so" "I am doing it automatically") are considered to diagnose stages, without the inclusion of time criteria (Lippke and Ziegelmann, 2006; Lippke, Ziegelmann, Schwarzer, and Velicer, 2007).

Further weaknesses of staging algorithms appear, if their quality of allocating persons to stages is tested (Adams and White, 2005; Littell and Girvin, 2002; Nigg, 2005). In line with theoretical postulations, persons in the inactive stages (i.e. *precontemplation*, *contemplation* or *preparation*) should exercise less than the defined criterion (i.e. at least 30min of exercise on seven day a week) and individuals in the active stages (i.e. *action* or *maintenance*) should exercise at least as often as the defined criterion (Nigg, 2005). However, studies showed repeatedly that the reality looks different: There are individuals, that assign themselves to inactive stages, even if they exercise to the extent of the criterion and others, that are allocated in the active stages and do not fulfill the requirements of exercise. This problem has two implications for future studies:

1) The amount of falsely diagnosed individuals should be assessed and considered as a measure of reliability when study results are interpreted (review see Nigg, 2005).

2) Available staging algorithms should be compared according to their quality in measuring stage affiliation (false and correct classifications). The best instrument for the targeted population and behavior should be chosen.

Such comparisons may reveal a need for new staging algorithms. However, most researchers are afraid of developing new instruments and try to apply validated instruments, as journal reviewers demand it. Even so, the development of a new staging algorithm is complex and time-consuming; it may pay off though, as the staging algorithm is the key to a well-elaborated examination of stages and to the development of successful stage-matched interventions.

How to Avoid Pseudo-Stages and Test for Discontinuity Patterns?

A typical topic, opponents of stage theories come up with, is whether stages have any advantage over continuum models. Do stage models subdivide a process that has a continuous nature in reality?

A continuous theory like the Theory of Planned Behavior assumes that people have higher or lower levels of intention (Ajzen, 1991). If an analogues staging algorithm would ask for the level of participant's intention and assign participants into several groups according to their level of intention, this would produce pseudo-stages as it can be assumed that these categories will not behave like true stages. This may also be the case for arbitrary time criteria, as these are continuous measures as well. The factors that promote pseudo-stage transitions will be the same for every pseudo-stage, as there are no qualitative differences between the stages. A single linear prediction equation that incorporates the same social-cognitive variables with the same weights will be sufficient to explain all possible pseudo-stage transitions.

On the contrary, real stages require separate stage-specific prediction equations as different factors are of different importance in each stage. Hence, pseudo-stages are arbitrary classifications of participants along a continuum of one variable. One example for the creation of pseudo-stages was demonstrated in a study by DeVries and Backbier (1994) that categorized *precontemplators* and *contemplators* by dichotomizing a 5-point scale to assess goals. Thus, it is necessary to consider several criteria in a staging algorithm (i.e. goals and behavior).

For statistical means this implies, that stages may be treated as variables on a nominal scale or at the most on an ordinal scale. Participant's answers to staging algorithms may not be treated as variables on an interval scale, as the stages are assumed qualitatively different. Therefore, it is not allowed to compare means of stage scores, as it has misleadingly been done in previous studies. For an example, Clark, Hampson, Avery and Simpson (2004) assessed a staging variable with an 11-point scale and reported the stage means and standard deviations on this measure for an intervention group and a control group at two points in time (pre- and post-treatment). The result of the MANOVA showed a significant group × time interaction. Hence, the staging algorithm in this study was rather used as measure for the intervention effect (i.e. probability of behavior implementation) than as a real staging algorithm. The analyzed variable, measured on an interval scale, rather assessed readiness to change than the affiliation to a certain stage.

The same statistical rules are undermined if stages are correlated with other variables. This occurred in a study by Courneya, Nigg and Estrabrooks (1998), in which the authors correlated the social-cognitive constructs of the Theory of Planned Behavior (Ajzen, 1991) with the TTM stages. Stages should furthermore be treated as moderators and not as mediators (Lippke, Nigg, and Maddock, 2007). In short: A correctly assessed staging variable may not be interpreted as continuous parameter, but as a variable measured on a categorical at the most on an ordinal scale. Readiness to change (on an interval scale) and a properly operationalized staging variable (qualitatively different conditions individuals are in) are completely different measures.

Hence, on the one hand, the operationalization and on the other hand the statistical utilization of stages have to be considered. Even if the stages are properly operationalized and none but feasible statistical analyses conducted, this does not defer the criticism of pseudo-stages. Do stages not simply disguise a linear process? This question would have to be answered positively, if variables (i.e. goals, self-efficacy or risk-perception) increased linearly, decreased linearly or remained stable across the stages (see panel A, B and C in Figure 7).

For this reason, Sutton proposed that stages should be tested empirically by searching for so-called discontinuity patterns (Sutton, 2000, 2005). If the stages of an hypothetical three-stage model (1, 2 and 3) are compared, discontinuity patterns are apparent if,

- variable A has a lower level in stage 1 than in stage 2, a higher level in stage 2 than in stage 3 and the stages 1 and 3 display a similar level (illustrated in Figure 8, panel D)
- variable B has a lower level in stage 1 than in stage 2, and a similar level in the stage 2 and 3 (illustrated in Figure 8, panel E)
- variable C has a similar level in the stage 1 and 2 and a lower or higher level in stage 3 (see Figure 8, panel F and G)

The same principles apply when more than three stages are compared.

Such discontinuity patterns may be tested statistically and with that the reproach of pseudo-stages disabled (c.f. Lippke and Plotnikoff, 2006; Sutton, 2005). One option is to conduct planned contrast analyzes, to compare the means of those variables that are considered to influence stage transitions. For example, it could be tested, whether variable A differs significantly between stage 1 and stage 2 and remains on a similar level between stage 2 and stage 3, whereas variable B shows a different pattern.

Another option to reveal discontinuity patterns is to test for statistical trends across the means. Hereby, the question is whether non-linear trends (quadratic, cubic etc.) may account for variance over the variance that is explained by linear trends (Sutton, 2000; Armitage and Arden, 2002). Only a small number of studies that examined stage characteristics also analyzed the trends across means.

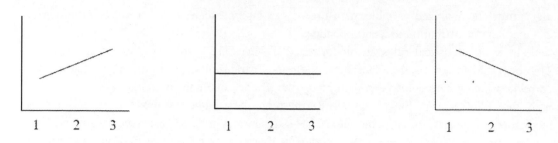

Figure 7. Possible linear patterns for theoretically relevant variables in a hypothetical three-stage model (Panel A; Panel B; and Panel C).

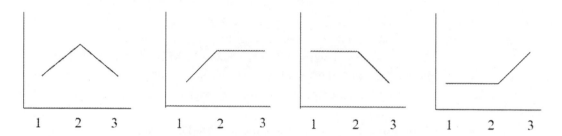

Figure 8. Possible discontinuity patterns for theoretically relevant variables in a hypothetical three-stage model (Panel D; Panel E; Panel F; and Panel G).

In the following, empirical studies that used the mentioned methods to detect discontinuity patterns will be summarized. A meta-analysis by Rosen (2000) on different behaviors focused on the detection of the processes of change in the TTM. Rosen aggregated the average level of cognitive-affective processes and behavioral processes in every stage over 12 studies in exercise domains. He showed that the cognitive-affective processes remained on a similar level over the five stages and the behavioral processes increased from stage to stage (Rosen, 2000). Hence, he found no discontinuity patterns for exercise.

Marshall and Biddle (2001) investigated the differences between adjacent stages in their meta-analysis in more detail, and analyzed the processes of change as well as the development of the social-cognitive variables and physical exercise across the TTM stages. Thereby they found that people in *precontemplation* and *contemplation*, and individuals in *preparation* and *action* differed more in their level of overall processes than people in *contemplation* and *preparation* and *action* and *maintenance*. Especially the comparison of *action* and *maintenance* revealed very little difference in use of processes.

For the behavioral measures the results showed, that *precontemplation* and *contemplation*, and *action* and *maintenance* were less different than *contemplation* and *preparation*, and *preparation* and *action*. That means that the processes are increasing mostly from the *precontemplation* to the *contemplation* and from the *preparation* to the *action stage*. The largest difference in behavior occurred between *contemplation* and *preparation*, and between *preparation* and *action*. Marshall and Biddle (2001) also found, consistent with the TTM that self-efficacy and pros increased and cons decreased across the stages.

These findings support the discontinuity thesis for pros and for the cognitive-affective processes, as there was a large mean difference between the *precontemplation* and *contemplation* stage, little to no difference between the *contemplation* and the *preparation stage* and again a difference between *preparation* and *action*. Furthermore, both types of processes increased more substantially from *preparation* to *action* than from *action* to *maintenance*. Marshall and Biddle (2001) interpreted these results for the TTM as support for discontinuity in the behavior change process.

One example for studies that investigated discontinuity patterns in the HAPA is a cross-sectional study of social-cognitive variables, which supported the predicted discontinuous levels of the according variables throughout the stages, see Figure 9 (Warner et al., 2007): Self-efficacy and goals increased linearly throughout the stages. Outcome expectancies and plans were lower in the *non-intentional stage* than in the *intentional* and *actional stage*. Risk-perception was higher in the *intentional stage* than in the other two stages (Warner et al., 2007).

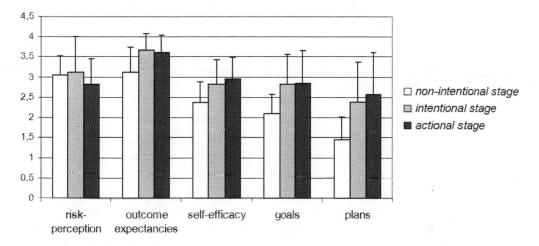

Note. Error bars are M + 1 SD.

Figure 9. Mean patterns of social-cognitive variables across the HAPA stages (Mean +1 Standard Deviation; Warner et al., 2007).

In a study on the BSM, Fuchs (2001) compared the levels of self-efficacy and social support across the BSM stages. Hereby, he found that both social-cognitive variables increased almost steadily from the *precontemplation* to the *habituation stage* and decreased rapidly if individuals were assigned to the *fluctuation* and *resumption stage*. Among individuals in the *resumption stage* the level of self-efficacy was even lower than among those in the *disposition stage* (Fuchs, 2001).

One of the few studies that included tests for linear and non-linear trends to detect discontinuity patterns has been conducted on the MSM (Lippke and Ziegelmann, 2006). This study found 73% of predicted discontinuity patterns across the MSM stages for goals, risk-perception, self-efficacy, pros, cons, planning and social support with regard to exercise behavior of rehabilitation patients confirmed. Additionally it tested linear trends against quadratic, cubic and 4th order trends that underlined the discontinuity in the behavior change process.

Another method to detect discontinuity patterns across stages is the prediction of *stage transitions*. In a field-study, Plotnikoff and colleagues (2001) examined which social-cognitive variables are capable of predicting stage-progressions in the TTM. An important assumption of stage models is that the social-cognitive variables should be of different importance for different stage-progressions and not all equally relevant in every stage. They found that self-efficacy was particularly important for individuals in the stages of *contemplation, action* and *maintenance* over a 6-month period: Those that progressed to a higher stage or prevented a relapse had higher levels of self-efficacy than those that regressed to stages more distal to behavior implementation. For individuals in the *precontemplation* or *preparation stages*, self-efficacy had no predictive power (Plotnikoff et al., 2001).

Studies on discontinuity patterns in the HAPA found that *non-intentional* individuals are more likely to set a goal, if they perceive risks; however, *intentional* individuals did not profit from risk-perception (Lippke et al., 2005). Another result supporting the HAPA derived from a study that found planning to be beneficial for rehabilitative patients in the *intentional* but not in the *non-intentional stage* (Lippke et al., 2004).

In sum, authors repeatedly noted that stage models have to defend themselves against the reproach of arbitrarily dividing a continuous process of behavior change into pseudo-stages. Only a small number of empirical studies explicitly integrated tests to answer this basic question and came to conflicting results. Further research is needed to bring this debate forward.

However, cross-sectional analyses and naturally occurring changes over time are only one way to test for the validity of stages and for discontinuity patterns (Nigg, 2005; Sutton, 2005): A promising alternative to validate stage models are experimental studies, that examine interventions to promote stage-progressions and with that physical exercise. Therefore, section 3.3 deals with this challenging design.

How to Test Stages Experimentally

Experimental studies exhibit the strictest testing of stage assumptions. Hereby, it is tested in experiments whether the theoretically relevant variables really show to be effective in those stages they are assumed to be. Ideally, these experiments are randomized controlled trials.

In order to demonstrate the principles of such experimental stage tests, a study by Weinstein, Lyon, Sandman and Cuite (1998) on the PAPM will be described. The authors assumed that individuals profit of different interventions depending on whether they were diagnosed to the pre-decisional or the post-decisional phase (see Figure 6): Pre-decisional individuals (*unaware, unengaged* and *deciding about acting*) should progress to higher stages if they received an intervention based on consciousness rising. The focus of this intervention lay on the communication of potential health threats. However, post-decisional participants (*decided to act*) should profit of an intervention that focused on plans of when were and how the behavior should be performed to actually progress to the action stage.

Figure 10 demonstrates those individuals that are in the pre-decisional stage (stage 1) and those that are in the post-decisional stage (stage 2). Stage 3 is assumed to be the acting stage. Intervention I aims at enhancing risk-perception and intervention II has the objective to increase planning. With other words, intervention I would be matched for participants in stage 1 and intervention II matched for participants in stage 2. However, intervention I would be mismatched for participants in stage 2 and intervention II mismatched for participants in stage 1.

	Intervention I	Intervention II
Stage-progression A: From stage 1 to stage 2	👍 matched/ effective	👎 mismatched/ ineffective
Stage-progression B: From stage 2 to stage 3	👎 mismatched/ ineffective	👍 matched/ effective

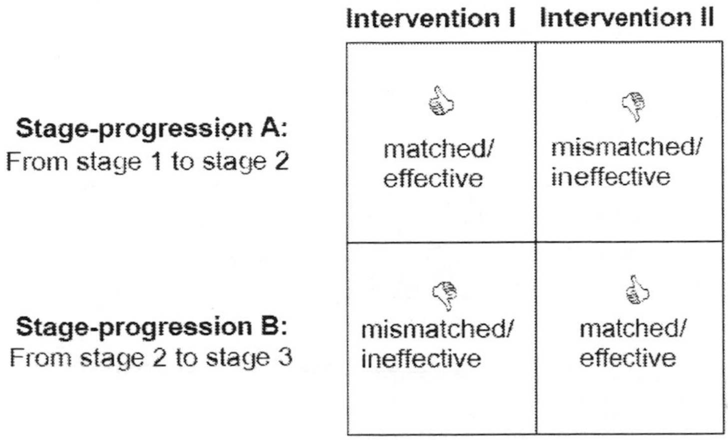

Figure 10. General design to test matched versus mismatched interventions.

Concerning the outcome measures, intervention I should be effective for persons in stage 1, but ineffective for persons in stage 2. Intervention II should show effects in criterion variables in the second stage but not the first stage. The authors set (a) stage-progressions and (b) changes in behavior as criterion-measures. Concerning criterion (a) the results were as hypothesized – participants in stage 1 (pre-decisional stage) that received intervention I (risk-intervention) progressed to higher stages with a higher probability than participants that were in stage 2 and received intervention I (31% more transition from stage 1 to stage 2 than from stage 2 to stage 3; c.f. Weinstein, Lyon et al., 1998). In other words – intervention I elicited a concrete decision to act in previously undecided participants, but did not induce acting in already decided participants.

The effectiveness of intervention II appeared in criterion (b): Participants in stage 2 (*decided to act*) that received intervention II (planning-intervention) acted significantly more often than participants in stage 1 that received intervention II (21% more progressions to the *action stage* in decided participants, cf. Weinstein and Lyon, et al., 1998). Hence, intervention II was able to induce acting in decided individuals but did not generate decisions in undecided individuals.

Even if this study has not been conducted in the area of physical exercise, several conclusions can be deduced:

1) Stage-matched and stage-mismatched interventions are existent.
2) It is important to consider meaningful criterion measures to evaluate the effectiveness of interventions (stage-progression and changes in behavior as discrete measures).
3) Not every criterion is meaningful to assess the effects of stage-specific interventions.

Along the line of Weinstein's results, the effectiveness of stage-matched strategic planning interventions could also be supported in a computer-based randomized controlled trail (software by Rademacher and Lippke, 2007). In this study on the HAPA, orthopedic patients were assisted to integrate self-instructed exercise into their daily routine, after having completed their medical rehabilitation programs (Lippke et al., 2004). The planning intervention resulted in higher levels of plans, whereas goals were not affected by the planning intervention in all three HAPA stages (expected stage-specific effect). Adherence rates to exercise recommendation did only increase in individuals in the *intentional stage* and slightly in the *actional stage*, too. Hence, a stage-specific effect of the planning-intervention could be confirmed, as it did neither affect the level of goals in none of the stages. Nor did it help *non-intenders* to increase their level of physical exercise as the intervention was designed to match the needs of *intenders* and *actors* (Lippke et al., 2004).

Further experimental studies that examine stage-specific effects by influencing only single variables in the context of physical exercise could not be found to date. More prevalent are studies that tailor their interventions extensively (by focusing on several variables) to the stages and compare the effectiveness in terms of stage-progressions or changes in behavior between matched versus mismatched or versus standard care interventions. Such extensive interventional studies will be dealt with in the next section.

4. Stage-Specific Interventions and Matched Versus Mismatched Designs

Whereas the preceding sections described the assumptions of stage models and some methodological problems, this section will focus on the implementation and development of stage-matched interventions to promote physical exercise.

Theoretical Assumptions of Stage-Matched Interventions

The increased popularity of stage models during the past 20 years lies in its implications for intervention designs in research and praxis of health promotion. This goes back to the assumed time- and cost-economy with a simultaneous increase in effectiveness.

The principle is easy: After having identified the stage a person belongs to (via the staging algorithm), only those factors have to be worked on that are assumed to be relevant in the diagnosed stage. Elaborated "packages" for each stage contain those aspects that are supposed to be effective for the particular stage. Marcus and Forsyth as well as Jordan and Nigg give detailed descriptions on how such packages can be designed according to the TTM for different populations in the context of physical exercise (cf. Marcus and Forsyth, 2003: for individuals: pp. 119-234; for groups: pp. 151-160; in companies: pp. 173-182 and in communities: pp. 194-205; and Jordan and Nigg; 2002, for elderly people: pp. 186-205).

In contrast to the theoretical principles of stage-specific interventions, the successful realization and evaluation of such programs is demanding. The question arises, which part of such intervention packages is the stage-specific one (do the packages not overlap across the stages?) and what accounts for the effectiveness of such interventions. It is a complex task to demonstrate the superiority of stage models over continuous models empirically. Hence, the next section focuses on giving an overview of the current state-of-research on stage-matched physical exercise promotion first and second goes into more detail on comparisons between standard care and stage-matched interventions.

Current State-of-Research of Stage-Matched Physical Exercise Promotion Programs

To date there are a number of successfully published studies that applied stage-matched interventions in the context of physical exercise. These studies may be classified into different categories:

(a) Studies that examine the effectiveness of stage-matched interventions over time. For example, this could be an intervention that conducts a stage-matched intervention in a company and analyses the *pre-interventional* and the *post-interventional* level of physical exercise. Such studies without a control group have only low chances of being published and are seldom included into reviews (such as those by Bridle et al., 2005; Adams and White, 2003).

(b) Studies that examine the effects of stage-matched interventions by comparing them to control groups. Either control groups get *no intervention at all* or they receive the intervention with some delay (also known as waiting control group). Napolitano and colleagues (2003) provided a three-month access for internet sites with stage-matched interventions for the experimental group. Participants in the experimental group were invited to visit these sites every week, whereas the waiting control group waited for the intervention to begin within these three months.

(c) Studies that compare stage-matched interventions to *placebo-interventions*. Hereby, the control group may be treated for other health issues, for example sun protection behavior as conducted in a study by Patrick et al. (2006).

(d) Studies that compare the effects of stage-matched versus *standard care* (one-size-fits-all) interventions. Standard care interventions focus on the same health issue with the exception that all participants get the same intervention regardless of their stage affiliation. An example for such a design is the study by Bolognesi, Nigg, Massarini and Lippke (2006).

(e) Studies that compare the effects of stage-matched versus stage-mismatched interventions. Such studies treat the mismatched group with stage-mismatched interventions, for example an individual in the first stage with an intervention designed for the last stage (e.g. Weinstein, Lyon et al., 1998; Figure 10)

(f) Studies that integrate characteristics of the designs a – e. One such study will be described in detail in the following.

In 2002, Blissmer and McAuley conducted a study on working place health promotion with the TTM as the basis for designing their stage-matched intervention. This study followed a complex design as it compared a stage-matched intervention group against three other groups over 16 weeks: (1) a placebo-group that got only general health information, (2) a standard care group in which all individuals got the same intervention to promote their physical exercise and (3) a stage-mismatched group. The authors found no advantages of the stage-matched over and above the standard care intervention. Both interventions lead to an increase in physical exercise, whereas the mismatched and the placebo-group did not change their exercising behavior. Hence, it did not make a difference whether participants got a stage-matched intervention that was falsely applied (mismatched) or whether they got no intervention at all: in both cases, participants did not change their behavior. The standard care and the stage-matched interventions outperformed equally good. That is, if there is a good standard care intervention, (Blissmer and McAuley applied a leaflet of the American Heart Association) its effects are similar to those of a stage-matched intervention.

Reviews of physical exercise (Adams and White, 2003) and other health behaviors (Bridle et al., 2005) come to similar conclusions. Bridle and colleagues differentiated studies that compared stage-matched interventions (based on the TTM) against individuals that received either a standard care intervention or no intervention at all. They analyzed six studies from the 1990s that compared a non-interventional group against a stage-matched intervention with regard to physical activity. Two out of these six studies additionally compared the stage-matched group against a standard care group with regard to their effects on physical exercise.

Three different groups emerged: The first group contained studies with better results for stage-matched interventions, the second group comprised studies that showed both positive and negative results, and the third group included only those studies that did not find any differences. For the comparison of stage-matched interventions against no interventions, only one out of six studies was identified as being in favor of stage-matched interventions (Peterson and Aldana, 1999), two were inconclusive (Harland, White, Drinkwater, Chinn, Farr and Howel, 1999; Cardinal and Sachs, 1996) and three showed no advantages over the control group (no-intervention group; Cash, 1997; Goldstein, Pinto, Marcus, Lynn, Jette and Rakowski, 1999; Graham-Clarke and Oldenburg, 1994). The results of the comparisons between stage-matched interventions and standard care interventions were even more disappointing: Of the two studies included in the analysis, there was one study with inconclusive findings (Peterson and Aldana, 1999) and one that did not reveal any advantages of stage-based interventions (Cash, 1997). Hence, with regard to the criterion of changes in physical exercise, stage-matched interventions do not seem to be better than no interventions or standard care interventions.

However, Bridle and colleagues did also account for *stage transitions* as criterion for intervention effects. Four studies reported stage transitions. One study (Peterson and Aldana,

1999) compared a stage-matched intervention against a standard care and a no-interventional group. Both comparisons resulted in clear advantages of the stage-matched intervention. The remaining three studies compared the effects of stage-based interventions against no-interventional groups. Only one supported the superiority of stage-based interventions to a non-interventional group (Braatz, Ames, Holmes-Rovner, King, McPhail, and Vogel, 1999), one was inconclusive (Goldstein et al., 1999) and the third (Cardinal and Sachs, 1996) found no significant differences.

Adams and White (2003) summarized physical exercise promotion studies based on the TTM that examined stage-progressions and changes in exercise behavior from 1982 to 2001. The authors found 16 studies that examined short-term effects (up to six months) and 7 studies that surveyed the participants again after more than six months (long-term effects). Among the 16 short-term studies, there were 11 effective interventions (69%). Among the long-term studies, only two out of seven showed to be effective. The authors concluded that even if long-term exercise promotion through TTM-stage-based interventions is not yet demonstrated, the results support the effectiveness of short-term interventions based on the TTM. In their discussion, they point out important methodological and logical issues: Stage-matched intervention packages should be designed for every stage of the underlying stage theory, so that every individual gets the intervention that suits his or her needs. Nevertheless, it may happen that the packages are more suitable for some groups than for others.

General conclusions that may be derived from this section are that stage-specific interventions assist the progression to higher stages. If the criterion is to increase the level of physical exercise, stage-matched interventions are no more effective than no interventions or one-size-fits-all interventions. This implies that if interventions are designed according to stage theories, a *stage-specific evaluation* should be applied, too. In other words, if different intervention-packages for different stages are applied, it is essential not only to search for changes in behavior or progressions from inactive to active stages but also to look for stage transition between all stages.

5. Summary

One appealing implication of stage models is that changes towards a healthy dose of physical exercise are apparent even if the target behavior is not yet performed. Along this line, success of health promotion programs may already be registered when persons progress to higher stages, for example if they become conscious of a health threat or decide to exercise more often in the future. These processes consist of qualitatively distinct developmental steps. Hence, there is no more-or-less or all-or-nothing principle in it. By examining stages, it is important to keep in mind that they are measured and used in analyses appropriately.

There are several stage theories and extensions of these. Empirical evidence supports the idea that changes in health behavior may take place in stages or steps. However, today it is not definite which factors are demonstrably effective and should be worked on in intervention packages. Contemporary stage models and stage-matched interventions provide room for further criticism and ameliorations. Therefore, further theory-based research in this field is strongly required as stage theories may be the key to successful and time-effective physical exercise promotion in the future if correctly investigated and applied.

References

Adams, J., and White, M. (2003). Are activity promotion interventions based on the transtheoretical model effective? A critical review. *British Journal of Sport Medicine, 37,* 106-114.

Adams, J., and White, M. (2005). Why don't stage-based activity promotion interventions work? *Health Education Research, 20* (2), 237-243.

Armitage, C. J., and Arden, M. A. (2002). Exploring discontinuity patterns in the transtheoretical model: An application of the theory of planned behaviour. *British Journal of Health Psychology, 7,* 89-103.

Ajzen, I. (1991). The Theory of Planned Behavior. *Organizational Behavior and Human Decision Processes, 50,* 179-211.

Bandura, A. (1997). Editorial: The anatomy of stages of change. *American Journal of Health Promotion, 12* (1), 8-11.

Biddle, S. J. H., Hagger, M. S., Chatzisarantis, N. L. D., and Lippke, S. (2007). Theoretical frameworks in exercise psychology. In G. Tenenbaum and R.C. Eklund (Eds.), *Handbook of Sport Psychology* (3rd ed, pp. 537-559). New York: Wiley.

Biddle, S. J. H., and Mutrie, N. (2001). *Psychology of physical activity: Determinants, well-being and interventions.* London: Routledge.

Blalock, S. J., DeVellis, R. F., Giorgino, K. B., DeVellis, B. M., Gold, D. T., Dooley, M. A., Anderson, J. J. B., and Smith, S. L. (1996). Osteoporosis prevention in premenopausal women: Using a stage model approach to examine the predictors of behavior. *Health Psychology, 15,* 84-93.

Blalock, S. J., DeVellis, B. M., Patterson, C. C., Campbell, M. K., Orenstein, D. R., and Dooley, M. A. (2002). Effects of an osteoporosis prevention program incorporating tailored education materials. *American Journal of Health Promotion, 16,* 146-156.

Blissmer, B., and McAuley, E. (2002). Testing the requirements of stages of physical activity among adults: The comparative effectiveness of stage-matched, mismatched, standard care, and control interventions. *Annals of Behavioral Medicine, 24* (3), 181-189.

Bolognesi, M., Nigg, C. R., Massarini, M., and Lippke, S. (2006). Reducing obesity indicators through brief physical activity counseling (PACE) in Italian primary care settings. *Annals of Behavioral Medicine, 31* (2), 179–185.

Braatz, J. S., Ames, B., Holmes-Rovner, M., King, S., McPhail, J., and Vogel, P. (1999). The effect of a physical activity intervention based on the transtheoretical model of changing physical-activity-related behavior on low-income elderly volunteers. *Journal of Aging and Physical Activity, 7,* 308–309.

Bridle, C., Riemsma, R. P., Pattenden, J., Sowden, A. J., Mather, L., Watt, I. S., and Walker, A. (2005). Systematic review of the effectiveness of health behavior interventions based on the transtheoretical model. *Psychology and Health, 20* (3), 283-301.

Brug, J., Conner, M., Harré, N., Kremers, S., McKellar, S., and Whitelaw, S. (2005). The transtheoretical model and stages of change: A critique. Observations by five commentators on the paper by Adams, J. and White, M. (2004) Why don't stage-based activity promotion interventions work? *Health Education Research, 20* (2), 244-258.

Cardinal, B. J., and Sachs, M. L. (1996). Effects of mail-mediated, stage-matched exercise behavior change strategies on female adults' leisure-time exercise behavior. *Journal of Sports Medicine and Physical Fitness, 36,* 100–107.

Cash, T. L. (1997). *Effects of different exercise promotion strategies and stage of exercise on reported physical activity, self-motivation, and stages of exercise in worksite employees* [EdD]: Philadelphia: Temple University.

Clark, M., Hampson, S. E., Avery, L., and Simpson, R. (2004). Effects of a brief tailored intervention on the process and predictors of lifestyle behaviour change in patients with type 2 diabetes. *Psychology, Health and Medicine, 9*, 440-449.

Courneya, K. S. (1995). Understanding readiness for regular physical activity in older individuals: An application of the Theory of Planned Behavior. *Health Psychology, 14*, 80-87.

Courneya, K. S., Nigg, C. R., and Estrabrooks, P. A. (1998). Relationships among the theory of planned behavior, stages of change, and exercise behavior in older persons over a three year period. *Psychology and Health, 13*, 355-367.

DiClemente, C. C, Prochaska, J. O., Fairhurst, S. K., Velicer, W. F., Velasquez, M. M., and Rossi, J. S. (1991). The process of smoking cessation: An analysis of precontemplation, contemplation, and preparation stages of change. *Journal of Consulting and Clinical Psychology, 59,* 295-304.

DiClemente, C. C., and Prochaska, J. O. (1998). Toward a comprehensive, transtheoretical model of change: Stages of change and addictive behaviors. In W. R. Miller and N. Heather (Eds.), *Treating addictive behaviours* (2nd ed., pp. 3-24). New York: Plenum.

Frey, D. (1986). Recent research on selective exposure to information. In L. Berkowitz (Ed.), *Advances in experimental social psychology* (Vol. 19, pp. 41–79). New York: Academic.

Fuchs, R. (1999). Psychology's contribution to the promotion of physical activity. In V. Hosek, P. Tilinger, and L. Bilek (Eds.), *Psychology of sport and exercise: Enhancing the quality of life* (pp. 20–28). Prague: Charles University.

Fuchs, R. (2001). Entwicklungsstadien zum sporttreiben [Developmental stages of exercise behavior]. *Sportwissenschaft, 31* (3), 255–281.

Fuchs, R. (2003). *Sport, Gesundheit und Public Health [Sport, health and public health].* Göttingen: Hogrefe.

Fuchs, R. (2005) Körperliche Aktivität [Physical activity]. In R. Schwarzer (Hrsg.). *Enzyklopädie der Psychologie. Gesundheitspsychologie* (S. 447–465). Göttingen: Hogrefe.

Goldstein, M. G., Pinto, B. M., Marcus, B. H., Lynn, H., Jette, A. M., and Rakowski, W. (1999). Physician-based physical activity counseling for middle-aged and older adults: A randomized trial. *Annals of Behavioral Medicine, 21*, 40–47.

Gollwitzer, P. M. (1999). Implementation intentions. *American Psychologist, 54,* 493-503.

Gollwitzer, P. M. and Sheeran, P. (2006). Implementation intentions and goal achievement: A meta-analysis of effects and processes. *Advances in Experimental Social Psychology, 38*, 69-119.

Graham-Clarke, P., and Oldenburg, B. (1994). The effectiveness of a general-practice-based physical activity intervention on patient physical activity status. *Behavior Change, 11*, 132–144.

Harland, J., White, M., Drinkwater, C., Chinn, D., Farr, L., and Howel, D. (1999). The Newcastle exercise project: A randomized controlled trial of methods to promote physical activity in primary care. *British Medical Journal, 319*, 828–832.

Jordan, P. J., and Nigg, C. R. (2002). Applying the transtheoretical model: Tailoring interventions to stages of change. Burbank, P. and Riebe, D. (Eds.) Promoting exercise and behavior change in older adults: Interventions with the transtheoretical model (pp. 181-208). New York: Springer.

Keller, S., Velicer, W., and Prochaska, J. (1999). Das Transtheoretische Modell - Eine Übersicht [The Transtheoreical Model – An overview]. In S. Keller (Hrsg.), *Motivation zur Verhaltensänderung - Das Transtheoretische Modell in Forschung und Praxis* (S. 17-44). Freiburg: Lambertus.

Kraft, P., Sutton, S. R., and McCreath-Reynolds, H. (1999). The Transtheoretical model of behaviour change: Are the stages qualitatively different? *Psychology and Health, 14*, 433–450.

Kreuter, M. W., Strecher, V. J., and Glassman, B. (1999). One size does not fit all: The case for tailoring print materials. *Annals of Behavioral Medicine, 21*, 276-283.

Lippke, S. (2004). *Changing health behaviour: Stages models and an intervention for adopting and maintaining a healthy lifestyle.* Doctoral dissertation. Berlin, Freie Universität Berlin. Retrieved June 1, 2007, from: http://userpage.fu-berlin.de/~slippke/Diss]

Lippke, S., Ziegelmann, J. P., and Schwarzer, R. (2004). Initiation and maintenance of physical exercise: Stage-specific effects of a planning intervention. *Research in Sports Medicine, 12*, 221-240.

Lippke, S., Sniehotta, F. F., and Luszczynska, A. (2005). Social cognitions across the stages of behavior change. A comparison of two stage models. *Polish Psychological Bulletin, 36* (1), 43-50.

Lippke, S., Ziegelmann, J. P., and Schwarzer, R. (2005). Stage-specific adoption and maintenance of physical activity: Testing a three-stage model. *Psychology of Sport and Exercise, 6*, 585-603.

Lippke, S., and Plotnikoff, R. C. (2006). Stages of change in physical exercise: A test of stage discrimination and non-linearity. *American Journal of Health Behavior, 30* (3), 290-301.

Lippke, S., and Ziegelmann, J. P. (2006). Understanding and modeling health behavior change: The multi-stage model of health behavior change. *Journal of Health Psychology, 11*, 37-50.

Lippke, S., Nigg, C. R., and Maddock, J. E. (2007). The Theory of Planned Behavior within the stages of the Transtheoretical Model - Latent structural modeling of stage-specific prediction patterns in physical activity. *Structural Equation Modeling: A Multidisciplinary Journal, 14*, 649-670.

Lippke, S., Ziegelmann, J. P., Schwarzer, R., and Velicer, W. F. (2007). Validity of stage assessment in the adoption and maintenance of physical activity and fruit and vegetable consumption. Manuscript submitted for publication.

Littell, J. H., and Girvin, H. (2002). Stages of change: A critique. *Behavior Modification, 26,* 223–273.

Janis, I.L, and Mann, L. (1977). *Decision making: A psychological analysis of conflict, choice, and commitment.* New York: Free Press.

Marcus, B. H., Rakowski, W., and Rossi, J. S. (1992). Assessing motivational readiness and decision-making for exercise. *Health Psychology, 11,* 257-261.

Marcus, B. H., Selby, V. C., Niaura, R. S., and Rossi, J. S. (1992). Self-efficacy and the stages of exercise behavior change. Research Quarterly for Exercise and Sport, 63, 60–66.

Marcus, B., and Forsyth, L. A. (2003). Using the stages model in community programs. In B. Marcus and L. A. Forsyth (Eds.). *Motivating people to be physically active* (pp. 183-207). Champaign, IL: Human Kinetics Publishers.

Marlatt, G. A., and Gordon, J. R. (Eds.) (1985). *Relapse prevention.* New York: Guilford.

Marshall, S. J., and Biddle, S. J. H. (2001). The transtheoretical model of behavior change: A meta-analysis of applications to physical activity and exercise. *Annals of Behavioral Medicine, 23* (4), 229-246.

McConnaughy, E. A., Prochaska, J. Q., and Velicer, W. F. (1983). Stages of change in psychotherapy: Measurement and sample profiles. *Psychotherapy, 20,* 368-375.

McConnaughy, E. A., DiClemente, C. C., Prochaska, J. Q., and Velicer, W. F. (1989). Stages of change in psychotherapy: A·follow-up report. *Psychotherapy, 26,* 494-503.

Napolitano, M. A., Fotheringham, M., Tate, D., Sciamanna, C., Leslie, E., Owen, N., Bauman, A., and Marcus, B. H. (2003). Evaluation of an internet-based physical activity intervention: A preliminary investigation. *Annals of Behavioral Medicine, 25,* 92-99.

Nigg, C. R. (2005). There is more to stages of exercise than just exercise. *American College of Sports Medicine, 33,* 32-35.

Nisbett, R., and Ross, L. (1980). *Human inference: Strategies and shortcomings of social judgment.* Englewood Cliffs, NJ: Prentice-Hall.

Patrick, K., Calfas, K. J., Norman, G. J., Zabinski, M. F., Sallis, J. F., Rupp, J., Covin, J., and Cella, J. (2006). Randomized controlled trial of a primary care and home-based intervention for physical activity and nutrition behaviors: PACE+ for adolescents. *Archives of Pediatrics and Adolescent Medicine, 160* (2), 128 - 136.

Peterson, T. R., and Aldana, S. G. (1999). Improving exercise behavior: An application of the stages of change model in a worksite setting. *American Journal of Health Promotion, 13,* 229–232.

Plotnikoff, R. C., Hotz, S. B., Birkett, N. J., and Courneya, K. S. (2001). Exercise and the transtheoretical model: A longitudinal test of a population sample. *Preventive Medicine, 33,* 441-452.

Prochaska, J. O., and DiClemente, C. C. (1982). Transtheoretical therapy: Toward a more integrative model of change. *Psychotherapy: Theory, Research and Practice, 20,* 161-173.

Prochaska, J. O., and DiClemente, C. C. (1983). Stages and processes of self-change of smoking : Toward an integrative model of change. *Journal of Consulting and Clinical Psychology, 51*, 390-395.

Prochaska, J. O., and DiClemente, C. C. (1985). Common processes of change in smoking, weight control, and psychological distress. In S. Shiftman and T. Wills (Eds.), *Coping and substance abuse* (pp. 345- 363). San Diego, CA: Academic Press.

Prochaska, J. O., and DiClemente, C. C. (1986). Toward a comprehensive model of change. In W. R. Miller and N. Heather (Eds.), *Treating addictive behaviors: Processes of change* (pp. 3-27). New \brk: Plenum Press.

Prochaska, J. O., and DiClemente, C. C. (1992). Stages of change in the modification of problem behaviors. In M. Hersen, R. M. Eisler, and P. M. Miller (Eds.), *Progress in behavior modification* (pp. 184-214). Sycamore, IL: Sycamore Press.

Prochaska, J. O., DiClemente, C. C., and Norcross, J. C. (1992). In search of how people change: Applications to addictive behaviors. *American Psychologist, 47*, 1102-1114.

Prochaska, J. O., Velicer, W. F., Rossi, J. S., Goldstein, M. G., Marcus, B. H., Rakowski, W., Fiore, C., Harlow, L. L., Redding, C. A., Rosenbloom, D., and Rossi, S. R. (1994). Stages of change and decisional balance for 12 problem behaviors. *Health Psychology, 13,* 39-46.

Prochaska, J. O., and Norcross, J. C. (2003). *Systems of psychotherapy: A transtheoretical analysis* (5th ed.). Pacific Grove, California: Brooks/Cole Publishing Company.

Rademacher, J. D. M., and Lippke, S. (2007). Dynamic online surveys and experiments with the free open source software dynQuest. *Behavior Research Methods.*

Richert, J. and Lippke, S. (2007). Theoretical approaches for evidence-based practice. In F. Columbus (Ed.), *Health knowledge, attitudes, and practices.* Hauppauge, NY: Nova Science Publishers.

Rosen, C. S. (2000). Is the sequencing of change processes by stage consistent across health problems? A meta-analysis. *Health Psychology, 19*, 593-604.

Schwarzer, R. (1992). Self-efficacy in the adoption and maintenance of health behaviours: Theoretical approaches and a new model. In R. Schwarzer (Ed.), Self-efficacy: Thought control of action (pp. 217-243). Bristol, PA: Taylor and Francis.

Schwarzer, R. (2001). Social-cognitive factors in changing health-related behaviors. *Current Directions in Psychological Science, 10* (2), 47-51.

Schwarzer, R. (2004). *Psychologie des Gesundheitsverhaltens. [Psychology of Health Behavior]* 3. Aufl. Göttingen: Hogrefe.

Schwarzer, R. (2008). Modeling health behavior change: How to predict and modify the adoption and maintenance of health behaviors. *Applied Psychology: An International Review, 57,* 1-29.

Schwarzer, R., and Lippke, S. (2005). Gesundheitsverhalten und Gesundheitsförderung [Health behavior and health promotion]. In D. Frey and G. Hoyos (Eds.), *Psychologie in Gesellschaft, Kultur und Umwelt* (pp. 149-155). Weinheim, Germany: Beltz-Verlag.

Sharp, K., and Thombs, D. (2003). A cluster analytic study of osteoprotective behavior in undergraduates. *American Journal of Health Behavior, 27,* 364-372.

Sutton, S. (2000). Interpreting cross-sectional data on stages of change. *Psychology and Health, 15,* 163-171.

Sutton, S. (2001). Back to the drawing board? A review of applications of the transtheoretical model to substance use. *Addiction, 96,* 175-186.

Sutton, S. (2005). Stage theories of health behaviour. In M. Conner and P. Norman (Eds.), *Predicting health behaviour: Research and practice with social cognition models* (2nd ed.). Buckingham, UK: Open University Press.

Warner, L. M., Lippke, S., Wiedemann, A. U., Reuter, T., and Ziegelmann, J. P. (2007). Theory-based investigation of the interplay of social-cognitive variables and stages of helath behavior change. Poster presented at the 8th Congress of Health psychology in Schwäbisch Gmünd; Germany, September 17-19.

Weinstein, N. D. (1988). The precaution adoption process. *Health Psychology, 7,* 355- 386.

Weinstein, N. D., Lyon, J. E., Sandman, P. M., and Cuite, C. L. (1998). Experimental evidence for stages of health behavior change: The precaution adoption process model applied to home radon testing. *Health Psychology, 17,* 445-453.

Weinstein, N. D., Rothman, A. J., and Sutton, S. R. (1998). Stage theories of health behavior: Conceptual and methodological issues. *Health Psychology, 17,* 290-299.

Weinstein, N. D., and Sandman, P. M. (1992). A model of the precaution adoption process: Evidence from home radon testing. *Health Psychology, 11,* 170-180.

Weinstein, N. D., and Sandman, P. M. (2002). Reducing the risks of exposure to radon gas: An application of the precaution adoption process model. In D. Rutter and L. Quine (Eds.), *Changing health behaviour: Intervention and research with social cognition models* (pp. 66-86). Buckingham, England: Open University Press.

Weinstein, N. D., and Sandman, P. M. (2002b). The precaution adoption process model. In K. Glanz, B. K. Rimer and F. M. Lewis (Eds.), *Health behavior and health education: Theory, research, and practice* (3rd ed., pp. 121-143). San Francisco: Jossey-Bass.

West, R. (2005). Time for a change: putting the Transtheoretical (Stages of Change) Model to rest. *Addiction, 100* (8), 1036-1039.

Ziegelmann, J. P. and Lippke, S. (2007). Planning and Strategy Use in Health Behavior Change: A Life Span View. *International Journal of Behavioral Medicine, 14,* 30–39.

Ziegelmann, J. P., Luszczynska, A., Lippke, S., and Schwarzer, R. (2007). Are goal intentions or implementation intentions better predictors of health behavior? A longitudinal study in orthopaedic rehabilitation. *Rehabilitation Psychology, 52,* 97–102.

In: Sport and Exercise Psychology Research Advances ISBN: 978-1-60456-157-9
Editors: M. P. Simmons, L. A. Foster, pp. 53-83 © 2008 Nova Science Publishers, Inc.

Chapter II

Facilitating Anxiety: Myth or Mislabeled? The Relationship between Interpretations of Competitive Anxiety Symptoms and Positive Affective States

Stephen D. Mellalieu[3] and Sheldon Hanton
Department of Sports Science, Swansea University, United Kingdom
Cardiff School of Sport, University of Wales Institute, Cardiff, United Kingdom

Abstract

Despite the wealth of productive research examining the concept of competitive anxiety, the notion of 'facilitating' or 'positive anxiety' has recently stimulated an exciting conceptual debate amongst researchers (Burton and Naylor, 1997; Hanton and Connaughton, 2002; Hardy, 1997, 1998; Jones and Hanton, 2001, Mellalieu, Hanton, and Jones, 2003). One perspective postulates that high levels of cognitive anxiety can be perceived as facilitating to performance (Hardy, 1997). The opposing view maintains that, such cognitive symptoms are purported to reflect positive expectations of coping and goal achievement and lead to positive emotions including 'challenge' or 'excitement' (Burton, 1998; Burton and Naylor, 1997). The purpose of the study therefore was to examine the suggestion that facilitating interpretations of symptoms associated with the competitive stress response may be representative of some other positive affective state other than anxiety. 322 competitive athletes, sampled from a range of team and individual sports aged 18-29 years ($M = 24.8$, $SD = 3.1$) completed the modified Competitive Trait Anxiety Inventory-2 (CTAI-2; Martens, Burton, Vealey, Bump, and Smith, 1990), the Positive and Negative Affect Schedule (Watson and Tellegen, 1988), and adapted from the work of Jones and Hanton (1996, 2001) a measure of feeling states, the Pre-Performance Feelings Scale (PPFS; Mellalieu, 2000). Three separate one-way MANOVA's were conducted with groups (debilitated versus facilitated) as the

3 Corresponding author: Stephen D. Mellalieu, Ph.D, Department of Sports Science, Swansea University, SA2 8PP, United Kingdom. Tel: 00-44-1792-513-101, E-mail: s.d.mellalieu@swan.ac.uk.

independent variable and performers' PPFS, PANAS and CTAI-2 subscales as the dependent variables respectively. All three MANOVA's were found to be significant with follow-up univariate analyses revealing differences between debilitators and facilitators of competitive trait anxiety for mental readiness, confidence and perception of physical state subscales of the PPFS and the positive and negative affect subscales of the PANAS. Correlation analyses revealed negative affect as more important in mediating competitive trait anxiety intensity, while positive affect was found to be more important in mediating competitive trait anxiety direction. Strong relationships were also found between the direction of competitive trait anxiety and positive and negative subscales of the PPFS. The findings indicate that sports performers' facilitative interpretations of symptoms associated with competitive anxiety responses may indeed be representative of some other positive affective state. Further, this positive affective state experienced in the precompetition period may therefore be more influential in determining successful sports performance than the existing belief that suggests competitive anxiety *per se* is the key factor in accounting for performance. Finally, the oxymoron of 'positive anxiety' is discussed in light of the study findings regarding the difference between true feelings of anxiety resulting in performance benefits versus the interpretation of associated symptoms having a similar positive influence. Practical implications and significant future recommendations for the practitioner are also offered.

Keywords: *Competitive trait anxiety, directional perceptions, positive affective states.*

Among the plethora of research areas pursued by the growing discipline of sport psychology, one of the most frequently investigated has been the concept of competitive anxiety. Indeed, the reasons as to why emotional and motivational factors associated with anxiety will cause one athlete to 'peak' during competition while a fellow competitor will 'choke', experiencing performance impairments, has been a fundamental question posed by any observer or participant of sport at one time or another (Smith, Smoll, and Wiechman, 1998).

"Competitive anxiety has long held a paradoxical fascination for sport psychologists, and coaches and athletes with whom they work. Because no other single psychological attribute can have such a debilitating effect on performance research on the causes and consequences of competitive anxiety as well as on how practitioners can reduce anxiety or more effectively cope with its effects has therefore been one of the most heavily researched topics in sport psychology."

(Burton, 1998, p.12)

The study of competitive anxiety has enjoyed a large prominence in sport psychology over the last 25 years since its origins in the social psychology of test anxiety (see Jones, 1995; Mellalieu, Hanton, and Fletcher, 2006; Tenenbaum and Bar-Eli, 1995; Woodman and Hardy, 2001 for a review). Research has been aided significantly by the evolution of a multidimensional approach to the construct that possesses separate cognitive and somatic components (Martens, Vealey, and Burton, 1990). This development, and that of its subsequent measurement instrument, the Competitive State Anxiety Inventory-2 (CSAI-2; Martens, Burton, et al., 1990) has allowed for a greater understanding of the competitive state anxiety response and a plethora of literature investigating the intensity of symptoms of sports performers and the relationship with performance (see Woodman and Hardy, 2001). Consequently, utilizing the CSAI-2 these separate cognitive and somatic components have been observed to differ prior to competition as a function of their antecedents (Jones, Swain, and Cale, 1990), temporal characteristics (Gould, Petlichkoff, and Weinberg, 1984; Jones, Swain, and Cale, 1991; Martens, Vealey, et al., 1990), performance consequences (Burton, 1988; Gould, Petlichkoff, Simons, and Vevera, 1987; Jones and Cale, 1989; Parfitt and Hardy, 1987), in response to interventions (Burton, 1990), together with situation variables such as sport type (Martens, Vealey, et al., 1990). Additional developments have included both retrospective and in-event methods to measure the construct (Butt, Weinberg, and Horn, 2003; Harger and Raglin, 1994; Krane, 1994), together with several theoretical attempts to explain the relationship with performance including multidimensional anxiety theory (Martens, Vealey, et al., 1990), catastrophe theory (Hardy, 1996; Hardy and Parfitt, 1991) and the individual zones of optimal functioning hypothesis (Hanin, 1989, 2000).

Anxiety Direction: Directional Perceptions of Symptom Interpretation

In the last decade, dissatisfaction has been expressed about the limitations of solely examining the intensity of the competitive anxiety response (Jones, 1991; Jones 1995; Parfitt, Jones, and Hardy, 1990). The CSAI-2 essentially assesses the 'intensity' of the response (certain cognitive and perceived physiological symptoms) which are purported to signify the presence of anxiety by the researchers responsible for developing the instrument. However, the inventory fails to measure what has been referred to by Jones (1991) and his colleagues as the 'directional perceptions' of the symptoms. Specifically, 'directional perceptions' refers to the extent to which individuals interpret the intensity of symptoms experienced in precompetitive situations as either facilitating or debilitating to performance (Jones, 1995; Jones and Hanton, 2001). For example, Jones (1991) indicates that one performer may be very concerned about an impending competition or game, to the extent that they are worried and in a near-panic, debilitative state. Another performer, however, who is 'very concerned' might view such a state as necessary, since it signals the importance of the event and means that they will invest effort in it (Eysenck, 1992; Eysenck and Calvo, 1992), thus constituting a motivated, facilitative state. Eysenck further proposed that anxiety effectively reduces working memory capacity due to task irrelevant cognitive activity or worry, as it impairs processing efficiency. He argued that this reduction in effective capacity could be countered by an increased effort. Therefore, while processing efficiency is impaired, performance effectiveness may be maintained or even enhanced under conditions of high anxiety but at the expense of utilizing a greater proportion of the available resources. Similarly, two athletes experiencing similar precompetition levels of physiological arousal might label their symptoms at opposite ends of the direction continuum. This process may be seen as a further level of cognitive appraisal that has the function of interpreting the meaningfulness of the cognitive and physiological symptoms experienced following earlier appraisal of the congruence between the situational demands and ability to meet those demands (Jones, 1995).

The 'intensity alone' approach to measuring competitive anxiety has prevailed in the sports psychology literature because the concept of anxiety has been viewed for a long time as invariably negative and detrimental to performance (Martens, Burton, et al., 1990). However, findings have suggested this is not the case and that competitive anxiety is not necessarily negative (i.e., debilitative), and can have positive effects that facilitate performance (Hardy and Parfitt, 1991; Jones and Cale, 1989; Jones, Swain, and Hardy, 1993; Mahoney and Avener, 1977; Parfitt and Hardy, 1987, 1993). The notion of debilitating and facilitating dimensions of the anxiety response has been prominent in the test anxiety literature for a number of years. Alpert and Haber distinguished between debilitating and facilitating anxiety as long ago as 1960, and found that a scale that measured both dimensions of anxiety (i.e., the Achievement Anxiety Test; AAT; Alpert and Haber, 1960) provided a significantly stronger predictor of academic performance than a conventional debilitating anxiety scale. Subsequent investigations employing the AAT have also supported the value of distinguishing between debilitating and facilitating anxiety (Carrier, Higson, Klimoski, and Peterson, 1984; Couch, Garber, and Turner, 1983; Gaeddert and Dolphin, 1981; Hudesman and Weisner, 1978; Munz, Costello, and Korabek, 1975).

Although the literature within the test anxiety context has provided the basis for important developments in anxiety research, its application to other areas, such as competitive anxiety, has been described as somewhat limited on two counts (Jones, Hanton, and Swain, 1994). First, it has examined the bi-directional model in the context of cognitive (i.e., academic) performance, so that there is a need for investigation in the area of motor performance. Second, the research on debilitating and facilitating anxiety has largely examined an undifferentiated, unidimensional 'test' anxiety state as opposed to the favored multi-component conceptualization of anxiety. Additionally, little research in the test anxiety literature has examined how individual difference variables may mediate an individual's interpretations of their cognitive symptoms.

Following on from this work, the notion of 'direction' of anxiety has been introduced into the sport psychology literature (Jones, 1991). Employing a directional version of the modified CSAI-2 (Jones and Swain, 1992) interpretation of reported symptoms has subsequently received considerable empirical attention. At a state level, directional perceptions have been examined as a function of both situational and individual difference variables including performance (Jones, et al., 1993; Swain and Jones, 1996); competitive orientation (Jones and Swain, 1992); the antecedents of competitive anxiety (Hanton and Jones, 1997); the temporal patterning of the anxiety response (Hanton, Thomas, and Maynard, 2004; Thomas, Maynard, and Hanton, 2004; Wiggins, 1998); goal attainment expectations (Jones and Hanton, 1996); and the use of psychological skills (Fletcher and Hanton, 2001). In a trait context, gender differences (Perry and Williams, 1998); the nature of the sport (Hanton, Jones, and Mullen, 2000); perceptions of control (Hanton, O'Brien, and Mellalieu, 2002); the personality trait of hardiness (Hanton, Evans, and Neil, 2003) and the relationship with state anxiety symptoms (Hanton, Mellalieu, and Hall, 2002) have been investigated. Collectively, from both a state and dispositional context, these studies support the value of distinguishing between the intensity and direction of symptoms experienced in competitive situations. In addition, the literature also suggests that 'direction' may actually be a more sensitive variable in distinguishing between group differences when compared with the intensity of the response (Jones and Hanton, 2001; Mellalieu, Hanton, and Jones, 2003; Swain and Jones, 1996; see also Mellalieu et al., 2006).

Understanding of the mechanisms by which the direction of symptoms is moderated has been furthered by Jones' (1995) control model of facilitative and debilitative anxiety. Based upon the initial model proposed by Carver and Scheier (1986, 1988) and other researchers in the test anxiety literature (e.g., Borkovec, Metzger, and Pruzinski, 1986; Rich and Woolever, 1988), Jones' model conceptualizes control as the cognitive appraisal of the degree of influence the performer is able to exert over both the environment and the self. Individuals who perceive themselves as being in control, able to cope with their anxiety, and achieve their goals are predicted to interpret competitive symptoms as facilitative to performance. However, those performers who perceive that they are not in control and possess negative expectancies regarding goal attainment are predicted to interpret these symptoms as debilitative (Jones, 1995). Preliminary support for the model's predictions and the latter work of Carver and Scheier (1998, 1999) has subsequently been provided in both empirical and qualitative investigations (e.g., Hanton and Connaughton, 2002; Hanton, Mellalieu, and Hall, 2004; Hanton et al., 2003; Jones and Hanton, 1996; Ntoumanis and Jones, 1998).

Anxiety Interpretation: The 'Positive Anxiety' Conceptual Debate

Despite the wealth of productive research, recent concern has been expressed by certain researchers in the sport psychology community regarding the concept of directional interpretations of anxiety symptoms. Continuing the points raised by Jones (1995), the notion of 'facilitating' or 'positive anxiety' has stimulated a conceptual debate (Burton and Naylor, 1997; Hardy, 1997, 1998; Jones and Hanton, 2001; Mellalieu et al., 2003; see also Mellalieu et al., 2006). The first view maintains that direction researchers have mistakenly mislabeled other positive emotions such as challenge and self-confidence as facilitating anxiety (Burton and Naylor, 1997; Burton, 1998). Specifically, in line with Lazarus' (1991) cognitive-motivational-relational model of emotion (cf. Lazarus, 2000), it is suggested that such cognitive symptoms are purported to reflect positive expectations of coping and goal achievement. These experiences are proposed to lead to positive emotions that include 'challenge' or 'excitement', beneficial for performance and not indicative of facilitative anxiety (Burton, 1998; Burton and Naylor, 1997). Subsequently, Burton and Naylor (1997) have commented that the measurement approach adopted by Hardy and colleagues appears to be confounding anxiety with other more positive emotions. Burton and colleagues further suggest that competitive anxiety theorists must therefore address the question of whether anxiety is really facilitating, or whether positive emotions such as challenge, excitement, or self-confidence simply have been mislabeled as facilitative anxiety.

The second perspective on the notion of 'positive anxiety' postulates that high levels of cognitive anxiety can be perceived as facilitating to performance (Hardy, 1997, 1998; Jones and Hanton, 2001). Specifically, Hardy and colleagues cite the tenets of processing efficiency theory (Eysenck and Calvo, 1992) which explains the impact of the motivational effects of cognitive anxiety upon performance through signaling to the performer the importance of the upcoming event, and the need to muster all available resources in order to perform the necessary actions on the field (Hardy, 1997). Furthermore, Hardy (1996) has argued that these negative cognitions may be precisely what are needed in order for performers to muster the very high levels of motivation and commitment that may be necessary in order to perform at the absolute limits of their capabilities. In light of this conceptual debate, Jones and Hanton (2001) have suggested that although commonalties of opinion exist within the dispute surrounding 'positive' anxiety, essentially researchers should accept that either a positive anxiety state for performance exists or reject this in support of another affective state previously labeled as anxiety.

Existing research investigating affect and the competitive stress response has provided some initial, albeit limited, guidance on this debate. For example, Jones, Swain, and Harwood (1996) found that Negative Affect (NA) was related to the intensity of cognitive and somatic anxiety response while Positive Affect (PA) was observed to play a more significant role than NA in the interpretation of both cognitive and somatic anxiety symptoms. However, the findings were limited in that the authors only compared participant's directional perceptions of cognitive anxiety and somatic anxiety direction to PA and NA separately and did not specifically compare the specific responses of facilitators (positive scores for both cognitive and somatic anxiety direction) or debilitators (negative scores for both cognitive and somatic anxiety direction). A further study by Treasure, Monson, and Lox (1996) examining the relationship between self-efficacy, PA and NA and competitive anxiety found self-efficacy to be positively related to PA, while being negatively relative to NA and intensity of cognitive and somatic anxiety. NA was also found to be strongly related to intensity of cognitive and somatic anxiety. Despite, the findings, however, the results were also somewhat limited in their extrapolation to the conceptual debate in that no examination of the direction of the competitive anxiety response was made.

In a specific attempt to advance the debate surrounding the notion of 'positive anxiety' Jones and Hanton (2001) conducted an exploratory study with elite swimmers to investigate directional interpretations of the intensity of competitive state anxiety symptoms and the nature of the preperformance emotional state experienced (i.e., positive or negative). Those swimmers who indicated symptoms identified on the CSAI-2 as facilitative to performance highlighted significantly higher scores for positive feeling state labels and lower scores on negative labels. Likewise, debilitators of symptoms associated with competitive anxiety indicated significantly higher scores on negative labels and lower scores on positive labels than the facilitators of competitive symptoms. Despite this attempt to advance the understanding of the conceptual debate, Jones and Hanton (2001) acknowledged that their findings were limited. The feeling state labels employed were pre-decided as either positive or negative from a pilot study with large athletic sample. The scale did not ask respondents to report the experience of affective states in regard to helping/hindering performance, positive feeling states reported were assumed to be facilitative to performance and negative feeling states debilitative. Conceptually, however, two performers may experience an intense feeling of aggression, one as positive, the other negative, yet it may not be differentiated so in such a scale. Cognitive labeling (i.e., facilitating/debilitating) of the affective state may therefore also be important (Hanin, 1997). In addition, the adjective checklist employed by Jones and Hanton (2001) utilized a composite measure of positive and negative feeling states that had limited psychometric properties. In an attempt to extend the work of Jones and Hanton (2001) and address some of these conceptual limitations, Mellalieu et al. (2003) examined differences in the precompetitive affective states of performers who reported facilitating or debilitating interpretations of symptoms associated with anxiety in both a state and dispositional context. Similar to the findings of Jones and Hanton (2001), facilitators of precompetitive anxiety symptoms reported experiencing significantly greater positive and lower negative feeling states than their debilitating counterparts with regard to their preparation for competition, and in respect of their actual upcoming performance. Additional descriptive analysis of the content of the feeling state responses labeled by performers revealed that 90% of labels listed were perceived as positive for preparation for, and actual performance by facilitators, compared with a mere 30% of labels for debilitators. These findings together with those of Jones and Hanton (2001) therefore suggest that the way athletes interpret the competitive stress response may affect the overall nature of the affective experience that the performer takes into competition (i.e., facilitating/debilitating). Despite providing some advancement to the conceptual debate surrounding the notion of 'positive' anxiety, however, the observations of these investigations are somewhat cautionary in that both studies have adopted relatively open-ended preliminary measures of affect with limited psychometric integrity. Indeed, Mellalieu et al. (2003) suggested that order to further explore the conceptual debate a consideration of the existing limitations of the measurement of affect in sport was required together with the design of sport-specific scale to measure the construct.

Affect Measurement in Sport

While the study of competitive anxiety has dominated the examination of the precompetition period sport psychology research has been suggested to be over-restrictive in its investigation of affective states by relying on constructs such as anxiety and arousal, which appear unnecessarily limiting and too narrow to account for the performers' precompetitive response that is proposed to encompass a recipe of emotions (Gould and Udry, 1994; Hanin, 1997; 2000; Jones, 1995; Tenenbaum and Bar-Eli, 1995). Indeed, for almost as long, there has been a call for a broader examination of affect in sport. This request began with researchers such as Vallerand (1983, 1984) and Silva and Hardy (1984, 1986) who viewed emotions and precompetitive affect as playing a significant role in athletic performance, with control of affective states viewed as a fundamental pre-cursor of consistent performance or athletic excellence (Silva and Hardy, 1986). More recently, this request has re-emerged with criticism of the pre-occupation with anxiety, and a call for an emphasis on the importance of other more functional emotions and affective responses in the preperformance period (Hanin, 1997, 2000; Jones, 1995; Kerr, 1997). This view accompanies that of other authors in the social psychology literature who have moved away from the examination of stress to one of cognition and emotion (e.g., Lazarus, 1991, 1999).

Specific research into the affective antecedents of performance in sport has however tended to prove less helpful in addressing this problem, with a lack of investigation into positive emotions. Instead, the focus has traditionally been on negative responses such as anxiety, aggression, and anger (cf. Hahn, 1991). Despite the lack of investigation, research has been conducted into related constructs, including mood (Lane and Terry, 2000; Prapavessis and Grove, 1994; Terry, 1995; Totterdell, 1999; Totterdell and Leach, 2001), cognition and affect (Gould, Eklund, and Jackson, 1992; Eklund, 1994; Jones et al., 1996; Robazza, Bortoli, and Nougier, 1998; Robazza, Bortoli, Nocini, Moser, and Arslan, 2000; Robazza, Bortoli, Zadro, and Nougier, 1998; Silva and Hardy, 1984, 1986) and emotional labeling and feeling states (Jones and Hanton, 2001; Mellalieu et al., 2003). Several normative measures of affect and mood have been in employed in the sport psychology literature to date including the Activation-Deactivation Checklist (ADCL; Thayer, 1989), the Multiple Affective Adjective Check List (MAACL; Zuckerman and Lubin, 1985), the Profile of Mood States (POMS; McNair, Lorr, and Dropleman, 1971) and the Positive and Negative Affect Scale (PANAS; Watson, Clark, and Tellegen, 1988). While the ADCL and MAACL have had little use with limited findings in the sporting domain the POMS has been employed in a large number of studies examining mental health in athletes via Morgan's (1980) 'iceberg profile' of successful performers (see Prapavessis, 2000; Terry, 1995 for a full review), and the PANAS has been used to examine the relationship of positive and negative affect with constructs such as self-efficacy and competitive anxiety (i.e., Jones et al., 1996; Treasure et al., 1997).

Despite some initial promise, the existing instruments utilized in sport psychology to measure affect tend to suffer from both conceptual and methodological limitations (see Jones, Mace, and Williams, 2000; Lane and Terry, 2000; Mellalieu, 2003). This lies with the fact that researchers in sport psychology have employed scales borrowed from other disciplines of psychology (i.e., social, clinical). Specifically, questions are raised regarding the relevance of some of these questionnaires' items to sport (Gauvin and Spence, 1998; McAuley and Courneya, 1994). Further, the majority of affect measurement scales originate or and have been borrowed from clinical psychology, and directly transferred to sport, with little or no allowance for population differences (Biddle, 1997; Brawley and Martin, 1995; Mellalieu, 2003). Hence, the content and construct validity of the scales designed in the clinical setting have not been fully tested in the sport domain. Indeed, Hanin (1997) has added that normative affective scales from non-sport settings with excellent psychometric characteristics may be functionally inadequate in the assessment of emotional experiences in sport. Any attempts to utilize these scales may therefore question the validity of the studies, further emphasizing the need for sport-specific measures of affect. Gauvin and Spence (1998) suggest that the use of sport-specific measures can be more sensitive to the stimulus properties of sport than can measures that gauge movement along broader dimensions of the human experience. Recent empirical investigation in sport psychology has gone some way to dealing with these problems by working towards the development of normative scales in sport (Prapavessis and Grove, 1992; Terry and Lane, 2000), however, limitations also exist with such scales pertaining to the credibility of measures designed for clinical use to the transfer to sport and their biased negativity (Gauvin and Spence, 1998; Kerr, 1997). Kerr (1997) for example, suggests that by concentrating on mood profiles, derived from instruments like the POMS that are biased towards negative moods and negative affect, and in particular anxiety, sport psychology researchers and practitioners are missing a major part of the mood and performance jigsaw by ignoring the positive experiences associated with sporting competition.

An additional problem with the measurement of affect is the fact that there has been a lack of clear definition in relation to distinguishing between mood, affect, emotion and feeling states (Diener, Smith, and Fujita, 1995; Ekman, 1994). Within sport and exercise psychology researchers have employed terms such as 'emotion', 'mood', and 'feeling' interchangeably, when indeed they are recognized as relatively distinct concepts (Lane and Terry, 2000; Mellalieu, 2003). Indeed, Gauvin and Spence (1998) suggest that one of the most daunting problems facing researchers interested in studying exercise-induced changes in psychological states is the difficulty associated with defining concepts of feeling states, mood and emotions. One solution to this problem comes from the work of Clore and associates, who describe affect in terms of feeling states (Clore, Ortorny, and Foss, 1987). The understanding here is that how a person feels will have a large influence on the emotions and moods experienced. This approach has been employed extensively by researchers in the exercise psychology setting, with scales such as the Subjective Experiences Exercise Scale (SEES; McAuley and Courneya, 1994), Feelings Scale (FS; Rejeski, Best, Griffith, and Kenney, 1987) and the Exercise Feelings Inventory (EFI; Gauvin and Rejeski, 1993). Research employing these measures has shown that while feelings are not directly indicative of emotions they are representative of an affective experience from which emotional states may emanate (see Rejeski et al., 1987; Gauvin and Spence, 1998 for a review). For the purposes of the current paper affective responses are therefore deemed characteristic of feeling states that refer to "those human experiences that include bodily reactions, cognitive appraisals, actual or potential instrumental responses, or some combination thereof" (Gauvin and Spence, 1998; p. 326). We have also adopted the traditional definition of anxiety for our research (Jones, 1990; Jones and Hanton, 2001; Lazarus, 1966; Mellalieu et al., 2006) that refers to anxiety as a negative, cognitive and perceived physiological response to uncertain appraisals of coping with the demands of a stressful situation (e.g., competition).

Summary and Study Overview

While the understudying of the precompetitive psychological response of sports performers has been advanced considerably by the study of the intensity, and in particular, the direction of the competitive anxiety response, researchers have recently criticized the notion of facilitating and debilitating anxiety. Subsequently, a conceptual debate has emerged surrounding the existence of 'positive anxiety' and whether facilitating interpretations of anxiety symptoms are a myth and represent positive interpretations of the competitive stress response or have been mislabeled and actually represent a distinct positive emotional episode (Burton, 1998; Burton and Naylor, 1997; Hardy, 1997, 1998; Jones and Hanton, 2001; Mellalieu et al., 2003). Accompanying this conceptual debate has been a growing dissatisfaction that the measurement of the precompetition response has been unnecessarily limited due to the restricted focus on solely symptoms associated with competitive anxiety thereby neglecting the broader picture of the affective response (Hanin, 2000; Mellalieu et al., 2003). The understanding of the precompetitive affective experience has also been further constrained by a lack of appropriate measurement of the construct. Specifically, there is a need to utilize a sport-specific scale, in addition to examining further utility of traditional scales from social psychology, which can be employed as a comprehensive measure of preperformance affect in competitive sports performers. Such inquiry will allow researchers to investigate issues such as the content of the precompetitive response and the conceptual debate surrounding positive anxiety (Mellalieu et al., 2003).

In light of the conceptual debate surrounding the notion of positive anxiety and the associated measurement issues in the assessment of the preperformance affective experience in sporting competition the primary propose of this study was to investigate sports performer's interpretations of competitive anxiety symptoms and the relationship with the subsequent affective states reported. Specifically, we aimed to address the limitations in existing studies concerning the conceptual debate and advance the understanding of the precompetitive affective experience by utilizing both traditional and sport-specific validated measures of precompetitive affect with desirable psychometric integrity. Several predictions were generated for the study. First, in line with previous investigations indicating relationships between competitive anxiety and affective states (Jones et al., 1996; Treasure et al., 1996) it was predicted that positive affect would correlate strongly with direction of competitive anxiety while negative affect would correlate strongly with the intensity of cognitive and somatic anxiety symptoms. Second, specific to the conceptual debate regarding symptom interpretation and the labeling of precompetitive symptoms (Jones and Hanton, 2001; Mellalieu et al., 2003) it was hypothesized that a strong positive relationship would be observed between facilitating interpretations of symptoms associated with competitive anxiety and performers' reported positive affective responses. Similarly, a positive relationship was predicted between debilitating symptom interpretation and negative affective states. Finally, performers who labeled their symptoms associated with precompetitive anxiety as facilitating to performance were predicted to report greater positive precompetitive affective experiences than their debilitating counterparts, who were expected to experience greater negative precompetitive affective responses than facilitators.

Methods

Participants

Data for the study were obtained from 322 competitive athletes ($n = 120$ males, $n = 97$ females), all of whom provided informed written consent. Participants were sampled at random and ranged in age from 18 to 34 years ($M = 21.83$, $SD = 3.12$) and competed in a variety of different activities ($n = 29$) including team sports such as rugby, cricket, and football and individual sports such as athletics, golf, and tennis. In order to be selected for the study, the participants had to be currently competing, or at least, have participated in some form of national competition or championship. Prior to taking part in the study, all participants provided informed written consent to the researcher. At the time of completing the study all participants were in competition or training for competition.

Measures

Measurement of Competitive Trait Anxiety

The Competitive State Anxiety Inventory-2 (CSAI-2; Martens, Burton, et al., 1990) was originally employed to measure the intensity of preperformance cognitive anxiety, somatic anxiety, and self-confidence, with nine items in each subscale. The response scale asked the participant to rate the intensity with which each symptom was being experienced on a continuum from 1 ("not at all") to 4 ("very much so"). Thus, possible intensity scores on each subscale ranged from 9 to 36. Cronbach's Alpha coefficients demonstrating internal consistency for the intensity responses have been reported ranging from .79 to .90 (Martens, Burton, et al., 1990). In addition, a direction scale developed by Jones and Swain (1992) was included for the cognitive and somatic anxiety items in which each participant rated the degree to which the experienced intensity of each symptom was either facilitative or debilitative to subsequent performance on a scale from -3 ("very debilitative") to +3 ("very facilitative"). Thus, possible direction scores on each subscale ranged from -27 to +27, where a positive score represented a state of facilitation, and a negative one debilitation. A score of zero was deemed an interpretation that intensity levels were unimportant to performance. Internal consistency for the direction scale has been reported with coefficients ranging from .80 to .89 for cognitive anxiety and .72 to .84 for somatic anxiety (Jones and Hanton, 1996, 2001; Swain and Jones, 1996). Although essentially a measure of state anxiety, the modified CSAI-2 test instructions have been successfully adapted by previous researchers to assess intensity and direction of trait anxiety (i.e., Hanton and Jones, 1999a, 1999b; Jones and Ntoumanis, 1998; Jones and Swain, 1995; Perry and Williams, 1998). Each item is converted in terms of how the participant *usually* feels so that a general or trait measure is created. Similar procedures have been successfully employed by a number of other developers of state-trait measures (e.g., Albrecht and Feltz, 1987; McNair, et al., 1971; Vealey, 1986). Internal consistency for the trait scale has been reported with coefficients of .78, .84, and .84 for cognitive anxiety intensity, somatic anxiety intensity, and self-confidence intensity respectively, and between .79 and .85 for cognitive anxiety direction and .73 and .83 for somatic anxiety direction (Mellalieu et al., 2003; Perry and Williams, 1998).

The Positive and Negative Affect Scale (PANAS)

The Positive and Negative Affect Scale (PANAS; Watson et al., 1988) consists of two 10-item scales to measure the independent affective constructs of Positive Affect (PA) and Negative Affect (NA; Watson and Clark, 1984, 1994; Watson and Tellegen, 1985). Items on the PA scale include "interested", "excited" and "alert"; while items on the NA scale include "distressed", "nervous" and "afraid". The participant is required to indicate to what extent s/he generally experiences the response on a five point scale ranging from 1 ("very slightly/not at all") to 5 ("extremely"). Thus, possible scores on both scales range from 10 to 50. Extensive reliability and validity have been reported on the scales (Watson and Clark, 1994; Watson et al., 1988; Watson and McKee-Walker, 1996). For example, Watson et al.

(1988) have shown the scales to be high on internal consistency (alpha = 0.86 to 0.90 for PA; 0.84 to 0.87 for NA), largely uncorrelated (intercorrelations ranging from -0.12 to -0.23) and stable over a two month period (test-retest reliability = 0.68 for PA, 0.71 for NA).

The Pre-Performance Feelings Scale (PPFS)

The PPFS (Mellalieu, 2000) is a sport-specific trait measure of preperformance affective states that consists of 40 adjectives describing how sports performers usually 'feel' prior to competing. The scale was constructed from the sampling of responses of competitive athletes (representing a range of over 15 team and individual sports) to an item pool of 600 labels derived from a list of 'feelings' taken from the affective lexicon (Clore et al., 1987), used to describe affective experiences, together with existing sport mood state measurement scales (e.g., POMS, McNair et al., 1971). The scale consists of 8 subscales (4 negative and 4 positive) each of 5 adjectives that describe common feelings for that subscale. The 8 subscales are mental readiness, anger, distress, confidence, joy, competitive anxiety, positive perceptions of physical state and negative perceptions of physical state. Each item on the scale has an intensity component that asks individuals to rate the extent to which they experienced the feeling on a scale of '1' 'Not at All' to '7' 'Extremely So'. Thus, possible subscale scores ranged from 5 to 35. Initial measures show internal consistency values of a moderate to high range (.72 to .92) which provide adequate support for the reliability of the scale (Mellalieu, 2000). Exploratory and confirmatory factor analysis procedures have confirmed the 8-factor structure of the scale and discriminant and convergent validity measures have also supported the scale as a valid measurement tool (Mellalieu, 2000).

Procedure

Participants were contacted and informed of the nature of the study and invited to take part. Demographic information and written informed consent regarding the study objectives was obtained from those individuals who agreed to participate. A suitable time and venue for the collection of the data was then arranged. In addition, permission was sought and granted from the relevant coaches and organizers of the respective performers (where appropriate) to involve the participants. All questionnaires were administered by the lead researcher who possessed over 10 years experience in the administration of psychometric instruments to sports performers. Specific verbal and written instructions regarding the content of the questionnaires or scales were then provided. In accordance with previous trait investigations (i.e., Hanton, Evans, et al., 2003) participants completed the PANAS, PPFS and CTAI-2 scales in random order away from the competitive environment in order to avoid any contextual influences (e.g., audience effects). All responses were completed within the time frame of the participants' competitive season. In order to counter any cognitive bias or judgment effects (i.e., attributional) no questionnaires were completed directly prior to or after major competitions. Before completing responses, performers were presented with respective anti-social desirability instructions based upon the recommendations of Watson and Clark (1994), Martens, Burton, et al. (1990), and Mellalieu (2000). These directions emphasized the confidentiality of the responses at an individual level, the need for honesty, and an indication of the thoughts and feelings the performer would *usually* experience just prior to competing in an important competition.

Data Analysis

Employing a moderate effect size, the sample size used gave a statistical power that exceeded the required value of .80 (Cohen, 1988). Data analysis was then divided into four stages. First, data screening procedures were conducted to investigate the accuracy of the data, and measure the influence of any potential covariates such as gender, age, sport type or skill level, as highlighted in previous anxiety-direction studies (e.g., Hanton et al., 2000; Perry and Williams, 1998). Second, internal consistencies for each of the subscales were conducted (Cronbach, 1951). Third, Correlation analysis was employed to examine the relationships within, and between, the subscales of the CTAI-2, PPFS and PANAS questionnaires. Finally, in accordance with procedures adopted by recent direction studies (Hanton and Jones, 1999a; Jones and Hanton, 2001; Jones et al., 1994; Mellalieu et al., 2003) participants were dichotomized into facilitated (positive scores for cognitive and somatic anxiety direction) and debilitated groups (negative scores for cognitive and somatic anxiety direction). Thus, the facilitated group comprised those participants who had positive scores on both cognitive and somatic anxiety direction ($n = 156$), and the debilitated group comprised those participants who had negative scores on both ($n = 144$). Participants who had a combination of a positive score and a negative score, or a negative and zero score or positive and zero score ($n = 22$) were omitted from the analysis. Multivariate Analyses of Variance (MANOVA) procedures were used to investigate any significant multivariate effects in relation to scoring on the subscales of the PPFS, PANAS and CTAI-2 subscales as a function of anxiety interpretation. Specifically, three separate one way MANOVA's were conducted with groups (debilitated versus facilitated) as the independent variable and performer's PPFS, PANAS and CTAI-2 subscale scores as the dependant variables in each MANOVA respectively. Univariate Analyses of Variance (ANOVA) with Bonferroni adjustments ($p < .01$) was employed for follow up analyses in the case of all significant MANOVA effects.

Results

Preliminary Data Analysis

Participants' scores on the CTAI-2, PPFS, and PANAS scales were examined for accuracy of data entry, missing values and fit between their distribution and the assumptions of multivariate analysis. No missing values were recorded and there were no univariate or multivariate within-cell outliers at $p = .001$. In accordance with recommendations of Tabachnick and Fidell (1996), the assumptions of normality, homogeneity of variance-covariance matrices, F (3, 26645) = 1.11, $p > .05$, linearity, and multicollinearity were also observed to be satisfactory. Additional analyses were performed to measure the influence of any potential covariates. Separate one-way MANOVAs were conducted to determine the possible effects of age, skill level, sport type and gender on the modified CTAI-2 scores with each covariate group acting as the independent variable and CTAI-2 intensity and direction subscale scores acting as the dependent variables. Non-significant effects were observed for gender, sport type, age, and skill level ($p > 0.05$). Internal consistency analyses were conducted on the CTAI-2 direction subscales with coefficients of .76 ($p < .01$) for cognitive anxiety direction and .75 ($p < .01$) for somatic anxiety direction respectively. For the PANAS subscales coefficients of .85 ($p < .01$) for PA and .87 ($p < .01$) for NA. For the PPFS subscales values of .80 ($p < .01$) were reported for mental readiness, .72 ($p < .01$) for anger, .83 ($p < .01$) for distress, .86 ($p < .01$) for confidence, .74 ($p < 0.01$) for joy, .84 ($p < .01$) competitive anxiety, .72 ($p < .01$) for positive perceptions of physical state, and .82 ($p < .01$) for negative perceptions of physical state. Values for the internal reliability of the three scales were therefore satisfactory (Nunnally and Burnstein, 1994) and similar to the results previously reported (i.e., Mellalieu, 2000; Mellalieu et al., 2003; Watson et al., 1988).

Correlation Analyses

Table 1 provides a summary of the analysis employed to examine the inter relationships between the subscales of the CTAI-2 and PANAS, and CTAI-2 and PPFS, questionnaires respectively. For the relationships between CTAI-2 and PANAS subscales the results agreed with the previous research of Jones et al. (1996). Therefore, Cognitive Anxiety Intensity (CAI) displayed a significant positive correlation with NA ($p < .01$), but no significant relationship emerged with PA. These results were replicated for Somatic Anxiety Intensity SAI ($p < .01$). A significant positive correlation was observed between PA and self-confidence ($p < .01$) and a significant negative correlation between NA and self-confidence ($p < .01$). For direction subscales, Cognitive Anxiety Direction (CAD) displayed a significant positive correlation with PA ($p < .01$), and a significant negative relationship with NA ($p < .01$). Somatic Anxiety Direction (SAD) displayed a significant positive correlation with PA ($p < .01$) and no significant relationship with NA. In addition, a moderate positive correlation ($p < .01$) of .23 was observed between Cognitive Anxicty Intensity (CAI) and Somatic Anxiety Intensity (SAI), and .13 between CAD and SAD, supporting previous research employing the CSAI-2 (Jones et al., 1991; Jones et al., 1996; Martens, Vealey, et al., 1990). Furthermore, very low, and non-significant correlations were observed between PA and NA, reinforcing the independent nature of the two affective dimensions (Watson et al., 1988).

For the correlations between CTAI-2 and PPFS intensity sub-scale scores the intensity of competitive anxiety (CAI and SAI), a significant positive relationship was observed for anger ($p < .05$), distress ($p < .05$ and $p < .05$ for CAI and SAI respectively) and competitive anxiety ($p < .01$) intensity subscales. A significant negative correlation was displayed for mental readiness and confidence subscales ($p < .05$). For direction of competitive anxiety (cognitive anxiety direction and somatic anxiety direction; CAD and SAD), a significant positive relationship was observed ($p <.05$) with each of the PPFS direction subscales except with competitive anxiety, and between CAD and anger and joy, and between SAD and anger.

For self-confidence, significant positive correlations were observed with mental readiness, confidence and positive perceptions of physical state ($p <.01$). Significant negative relationships were also observed between self-confidence and distress ($p <.01$) and competitive anxiety subscales ($p <.05$).

Table 1. Correlations between CTAI-2, PPFS and PANAS sub-scale scores

	Cognitive anxiety intensity	Somatic anxiety intensity	Self-confidence	Cognitive anxiety direction	Somatic anxiety direction
PPFS					
Mental readiness	-.19*	-.15*	.54**	.28**	.41**
Anger	.20*	.18*	.08	-.02	.10
Distress	.22**	.21*	-.17*	-.17*	-.11
Confidence	-.27**	-.17*	.63**	.38**	.42**
Joy	-.03	.03	.40**	.04	.17*
Competitive anxiety	.50**	.51**	-.24**	-.16	-.16
Positive physical state	-.13	-.12	.49**	.27**	.45**
Negative physical state	.12	.12	-.13	-.19*	-.22**
PANAS					
Positive Affect	-.05	-.005	.42**	.31**	.42**
Negative Affect	.38**	.37**	-.28**	-.13**	-.15

*$p < .05$, **$p < .01$

Table 2. Means, Standard deviations and One-way analysis of variance for CTAI-2, PANAS and PPFS subscales as a function of facilitators / debilitators

	Facilitators ($n = 156$)		Debilitators ($n = 144$)	
	M	SD	M	SD
CTAI-2				
Cognitive Anxiety Intensity	19.21	3.33	22.3*	2.87
Somatic Anxiety Intensity	22.50	2.65	19.00	3.54
Self-Confidence	22.70	4.21	19.50**	1.65
Cognitive Anxiety Direction	7.00	0.78	-6.00**	1.23
Somatic Anxiety Direction	8.00	0.98	-4.60**	1.09
PANAS				
Positive Affect	38.2	4.67	33.3**	2.67
Negative Affect	17.8	3.24	19.8**	3.39
PPFS				
Mental readiness	24.9	2.34	21.82**	3.54
Anger	11	7.98	12	2.65
Distress	6.1	9.76	6.2	7.56
Confidence	23.2	2.43	18.5**	3.3
Joy	18.1	1.23	17.2	2.34
Competitive anxiety	16.1	3.2	17.3	1.2
Positive physical state	23.2	4.2	20.3**	6.45
Negative physical state	8.4	2.1	9.5	5.34

*$p < .05$, **$p < .01$

Ppfs, Panas, CTAI-2 Scores as a Function of Facilitators / Debilitators

Three separate one way MANOVA's were conducted with groups (debilitated versus facilitated) as the independent variable and performer's PPFS, PANAS and CTAI-2 subscale scores as the dependant variables in each MANOVA respectively. Mean scores and results for univariate analyses are shown in Table 2.

For the relationship between anxiety interpretation and CTAI-2 subscale responses a one-way MANOVA was conducted with groups (debilitated versus facilitated) as the independent variable and scores for the performers' CTAI-2 sub-scales as the dependent variables. The MANOVA was significant (Wilks' Lambda = .98, F (2,298) = 12.4; p <.01, ES = .25). For intensity of competitive anxiety, significant differences between facilitators and debilitators in terms of cognitive anxiety (p <.05, ES = .11) and self-confidence (p <.01, ES = .21) were observed. No significant differences emerged for somatic anxiety. For direction, significant differences were observed between facilitators and debilitators for both cognitive (p <.01, ES = .19) and somatic anxiety (p <.01, ES = .26). These results partially support the research of Jones and Swain (1992) that observed no differences in intensity of cognitive and somatic trait anxiety symptoms experienced between facilitators and debilitators. For PANAS scores as a function of facilitators/debilitators, a one-way MANOVA was conducted with groups (debilitated versus facilitated) as the independent variable and performers' PA and NA scales as the dependent variables. The MANOVA was significant (Wilks' Lambda = 0.87, F (2,298) = 8.45; p <.01, ES = .21).

Follow-up univariate analysis revealed facilitators were significantly higher on PA (p <.01, ES = .33) and lower on NA (p <.01, ES = .20) than their debilitating counterparts.

For the relationship between anxiety interpretation and PPFS subscale responses a one way MANOVA was conducted with groups (debilitated versus facilitated) as the independent variable and scores for the performers' PPFS sub-scales as the dependent variables. A significant difference was demonstrated (Wilks' Lambda = .83, F (2,298) = 5.67; p <.01, ES = .33). Follow-up ANOVAs indicated that facilitators were significantly higher on intensity subscales for mental readiness (p <.01, ES = .27), confidence (p <.01, ES = .28) and positive perceptions of physical states (p <.01, ES = .16) than their debilitating counterparts (p <.01).

Discussion

Summary of Findings

The present study examined the conceptual debate surrounding the notion of 'Positive Anxiety' (Burton, 1998; Burton and Naylor, 1997; Hardy, 1997, 1998; see also Mellalieu et al., 2006) and whether facilitating interpretations of competitive trait anxiety symptoms were indeed a 'myth' or merely representative of some other affective experience other than anxiety as a result of 'mislabeling' by existing measurement scales. The findings revealed that a strong positive relationship existed between directional interpretations of symptoms associated with competitive anxiety and the various measures of positive affect. Significant positive relationships were found between the intensity of the anxiety response and the measures of negative affect. The results also showed that facilitating interpretations of competitive trait anxiety correlated significantly with the various measures of positive affective states. Further, those individuals who were labeled as facilitators (i.e., positive interpretations of symptoms) were found to be report significantly higher scores on the positive subscales of the PPFS and PANAS scales and lower scores on the accompanying negative affective scales than their debilitating counterparts. The findings would therefore appear to indicate that while it appears there may be some 'mislabeling' of anxiety symptoms those individuals who interpret symptoms associated with the competitive stress response in a positive or facilitating way with respect to forthcoming performance experience a greater overall positive emotional state prior to competition than their debilitating counterparts (Jones and Hanton, 2001; Mellalieu et al., 2003).

In the conceptual debate, one of the central arguments against positive anxiety is concerned with the measurement instrument of the construct, the CSAI-2. Specifically, the suggestion that directional perceptions of anxiety symptoms may not actually be measuring what they are purported to due to the wording of the questions employed in the scale. Burton and Naylor (1997) suggested that many symptoms are worded neutrally so they are not only characteristic of anxiety states but also representative of other more positive affective states. The authors cite the example of such CSAI-2 questions as 'I feel nervous' or 'I am concerned about this competition' and claim that they may be perceived as negative and debilitating to some, whereas to others they may be seen an indication of positive excitement and effective mental readiness. Consequently, if athletes report they are experiencing such symptoms intensely, they are scored high on cognitive and somatic anxiety, and deemed to experience debilitating effects in accordance with multidimensional anxiety theory (Martens et al., 1990) which purports that intensities of symptoms are always negative to performance. Burton and Naylor (1997) further conclude that positive emotions such as challenge, excitement, and self-confidence have therefore been mislabeled as facilitating or positive anxiety. This would account for the previous research findings that have shown direction of competitive anxiety to be mediated by positive affect, and intensity of competitive anxiety to be mediated by negative affect (Jones and Hanton, 2001; Jones et al. 1996; Treasure et al. 1996). In the current study, strong correlations were observed between cognitive and somatic anxiety direction and the positive subscales of the PPFS, such as mental readiness, confidence, and positive perceptions of physical state and the PA subscale of the PANSA. Likewise, positive correlations were observed between cognitive and somatic anxiety intensity responses and the various measures of negative affect. The findings would appear to suggest that facilitating interpretations of symptoms associated with competitive anxiety may be representative of, or closely linked to, positive affective states and feelings. Indeed, Jones himself has indicated 'a state in which cognitive and physiological symptoms, however intense, are interpreted as being facilitative to performance are unlikely to represent 'anxiety'...it will be probably be labeled by the performer as 'excitement', 'psyched up', 'motivated', etc.' (Jones et al., 1994, p. 13).

The findings of the current investigation, however, would also appear to support the suggestions of Jones, Hanton and colleagues that the overall precompetitive affective one is positive for individuals who view symptoms associated with competitive anxiety as facilitative towards performance. Specifically, in the current study, the top five highest mean subscale scores of the PPFS scale consisted of 'positive feelings' subscales (i.e., mental readiness, confidence, joy, positive perception of physical state). These results confirm the findings of Jones and Hanton (2001) and Mellalieu et al. (2003), that from a situational and dispositional context, positive affective experiences can exist alongside symptoms of competitive anxiety in the preperformance period. The findings also reinforce the view that the precompetitive stress response is not necessarily entirely negative and characterized solely by anxiety (cf. Eysenck and Calvo, 1992; Hardy, 1997) and that a multitude of emotional states, including anxiety, influence athletic performance (Hanin, 2000; Jones, 1995; Kerr, 1997). Furthermore, findings from qualitative investigations examining precompetition affect and cognitions support the notion of the precompetition experience as one that in the majority can be experienced in a positive mental state (Eklund, 1994; Gould et al., 1992; Hanton, Mellalieu, and Young, 2002). Specifically, certain performers may label their overall psychological state as 'excited' or 'motivated' or a combination of these (cf. Gould and Udry, 1994; Hanin, 1997), but may also simultaneously experience negative anxiety symptoms during a stressful competitive situation. One possibility is that the negative anxiety symptoms experienced by these individuals may be over-ridden by the positive feelings. Because both the facilitators and debilitators report being anxious prior to competition, then anxiety *per se* may not be the central variable that researchers assume it to be (cf. Jones, 1995; Mellalieu, 2003). Some individuals therefore appear to experience a highly complex state prior to competition that may predominantly be positive but also includes negative aspects. Interestingly, Hanton and Jones' (1999a) qualitative study with world class swimmers established that a fine line existed between 'anxiety' and 'excitement' with optimum athletic performance occurring when the individual was very close to the line and potentially experiencing both (cf. Apter, 1982; Kerr, 1997). Therefore, these individuals may need to be 'on the edge' or 'on the limit' while remaining in control to perform at their best (cf. Carver and Scheier, 1988, 1998; Hanton and Connaughton, 2002; Jones and Hanton, 1996).

The conceptual paradox of experiencing facilitative interpretations of symptoms and 'anxiety' concurrently may be partially explained by the self-confidence findings of this study where all ANOVAs reached significance between the interpretation groups. These results provide further evidence to confirm that self-confidence is a moderating variable in the directional interpretation of symptoms experienced in pressure situations (Bandura, 1982, 1997; Hanton and Connaughton, 2002). Hardy (1996) has attempted to explain the role of self-confidence in the anxiety-performance relationship via the five-dimension butterfly catastrophe model which suggests self-confidence moderates the effects of cognitive anxiety and physiological arousal upon performance. Specifically, self-confidence is purported to increase the probability that cognitively anxious performers can tolerate higher levels of arousal before experiencing a decrement in performance (Hardy, 1990). Subsequently, participants who experience high intensities of anxiety and confidence simultaneously may still perform successfully, while performers who experience high anxiety intensities without the accompanying feelings of confidence may suffer performance decrements. Self-confidence is therefore suggested to influence performance over and above that exerted by cognitive anxiety and physiological arousal (Hardy et al., 1996), and has the ability to discriminate between anxiety interpretations (Hanton and Connaughton, 2002; Jones and

Hanton, 2001; Jones et al., 1994). However, despite these suggestions, tentative explanations exist for the exact mechanism by which self-confidence may protect against the harmful effects of symptoms associated with competitive anxiety. Jones et al. (1994), for example, suggested that elite athletes who experience potentially debilitating anxiety symptoms may be able to maintain self-confidence levels and keep a subsequent positive outlook towards performance by the use of effective cognitive strategies. Indeed, high confidence may facilitate coping resources (e.g., rationalization of thoughts and feelings) to deal with competitive anxiety resulting in the performers perceiving that they can remain in control in the pressure environment of competition (cf. Carver and Scheier, 1988, 1998; Hanton and Connaughton, 2002; Hanton et al., 2004; Jones and Hanton, 1996). Therefore, it is possible that participants who experience high intensities of anxiety and confidence simultaneously will still perform successfully. Conversely, performers who experience high anxiety intensities without the accompanying feelings of confidence may suffer performance decrements. The absence of self-confidence in stressful competitive situations may therefore be the critical factor potentially due to its additional motivational properties along with experiencing anxiety symptoms (cf. Eysenck and Calvo, 1992). Jones and Hanton (2001) have provided some empirical support for these proposals, such that, in the presence of increasing physiological arousal and cognitive symptoms, athletes are able to protect their level of self-confidence and maintain positive affective states. The identification of the underlying protection mechanisms by which this may occur has recently been explored in a qualitative investigation by Hanton et al. (2004) which found that elite performers reported using cognitive strategies, including thought stopping, positive self-talk and mental rehearsal, that functioned to remove, reduce, or control any negative thoughts or images experienced. This protective mechanism was reported to allow the athlete to adopt a positive outlook (i.e., confident coping) towards the symptoms experienced and, assisted by enhanced effort and motivation (cf. Eysenck and Calvo, 1992), maintain a positive perception of control and subsequent facilitating interpretations of symptoms experienced with regard to successful forthcoming performance. In the current study, therefore, it could be suggested that the 'facilitators' have learned to utilize or employ such cognitive strategies to serve as a confidence protection function. Subsequently these strategies reduce, remove, or alter the negative 'doubting' cognitions experienced from one of a negative state to a more positive confident outlook towards forthcoming competition and performance and report a greater positive precompetitive affective state overall (Hanton and Jones, 1999a, 1999b). Those individuals low in confidence do not appear to have control over thoughts and cognitions and subsequently experience an enhanced overall negative affective state in conjunction with debilitating interpretations of symptoms associated with competitive anxiety.

In summary, therefore, given that the findings regarding the conceptual debate suggesting that the overall precompetitive stress response to competition is a complex interaction of the interpretation anxiety symptoms together with a combination of other positive and negative affective responses the central tenets of the authors' position are as follows: 1) Anxiety is by definition a negative emotional response to appraisal mechanisms (Lazarus, 1991); 2) The CSAI-2 may not directly measure competitive anxiety but only symptoms commonly associated with the response; 3) Finally, but importantly, experiencing competitive anxiety can result in positive performance consequences if the individual remains in control and 'on the edge'.

While some additional light has been shed on the conceptual debate surrounding the notion of positive anxiety it is important to note that the data analysis procedures adopted in the current study (i.e., correlations) only indicate relationships between variables and do not indicate causality. Further, as the study also only measures trait responses, asking respondents to recall how they usually feel away from the competitive environment brings with it its own problems. Specifically, recalling the entire range of the intensity of feelings and responses may be more difficult for individuals in retrospect. There is considerable evidence, however, to support the use of such methods from the eyewitness memory account literature. Studies of real-life events appear to suggest that highly emotional or arousal inducing events (such as that of major competitions or matches) are very well retained over time, especially with respect to detailed information directly associated with the event (e.g., Christianson, 1992). Similar evidence exists within in sport psychology to support the use of retrospective recall procedures to assess performers affective responses (see Brewer, Van-Raalte, Linder, and Van-Raalte, 1991; Hanin, 2000; Harger and Raglin, 1994; Rychta, 1982). Further research is therefore required to examine links between state and trait measures of anxiety, affect, and feeling. This will provide additional evidence regarding the proposed role of facilitating anxiety in sport performance, together with the influence of other cognitions and affective responses (Mellalieu, 2003; Mellalieu et al., 2006). Research may also provide some indication of the salience of affective responses other than anxiety, such as self-confidence, in the performance spectrum. By employing alternative methods of inquiry, such as in-depth interviews, it is possible to further examine, in detail, the proposed links between directional perceptions of anxiety and athletes feelings in detail.

One particular area for exploration is the temporal nature of the anxiety response experienced over the competition period. Lazarus (1991) posits that stress before achievement situations or competition, termed anticipatory stress, is often viewed as preparatory and facilitating by individuals, while stress during such contexts may be seen as debilitating to performance. This presents the case of performance versus preparatory anxiety (Burton and Naylor, 1997). Support for this contention comes from Mellalieu et al.'s (2003) study that found performers' cognitive perceptions of the precompetitive affective response changed in the time period before performance. Specifically, a number of the athletes experienced some symptoms associated with competitive anxiety as 'functional' and facilitating to their preparation for performance as they elicited the required effort and motivation to mentally and physically prepare the necessary resources for competition (Hanin, 2000). However, such symptoms that were used by the athlete to enhance preparation for performance were then considered 'dysfunctional' and debilitating for actual performance. Understanding of the athletes' cognitive interpretation and labeling of such responses will aid the psychologist in providing a clearer rationale to intervene and implement intentional and planned change (Cerin, Szabo, Hunt, and Williams, 2000). The idiosyncratic nature of these 'changes' in anxiety and emotional state interpretation with regard to preparation for, and actual performance identified by Mellalieu et al.'s (2003) study reinforces the emphasis on the need for the practitioner to adopt more sensitive intra-individual methods of assessment and intervention (see Hanin, 1997, 2000; Thomas, Hanton, and Jones, 2002). Here, qualitative investigations may prove a rich and valuable source of information that will allow researchers to pinpoint exactly what affective state athletes are experiencing and how they view their symptoms with regard to performance (Hanton, Mellalieu, et al., 2002).

A further issue in the contemporary competitive anxiety literature concerns the validity of the CASI-2 scale, particularly the factor structure, to assess the intensity and direction of the anxiety construct. While coefficient alphas provide some evidence for this structure, we cannot rely upon these as the sole indicators of subscale homogeneity. Using confirmatory analysis techniques researchers have produced findings to question the three-factor structure of the intensity component of the scale (e.g., Lane, Sewell, Terry, Bartram, and Nesti, 1999). Similar techniques are therefore required to investigate the integrity of the proposed two-factor structure of the direction dimension. Research should also consider the criteria by which performers are labeled as debilitators or facilitators of symptoms associated with competitive anxiety. Under Jones and Swain's (1992) criteria individuals are only considered for analysis if they score both negative and both positive on the CSAI-2 direction subscales. This leaves a percentage of individuals unaccounted for, who, for example, may score positive for cognitive anxiety direction and negative for somatic anxiety direction. In addition, some respondents may score an overall total of zero on either of the direction subscales, indicating that intensity levels experienced are unimportant to performance, yet are omitted from analysis. This is despite the fact they may interpret some anxiety symptoms as debilitative or facilitative to performance. In order to assess more sensitive measures of anxiety interpretation, future studies should consider examining not only participants' combined cognitive and somatic anxiety direction scores, but also separate totals for cognitive and somatic anxiety direction (cf. Jones and Hanton, 2001).

A final conceptual and methodological problem surrounding developments in the area of mood and affect has been the lack of sport-specific measures to describe the precompetition experience in the sport psychology literature (Gauvin and Spence, 1998; Kerr, 1998). As highlighted earlier, current mood/emotion questionnaires employed in sport are drawn from clinical and social psychology (i.e. POMS, PANAS). Intuitively, scales developed for testing on clinical patients are hardly likely to predict athletic performance as effectively as sport-specific instruments due to a prejudiced bias towards negative moods or emotions and the ignorance of participants' perceptions of physical symptoms (Clore et al., 1987). This has brought criticism regarding the 'borrowing' of ideas directly from social psychology (Biddle, 1997; Brawley and Martin, 1995; Mellalieu, 2003) and could further explain why existing research has been unable to predict significant performance variance employing current scales. Recent research, however, has made some advancement into dealing with these issues with the development of normative mood scales for sporting populations (Terry and Lane, 2000). Compounding this issue there exists the continuing debate over the actual structure of affect (Feldman, Barret, and Russell, 1998; Green, Goldman, and Salovey, 1993; Watson and Clark, 1997) together with a lack of clear definition in relation to distinguishing between mood, affect, emotion, and even feeling states (Ekman, 1994). This has led to some authors unwisely using the terms interchangeably. Distinctive differences exist between these structures and if research is to measure affect or mood then appropriate clarifications of definitions are required. The current study overcomes some of these problems by adopting a scale designed to measure a sport-specific measurement scale of feelings drawn from a lexicon of feeling states, chosen by a population of competitive sports performers (Mellalieu, 2000). Equally, this scale is designed in the context of feelings states, which have been suggested as strong antecedents of mood and emotional states (Gauvin and Rejeski, 1993; Rejeski et al., 1987). Future research in the area of affect measurement therefore requires acknowledgement of the distinct difference in affective states such as moods, feelings, and emotions. Specifically, the positive affective states performers experience prior to competition requires investigation in more detail, with measurement scales that are sport-specific in nature, and can overcome existing conceptual and measurement limitations (Gauvin and Spence, 1998; Mellalieu, 2003). While the initial findings reported here provide some support for both the PPFS and PANAS scales, however, there is a need to further examine the construct and test validity of the scales across specific demographic populations, situation, and person variables (e.g., age, sport type, skill level). Finally, in response to the call for a more holistic approach to investigation in sport psychology (Hardy, Jones, and Gould, 1996), it may be wise for future areas of investigation to examine the performer's precompetitive mental state as a whole. The fact may be that cognitions, thoughts, or emotions alone may not sufficiently describe the precompetition period. One factor or affective response may be more salient in determining a performer's precompetition states and mental readiness (Mellalieu, 2003; Robazza, et al., 1998; Robazza et al., 2000; Robazza, Bortoli, Zadro, et al., 1998). The movement towards this understanding and the development of a scale to measure preperformance competitive affect will not only assist in predicting performance but, as Silva and Hardy (1986) acknowledged nearly two decades ago such knowledge·will allow clinicians to utilize an objective technique by which interventions can be advanced to optimize performance by removing or replacing habitual patterns of dysfunctional precompetitive affect. Such an approach may strengthen the scientific basis of applied sport psychology and intervention prescriptions.

Practical Implications

The practical implications of the study suggest that the broader precompetitive affective response, particularly, the athletes' interpretation and cognitive labeling of such experiences, may be more salient in assisting achievement of optimal preperformance mental states (Mellalieu et al., 2003). The same intensity of thoughts and feelings may be interpreted very differently by individual performers, particularly when accounting for the overall labeling of the psychological state as positive or negative. Practitioners need to be cognizant that traditional negative or positive emotions reported may not necessarily debilitate/facilitate preparation for, or actual forthcoming performance. We recommend the use of cognitive restructuring techniques that focus upon changing perceptions of the individuals' affective state, rather than attempting to reduce the emotion, mood or feeling via relaxation strategies as this may lead to a lowered and ineffective activation state (Hanton and Jones, 1999b). Also, there appears to be a central role played by perceived feelings of self-confidence in stressful situations. Individualized cognitive restructuring programs may be beneficial for performers who clearly do not interpret pre-event symptoms as facilitative as opposed to anxiety reduction interventions. For example, Hanton and Jones (1999b) found that restructuring debilitative thoughts and feelings via an intervention using goal setting, imagery, and self-talk was accompanied by considerable increases in self-confidence and also improvements in swimming performance.

Conclusion

In conclusion, the results of the current study provide further detail regarding the conceptual debate surrounding the notion of 'positive anxiety'. Specifically, the findings provide some support for Burton and associates (Burton, 1998; Burton and Naylor, 1997) and the original proposals of Jones (1995) that symptoms associated with competitive anxiety may be mislabeled by the measures currently available. Subsequently, symptoms perceived as facilitating to competition are being mislabeled purely as anxiety symptoms when indeed they appear to indicate some broad affective response to the stressor of competitive sport that signifies readiness/preparation to perform. In addition, however, the findings also support the beliefs of Hanton and colleagues (Jones and Hanton, 2001; Mellalieu et al., 2003) in that that the experiences of competitive anxiety symptoms occur alongside more traditional positive emotional responses. In this respect, the study reinforces the growing body of literature that suggests anxiety is one of many affective responses experienced by performers in the precompetition period, and these other mental states identified in the current study, specifically the positive affective experiences, may be more salient in enabling researchers to predict sporting performance than the existing narrow focus on the construct of competitive anxiety.

Acknowledgment

The authors would like to express their appreciation to David Fletcher for his insightful and helpful comments in the preparation of this manuscript.

References

Albrecht, R.R., and Feltz, D.L. (1987). Generality and specificity of attention related to competitive anxiety and sport performance. *Journal of Sport Psychology*, *9*, 231-248.

Alpert, R., and Haber, N.N. (1960). Anxiety in academic achievement situations. *Journal of Abnormal Social Psychology*, *61*, 207-215.

Apter, M.J. (1982). *The experience of emotion: The theory of psychological reversals.* London: Academic Press.

Bandura, A. (1982). Self-efficacy mechanism in human agency. *American Psychologist, 377,* 122-147.

Bandura, A. (1997). *Self-efficacy: The exercise of control.* New York: Freeman.

Biddle, S.J.H. (1997). Current tends in sport and exercise psychology research. *The Psychologist, 46,* 63-69.

Borkovec, T.D., Metzger, R.L., and Pruzinsky, T. (1986). Anxiety, worry and self. In L.M. Hartman and K.R. Blankenstein (Eds.), *Perception of self in emotional disorder and psychotherapy* (pp. 200-234). New York: Plenum.

Brawley, L.R., and Martin, K.A. (1995). The interface between social and sport psychology. *The Sport Psychologist, 9,* 469-497.

Brewer, B.W., Van-Raalte, J.L., Linder, D.E., and Van-Raalte, N.S. (1991). Peak performance and the perils of retrospective introspection. *Journal of Sport and Exercise Psychology, 13,* 227-238.

Burton, D. (1988). Do anxious swimmers swim slower? Re-examining the elusive anxiety-performance relationship. *Journal of Sport and Exercise Psychology, 10,* 45-61.

Burton, D. (1990). Multidimensional stress management in sport: Current status and future directions. In G. Jones and L. Hardy (Eds.), *Stress and performance in sport* (pp. 171-201). Chichester: Wiley.

Burton, D. (1998). Measuring competitive state anxiety. In J. Duda. (Ed.), *Advances in sport and exercise psychology measurement* (pp. 129-148). West Virginia: Fitness Information Technology.

Burton, D., and Naylor, S. (1997). Is anxiety really facilitating? *Journal of Applied Sport Psychology, 9,* 295-302.

Butt, J., Weinberg, R., and Horn, T. (2003). The intensity and directional interpretation of anxiety: Fluctuations throughout competition and relationship to performance. *The Sport Psychologist, 17,* 35-54.

Carrier, C., Higson, V., Klimoski, V., and Peterson, E. (1984). The effects of facilitative and debilitative achievement anxiety on note taking. *Journal of Education Research, 77,* 133-138.

Carver, C.S., and Scheier, M.F. (1986). Functional and dysfunctional responses to anxiety: The interaction between expectancies and self-focused attention. In R. Schwarzer (Ed.), *Self-related cognitions in anxiety and motivation* (pp. 111-141). Hillsdale, New Jersey: Erlbaum.

Carver, C.S., and Scheier, M.F. (1988). A control-process perspective on anxiety. *Anxiety Research, 1,* 17-22.

Carver, C.S., and Scheier, M.F. (1998). *On the self-regulation of behavior.* New York: Cambridge University Press.

Carver, C.S., and Scheier, M.F. (1999). Stress, coping, and self-regulatory processes. In L.A. Pervin and O.P. John (Eds.), *Handbook of personality: Theory and research (2nd ed.)* (pp. 553-575). New York: Guilford Press.

Cerin, E., Szabo, A., Hunt, N., and Williams, C. (2000). Temporal patterning of competitive emotions: A critical review. *Journal of Sports Sciences, 18,* 605-626.

Christianson, S.A. (1992). Emotional stress and eyewitness memory. *Psychological Bulletin, 112,* 284-309.

Clore, G.L., Ortorny, A., and Foss, M. (1987). The psychological foundations of the affective lexicon. *Journal of Personality and Social Psychology, 53,* 751-766.

Cohen, J. (1988). *Statistical power analysis for the behavioural sciences*. Hillsdale, New Jersey: Earlbaum.

Couch, J.V., Garber, T.B., and Turner, W.E. (1983). Facilitating and debilitating test anxiety and academic achievement. *The Psychological Record, 33*, 237-244.

Cronbach, L. (1951). Coefficient alpha and internal structure of tests. *Psychometrika, 16*, 297-234.

Diener, E., Smith, H., and Fujita, F. (1995). The personality structure of affect. *Journal of Personality and Social Psychology, 69*, 130-141.

Eklund, R.C. (1994). A season long investigation of competitive cognition in collegiate wrestlers. *Research Quarterly for Exercise and Sport, 65*, 169-183.

Ekman, P. (1994). Moods, emotions, and traits. In P. Ekman and R.J. Davidson (Eds.), *The nature of emotion: Fundamental research questions* (pp. 56-58). New York: Oxford University Press.

Eysenck, M.W. (1992). *Anxiety: The cognitive perspective*. London: Lawrence Erlbaum.

Eysenck, M.W., and Calvo, M.G. (1992). Anxiety and performance: The processing efficiency theory. *Cognition and Emotion, 6*, 409-434.

Feldman, A., Barret, F., and Russell, D. (1998). Independence and bipolarity in the structure of current affect. *Journal of Personality and Social Psychology, 74*, 967-984.

Fletcher, D., and Hanton, S. (2001). The relationship between psychological skills usage and competitive anxiety responses. *Psychology of Sport and Exercise, 2*, 89-101.

Gaeddert, W.P., and Dolphin, W.D. (1981). Effects of facilitating and debilitating anxiety on performance and study effort in mastery-based and traditional courses. *Psychological Reports, 48*, 827-833.

Gauvin, L., and Rejeski, W.J. (1993). The exercise feeling inventory: Development and initial validation. *Journal of Sport and Exercise Psychology, 15*, 403-423.

Gauvin, L., and Spence, J.C. (1998). Measurement of exercise induced changes in feeling states, affect, mood, and emotions. In J. Duda. (Ed.), *Advances in sport and exercise psychology measurement* (pp. 325-336). West Virginia: Fitness Information Technology.

Gould, D., Eklund, R.C., and Jackson, S.A. (1992). 1988 U.S. Olympic wrestling excellence: II Thoughts and affect occurring during competition, *The Sport Psychologist, 6*, 358-362.

Gould, D., Petlichkoff, L., Simons, J., and Vevera, M. (1987). Relationships between competitive state anxiety inventory-2 subscales scores and pistol shooting performance. *Journal of Sport Psychology, 9*, 33-42.

Gould, D., Petlichkoff, L., and Weinberg, R.S. (1984). Antecedents of temporal changes in and relationships between CSAI-2 components. *Journal of Sport Psychology, 6*, 289-304.

Gould, D., and Udry, E. (1994). Psychological skills for enhancing performance: Arousal regulation strategies. *Medicine and Science in Sports and Exercise, 26*, 478-485.

Green, P.G., Goldman, S.L., and Salovey, P. (1993). Measurement error masks bipolarity in affect ratings. *Journal of Personality and Social Psychology, 64*, 1029-1041.

Hahn, E. (1991). Emotions in sports. In D. Hackfort and C.A. Spielberger (Eds.). *Anxiety in sports: An international perspective* (pp. 153-162). New York: Hemisphere.

Hanin, Y.L. (1989). Interpersonal and intergroup anxiety in sports. In D. Hackfort and C.D. Spielberger (Eds.), *Anxiety in sports: An international perspective* (pp.19-28). New York: Hemisphere.

Hanin, Y.L. (1997). Emotions and athletic performance: Individual zones of optimal functioning model. In R. Seiler (Ed.) *European yearbook of sport psychology* (pp. 29-72). St. Augustin, Germany: Academia.

Hanin, Y.L. (2000). *Emotions in sport.* Champaign, IL: Human Kinetics.

Hanton, S., and Connaughton, D. (2002). Perceived control of anxiety and its relationship to self-confidence and performance: A qualitative inquiry. *Research Quarterly for Exercise and Sport, 73,* 87-97.

Hanton, S., Evans, L., and Neil, R. (2003). Hardiness and the competitive anxiety response. *Anxiety, Stress and Coping, 16,* 167-184.

Hanton, S., and Jones, G. (1997). Antecedents of intensity and direction dimensions of competitive anxiety as a function of skill. *Psychological Reports, 81,* 1139-1147.

Hanton, S., and Jones, G. (1999a). The acquisition and development of cognitive skills and strategies. I: Making the butterflies fly in formation. *The Sport Psychologist, 13,* 22-41.

Hanton, S., and Jones, G. (1999b). The effects of a multimodal intervention program on performers. II: Training the butterflies to fly in formation. *The Sport Psychologist, 13,* 22-41.

Hanton, S., Jones, G., and Mullen, R. (2000). Intensity and direction of competitive anxiety as interpreted by rugby players and rifle shooters. *Perceptual and Motor Skills, 90,* 513-521.

Hanton, S., Mellalieu, S.D., and Hall, R. (2002). Re-examining the competitive anxiety trait-state relationship. *Personality and Individual Differences, 33,* 1125-1136.

Hanton, S., Mellalieu, S.D., and Hall, R. (2004). Protection mechanisms: Self-confidence and anxiety interpretation: A qualitative investigation. *Psychology of Sport and Exercise, 5,* 379-521.

Hanton, S., Mellalieu, S.D., and Young, S. (2002). A qualitative investigation into the temporal patterning of the pre-competitive anxiety response. *Journal of Sports Sciences, 20,* 911-928.

Hanton, S., O'Brien, M., and Mellalieu, S.D. (2002). Individual differences, perceived control and competitive trait anxiety. *Journal of Sport Behavior, 26,* 39-56.

Hanton, S., Thomas, O., and Maynard, I. (2004). Time-to-event changes in the intensity, directional perceptions and frequency of intrusions of competitive anxiety. *Psychology of Sport and Exercise, 15,* 169-181.

Hardy, L. (1990). A catastrophe model of performance in sport. In G. Jones and L. Hardy (Eds.), *Stress and performance in sport* (pp. 81-106). Chichester, UK: Wiley.

Hardy, L. (1996). A test of catastrophe model of anxiety and sports performance against multidimensional anxiety theory models using the methods of dynamic differences. *Anxiety, Stress, and Coping, 9,* 69-86.

Hardy, L. (1997). The Coleman Roberts Griffiths address: Three myths about applied consultancy work. *Journal of Applied Sport Psychology, 9,* 277-294.

Hardy, L. (1998). Responses to reactants on three myths in applied consultancy work. *Journal of Applied Sport Psychology, 10,* 212-219.

Hardy, L., Jones, G., and Gould, D. (1996). *Understanding psychological preparation for sport: Theory and practice of elite performers.* Chichester, UK: Wiley.

Hardy, L., and Parfitt, G. (1991). A catastrophe model of anxiety and performance. *British Journal of Psychology, 82*, 163-178.

Harger, G.H., and Raglin, J.S. (1994). Correspondence between actual and recalled affect and pre competition anxiety in collegiate track and field athletes. *Journal of Sport and Exercise Psychology, 16*, 206-211.

Hudesman, J., and Weisner, E. (1978). Facilitating and debilitating test anxiety among college students and volunteers for desensitization workshops. *Journal of Clinical Psychology, 34*, 484-486.

Jones, G. (1990). A cognitive perspective on the processes underlying the relationship between stress and performance in sport. In G. Jones and L. Hardy (Eds.), *Stress and performance in sport* (pp. 171-201). Chichester, England: Wiley.

Jones, G. (1991). Recent issues in competitive state anxiety research. *The Psychologist, 4*, 152-155.

Jones, G. (1995). More than just a game: Research developments and issues in competitive state anxiety in sport. *British Journal of Psychology, 86*, 449-478.

Jones, G., and Cale, A. (1989). Relationships between multidimensional competitive state anxiety and motor subcomponents of performance. *Journal of Sports Sciences, 7*, 129-140.

Jones, G., and Hanton, S. (1996). Interpretation of anxiety symptoms and goal attainment expectations. *Journal of Sport and Exercise Psychology, 18*, 144-157.

Jones, G., and Hanton, S. (2001). Precompetitive feeling states and directional anxiety interpretations. *Journal of Sports Sciences, 19*, 385-395.

Jones, G., Hanton, S., and Swain, A.B.J. (1994). Intensity and interpretations of anxiety symptoms in elite and non-elite sports performers. *Personality and Individual Differences, 17*, 657-633.

Jones, G., and Ntoumanis, N. (1998). Interpretation of competitive trait anxiety symptoms as a function of self-control beliefs. *International Journal of Sport Psychology, 29*, 99-114.

Jones, G., and Swain, A.B.J. (1992). Intensity and direction dimensions of competitive state anxiety and relationships with competitiveness. *Perceptual and Motor Skills, 74*, 467-472.

Jones, G., and Swain, A.B.J. (1995). Predispositions to experience facilitating and debilitating anxiety in elite and non elite performers. *The Sport Psychologist, 9*, 201-211.

Jones, G., Swain, A.B.J., and Cale, A. (1990). Antecedents of multidimensional competitive state anxiety and self-confidence in elite inter collegiate middle-distance runners, *The Sport Psychologist, 4*, 107-118.

Jones, G., Swain, A.B.J., and Cale, A. (1991). Gender differences in precompetition temporal patterning and antecedents of anxiety and self-confidence. *Journal of Sport and Exercise Psychology, 13*, 1-15.

Jones, G., Swain, A.B.J., and Hardy, L. (1993). Intensity and direction dimensions of competitive state anxiety and relationships with performance. *Journal of Sports Sciences, 11*, 533-542.

Jones, G., Swain, A.B.J., and Harwood, C. (1996). Positive and negative affect as predictors of competitive anxiety. *Personality and Individual Differences, 20*, 109-114.

Jones, M.V., Mace, R.D., and Williams, S. (2000). Relationship between emotional state and performance during international field hockey matches. *Perceptual and Motor Skills, 90,* 691-701.

Kerr, J.H. (1997). *Motivation and emotion in sport.* East Sussex: Psychology Press.

Krane, V. (1994). The mental readiness form as a measure of competitive state anxiety. *The Sport Psychologist, 8,* 189-203.

Lane, A.M., Sewell, D.F., Terry, P.C., Bartram, D., and Nesti, M.S. (1999). Confirmatory factor analysis of the competitive state anxiety inventory-2. *Journal of Sports Sciences, 17,* 505-512.

Lane, A.M., and Terry, P.C. (2000). The nature of mood: Development of a conceptual model with a focus on depression. *Journal of Applied Sport Psychology, 12,* 16-33.

Lazarus, R. (1966). *Psychological stress and the coping process.* New York: McGraw-Hill.

Lazarus, R. (1991). *Emotion and adaptation.* New York: Oxford University Press.

Lazarus, R.S. (1999). *Stress and emotion: A new synthesis.* London: Free Association Books.

Lazarus, R. (2000). How emotions influence performance in competitive sports. *The Sport Psychologist, 14,* 229-252.

Mahoney, M.J., and Avener, M. (1977). Psychology of the elite athlete: An exploratory study. *Cognitive Therapy and Research, 1,* 135-141.

Martens, R., Burton, D., Vealey, R.S., Bump, L., and Smith, D.E. (1990). Development and validation of the Competitive State Anxiety Inventory-2 (CSAI-2). In R. Martens, R.S. Vealey, and D. Burton (Eds.), *Competitive anxiety in sport* (pp. 117-213). Champaign, IL: Human Kinetics.

Martens, R., Vealey, R.S., and Burton, D. (1990). *Competitive anxiety in sport.* Champaign, IL: Human Kinetics.

McAuley, E., and Courneya, K.S. (1994). The Subjective Exercise Experiences Scale (SEES): Development and preliminary validation. *Journal of Sport and Exercise Psychology, 16,* 163-177.

McNair, D.M., Lorr, M., and Dropleman, L.F. (1971). *Profile of Mood States Manual.* San Diego, CA: Educational and Industrial Testing Services.

Mellalieu, S.D. (2000). Identification and enhancement of preperformance mental states in elite rugby union players. *Unpublished Doctoral thesis.* Leicestershire, UK: Loughborough University.

Mellalieu, S.D. (2003). Mood matters, but how much? A response to Lane and Terry 2000. *Journal of Applied Sport Psychology, 15,* 99-114.

Mellalieu, S. D., Hanton, S., and Fletcher, D. (2006). A competitive anxiety review: Recent directions in sport psychology research. In S. Hanton and S. D. Mellalieu (Eds.), *Literature reviews in sport psychology* (pp. 1-45). Hauppage, NY: Nova Science.

Mellalieu, S.D., Hanton, S., and Jones, G. (2003). Emotional labeling and competitive anxiety in preparation and competition. *The Sport Psychologist, 17,* 157-174.

Morgan, W.P. (1980). The trait psychology controversy. *Research Quarterly for Exercise and Sport, 51,* 50-76.

Munz, D.C., Costello, C.T., and Korabek, K. (1975). A further test of the inverted-U relating achievement anxiety and academic test performance. *Journal of Psychology, 89,* 39-47.

Ntoumanis, N., and Jones, G. (1998). Interpretation of competitive trait anxiety symptoms as a function of self-control beliefs. *International Journal of Sport Psychology, 29*, 99-114.

Nunnally, J.C., and Burnstein, I.H. (1994). *Psychometric theory* (3ʳᵈ ed.). New York: McGraw-Hill.

Parfitt, C.G., and Hardy, L. (1987). Further evidence for the differential effect of competitive anxiety on a number of cognitive and motor sub-systems. *Journal of Sports Sciences, 5*, 517-524.

Parfitt, C.G., and Hardy, L. (1993). The effects of competitive anxiety on the memory span and rebound shooting tasks in basketball players. *Journal of Sports Sciences, 11*, 517-524.

Parfitt, C.G., Jones, G., and Hardy, L. (1990). Multidimensional anxiety and performance. In G. Jones and L. Hardy (Eds.), *Stress and performance in sport* (pp. 43-81). Chichester: Wiley.

Perry, J.D., and Williams, J.M. (1998). Relationship of intensity and direction of competitive trait anxiety to skill level and gender in tennis. *The Sport Psychologist, 12*, 169-179.

Prapavessis, H. (2000). The POMS and sport performance: A review. *Journal of Applied Sport Psychology, 12,* 34-38.

Prapavessis, H., and Grove, J.R. (1992). Preliminary evidence for the reliability and validity of an abbreviated profile of mood states. *International Journal of Sport Psychology, 23*, 93-109.

Prapavessis, H., and Grove, J.R. (1994). Personality variables as antecedents of precompetitive mood state temporal patterning. *International Journal of Sport Psychology, 22*, 347-365.

Rejeski, W.J., Best, D., Griffith, P., and Kenney, E. (1987). Sex-role orientation and the responses of men to exercise stress. *Research Quarterly for Exercise and Sport, 58*, 260-264.

Rich, A.R., and Woolever, D.K. (1988). Expectancy and self-focused attention: Experimental support for the self-regulation model of test anxiety. *Journal of Social and Clinical Psychology, 7,* 246-259.

Robazza, C., Bortoli, L., and Nougier, V. (1998). Performance-related emotions in skilled athletes: Hedonic tone and functional impact. *Perceptual and Motor Skills, 87,* 547-564.

Robazza, C., Bortoli, L., Nocini, F., Moser, G., and Arslan, C. (2000). Normative and idiosyncratic measures of positive and negative affect in sport. *Psychology of Sport and Exercise, 1,* 103-116.

Robazza, C., Bortoli, L., Zadro, I., and Nougier, V. (1998). Emotions in track and field athletes: A test of the individual zones of optimal functioning model. *European Yearbook of Sport Psychology, 2,* 94-123.

Rychta, T. (1982). Sport as a human personality development factor. In T. Orlick, J. Partington, and J. Salmela (Eds.), *Mental Training for coaches and athletes* (pp. 101-102). Coaching Association of Canada.

Silva, J.M., and Hardy, C.J. (1984). Precompetitive affect and athletic performance. In W.F. Straub, and J.M. Williams (Eds.), *Cognitive sport psychology* (pp. 79-88). Lansing, NY: Sport Science Associates.

Silva, J.M., and Hardy, C.J. (1986). Discriminating between contestants at the US Olympic marathon trials as a function of precompetitive affect. *International Journal of Sport Psychology, 17*, 100-109.

Smith, R.E., Smoll, F.L., and Weichman, S.A. (1998). Measurement of trait anxiety in sport. In J. Duda. (Ed.), *Advances in sport and exercise psychology measurement* (pp. 129-148). West Virginia: Fitness Information Technology.

Swain, A.B.J., and Jones, G. (1996). Explaining performance variance: The relative contributions of intensity and direction dimensions of competitive state anxiety. *Anxiety, Stress and Coping, 9*, 1-18.

Tabachnick, B.G., and Fidell, L.S. (1996). *Using multivariate statistics* (3rd ed.). New York: Harper Collins.

Tenenbaum, G., and Bar-Eli, M. (1995). Contemporary issues in exercise and sport psychology research. In S.J. Biddle (Ed.) *European perspectives in sport and exercise psychology* (pp. 290-323). Chichester: Wiley.

Terry, P. (1995). The efficacy of mood state profiling with elite performers: A review and synthesis. *The Sport Psychologist, 9*, 309-324.

Terry, P.C., and Lane, A.M. (2000). Normative values for the profile of mood states for use with athletic samples. *Journal of Applied Sport Psychology, 12,* 70-93.

Thayer, P. (1989). *Biophysiology of mood and arousal.* Oxford: Oxford University Press.

Thomas, O., Hanton, S. and Jones, G. (2002). An alternative approach to short-form self-report assessment of competitive anxiety: A research note. *International Journal of Sport Psychology, 33,* 325-336.

Thomas, O., Maynard, I., and Hanton, S. (2004). Temporal aspects of competitive anxiety and self-confidence as a function of anxiety perceptions. *The Sport Psychologist, 18,* 172-188.

Totterdell, P. (1999). Mood scores: Mood and performance in professional cricketers. *British Journal of Psychology, 90,* 317-332.

Totterdell, P., and Leach, D. (2001). Negative mood regulation expectancies and sports performance: An investigation involving professional cricketers. *Psychology of Sport and Exercise, 2,* 249-265.

Treasure, D.C., Monson, J., and Lox, C.L. (1996). Relationship between self-efficacy, wrestling performance, and affect prior to competition. *The Sport Psychologist, 10,* 73-83.

Vallerand, R.J. (1983). On emotion in sport: Theoretical and social perspectives. *Journal of Sport Psychology, 5,* 197-215.

Vallerand, R.J. (1984). Emotion in sport: Definitional, historical, and social psychological perspectives. In W.F. Straub and J.M. Williams (Eds.), *Cognitive Sport Psychology* (pp. 65-78). Lansing, NY: Sport Science Associates.

Vealey, R.S. (1986). Conceptualisation of sport confidence and competitive orientation: Preliminary investigation and instrument development. *Journal of Sport Psychology, 8,* 221-246.

Watson, D., and Clark, L.A. (1984). Negative affectivity: The disposition to experience aversive emotional states. *Psychological Bulletin, 96,* 219-235.

Watson, D., and Clark, L.A. (1994). *Manual for the Positive and Negative Affect Schedule (expanded form).* San Diego, CA: Educational and Industrial Testing Services.

Watson, D., and Clark, L.A. (1997). Measurement and mis-measurement of mood: Recurrent and emergent issues. *Journal of Personality Assessment, 68,* 267-296.

Watson, D., Clark, L.A., and Tellegen, A. (1988). Development and validation of brief measures of positive and negative affect: The PANAS scales. *Journal of Personality and Social Psychology, 54,* 1063-1070.

Watson, D., and McKee-Walker, L. (1996). The long term stability and predictive validity of trait measures of affect. *Journal of Personality and Social Psychology, 70,* 567-577.

Watson, D., and Tellegen, A. (1985). Toward a consensual structure of mood. *Psychological Bulletin, 98,* 219-235.

Wiggins, M.S. (1998). Anxiety intensity and direction: Preperformance temporal patterns and expectations in athletes. *Journal of Applied Sport Psychology, 10,* 201-211.

Woodman, T., and Hardy, L. (2001). Stress and anxiety. In R. Singer, H.A. Hausenblas, and C.M. Janelle (Eds.), *Handbook of research on sport psychology* (pp. 290-318). New York: Wiley.

Zuckerman, M., and Lubin, B. (1985). *Manual for the MAACL: The multiple affect adjective check list revised.* San Diego, CA: Educational and Industrial Testing Service.

In: Sport and Exercise Psychology Research Advances   ISBN: 978-1-60456-157-9
Editors: M. P. Simmons, L. A. Foster, pp. 85-109   © 2008 Nova Science Publishers, Inc.

Chapter III

Researching Social Goals in Sport and Exercise: Past, Present and Future

Justine B. Allen[4]
School of Physical Education, University of Otago, New Zealand

Abstract

The study of motivation has a long history in sport and exercise psychology research. Almost as long is the inclusion of social goals in relation to motivation (e.g., Ewing, 1981). Despite this inclusion of social goals, they have not received the same attention as other ability focused goals. In this article the 'past' and 'present' research that has included social goals in sport and exercise is reviewed. Drawing on this research, as well as related research from education and social psychology, a discussion of the possibilities to further develop this area of motivation research is presented. Review of the social goal research revealed the lack of a sustained systematic examination of social aspects of motivation, and specifically social goals. Furthermore, that this maybe due to a narrow focus of on just one social goal, social approval (e.g., Ewing, 1981; Whitehead, 1995). The social approval goal was conceptualised within achievement motivation theory (Maehr and Nicholls, 1980) as a universal view of success and was defined as aiming to maximize the probability of gaining others' approval. Despite attempts to operationalize and assess this social approval goal orientation questions remain regarding the measurement, consequences of holding a social approval orientation and its utility in furthering our understanding of motivation. Recently, however, a number of researchers in sport, education, and social psychology have begun to explore multiple social goals (e.g., Allen, 2003; Anderman, 1999; Ryan, Frederick, Rubio, and Sheldon, 1997; Stuntz and Weiss, 2003; Urdan and Maehr, 1995; Wentzel, 1999). An examination of this literature revealed a variety of conceptualizations of social goal constructs including what individuals are striving for and why individuals are striving. Therefore, despite this advance in social goal research, how social goals are conceptualised, assessed, and related to motivation remains unclear. Based on this review of past and present social

4 Contact information: Justine Allen,School of Physical Education.University of Otago, PO Box 56,Dunedin, New Zealand, Email: justine.allen@otago.ac.nz , Phone: +64 3 479 7746.

goal research, possibilities for future development of social goal research are discussed. The focus of this discussion is on developing conceptual clarity with regard to how many, what content, and what level of goals are necessary to adequately capture socially focused motivation, as well as the meaning of social goal pursuit.

Introduction

Initiating participation in sport or exercise for the first time, trying to make friends, co-operating with teammates, or giving up when faced with a challenge are all examples of motivated behavior. Of interest to sport and exercise psychology researchers is what drives individuals to behave in these ways. Social cognitive perspectives (e.g., Deci and Ryan, 1985; Dweck, 1999; Harter, 1978; Nicholls, 1989; Vallerand, 1997; Wigfield and Eccles,1992) have proved to be useful frameworks for explaining motivated behavior in several domains, including education and physical activity (see Eccles, Wigfield, Schiefele, 1998; Roberts, 2001 for reviews). Researchers have predominantly focused on achievement motivation frameworks in which the need for competence, academic or physical competence-related goals (i.e., task and ego goals), and perceptions of academic or physical competence are the central constructs for understanding individuals' thoughts, feelings, and actions in these domains (e.g., Duda and Whitehead, 1998; Dweck, 1999; Duda and Nicholls, 1992; Roberts, 2001). However, several researchers in sport and exercise psychology have suggested that approaches to motivation that focus solely on the goals of increasing one's ability or proving the adequacy of one's ability are limited (Allen, 2003; Hayashi, 1996; Stuntz and Weiss, 2003). Furthermore, the need for competence is not the only need, nor is the perception of competence the only perception, researchers have associated with cognition, affect, and motivated behavior in sport and exercise (e.g., Allen, 2006; Vallerand, 1997; Ingledew and Markland, 2007). This has led several of these researchers to examine social goals including social approval, social development, and social relationship goals, and social needs such as the needs for social competence, relatedness and belonging.

Research on sport participation motivation also indicates individuals have a variety of reasons for engaging in sport and exercise including social reasons. Social motives such as to be with friends or make new friends, to be part of a group or team, and gain approval from significant others are commonly reported reasons for sport participation (Weiss and Ferrer-Caja, 2002). Similarly, research examining exercise participants' motives reports social motives such as affiliation, being with others, and recognition as common reasons for their involvement in exercise (e.g., Duda and Tappe; 1989; Ingledew, Markland, and Medley, 1998; Markland and Hardy, 1993; Ryan, Frederick, Lepes, Rubio, and Sheldon, 1997). These motives reflect individuals' desires to engage in social activity in conjunction with physical activity participation. From this literature is it clear that individuals believe sport and exercise provide opportunities to pursue goals other than physical ability goals such as social goals. Despite recognition of social participation motives and more recent interest in social goals, the relative importance of social goals and the contribution they have for explaining and predicting motivation, cognitions, affect, and behavior in physical activities is not well understood. This paper explores the history of social motivation research, examines the current state of research on social goals and discusses the potential for future developments in this area.

Social Goals: A Brief History

Whether it is among team-mates, between opponents, with coaches, or workout partners many physical activities are social contexts. Interpersonal interactions are commonplace, they are often desired, and frequently inevitable occurrences within sport and yet relatively little is known about the implications for motivation and the quality of sport and exercise experience (Wylleman, 2000). Social goals are not new to motivation research, however, they have received only limited attention in sport and exercise psychology research. In this section, a brief examination of the history of motivation research provides two possible explanations for the paucity of research on social goals.

Social Motivation: A Neglected Area

Social motivation, the desire to develop and maintain social bonds or connections with others has a long history in theories of human motivation. It has been referred to as the need for affection between people (Murray, 1938), the need for positive regard from others (Rogers, 1951), belongingness (Maslow, 1954, Baumeister and Leary, 1995), affiliation motivation (McClelland, 1987), and the need for relatedness (Deci and Ryan, 1985, Ryan, 1993). Rogers suggested that in addition to individuals' propensity toward self-actualisation, individuals developed a need for positive regard from others. In contrast, Maslow proposed that although lower needs such as food and safety would be satisfied first, individuals' need to belong would need to be satisfied before other higher needs such as esteem (i.e., achievement), or self-actualisation could be met. Furthermore, in his discussion of competence motivation, White (1959) also alluded to a desire to interact effectively with others. His discussion focused on individuals' innate and learned desire to interact effectively with inanimate objects in the environment, however, he suggested that "It applies equally well ... to transactions with animals and with other human beings" (p. 327). Each of these theorists recognised the importance of the social world and an innate need to be part of and function effectively within it.

Although, an acknowledged aspect of motivation, social motivation has received less empirical attention compared with other aspects of motivation such as competence motivation. One possible explanation for this lack of attention comes from Bernard Weiner's (1996) reflection on the history of motivation research. He suggested that individuals' reactions to experimental manipulations of affiliation motivation have been avoided because the connection with others is so important to participants that the consequences of experimentation are potentially devastating to them. Weiner came to this conclusion after noting that motivation researchers focused on the study of achievement first because it lent itself to experimental manipulations and that an instrument to assess achievement motivation was the first to be developed (i.e., Thematic Apperception Test). In contrast, initial research investigating affiliation, where individuals were placed in socially evaluative situations in an attempt to arouse the affiliative motive, were so devastating to participants that researchers concluded that affiliation motivation did not lend itself to experimental investigation. Weiner suggested that this led researchers to think of achievement and affiliation "as very distinct motivations" and that "their interactions and interplay were not considered" (1996, p. xiv).

Weiner's (1996) interpretation of the events in motivation history helps to explain the relatively limited examination of social goals. It is not that competence is necessarily the most important motivational concept nor is it that social or affiliative motivation has no contribution to make to understanding human motivation. Rather, social motivation was neglected because competence was examined first and the development and maintenance of social bonds did not appear as straightforward to investigate. However, as Weiner (1996) suggests, the motivation to be and feel connected with others may be so important to individuals that it may be at the very core of a general theory of motivation.

Physical Competence: A Narrow Perspective

Another possible explanation for the limited empirical attention to social goals, which is more specific to sport and exercise psychology research, is related to an emphasis in the field on physical ability. Goal-related research in sport psychology, in particular, has been heavily influenced by the theorising of Maehr and Nicholls (Maehr and Nicholls, 1980; Maehr, 1984; Nicholls, 1984; 1989). Central to their achievement goal perspective is the emphasis on perceptions of ability and two ability-related goal orientations, task and ego (e.g., Duda and Whitehead, 1998; Roberts, 2001). Furthermore, Nicholls conceptualised achievement motivation in terms of "a desire to develop or demonstrate ability - to self or others - and avoid demonstrating low ability" (Nicholls, 1984, p. 328). Although Nicholls was referring to intellectual ability in the classroom, this conception of ability has been adopted by many sport psychology researchers to understand motivation in the physical domain, with the emphasis on physical ability. As a result, a substantial body of research exists examining correlates of task and ego goals orientations (see Duda and Whitehead, 1998; Duda and Hall; 2001; Roberts 2001 for reviews).

Taking the perspective that sport is a physical achievement context, and emphasising physical competence goals and physical perceptions is limiting. By adopting this narrow perspective researchers are assuming that all participants view sport as an opportunity to develop or demonstrate physical competence and that all participants value physical competence to the same extent. Although competence may be a concern some of the time, as Maehr (1984) argued with regard to achievement goals in school "other goals, other intentions, other attractions, continually intrude." (p. 116). Just as children may have different agendas for school, individuals may have concerns other than physical competence in sport and exercise. That is, the goals individuals have for involvement in physical activities may not always be related to demonstrating or developing physical ability. For example, an individual may engage in physical activities and feel successful when he or she gains approval from a parent, teacher, or coach. Equally, he or she may want to be part of a group for the inherent pleasure or enjoyment of the social interaction and feelings of connection with friends.

This brief history of social motivation research reveals that social aspects of motivation are fundamental to understanding motivation. They have, however, received less attention than other aspects of motivation perhaps due to difficulties in assessment and an overemphasis on physical competence. This has not stopped some researchers from continuing to explore social goals. In the next section the current status of social goal research is examined.

Social Goals in Sport and Exercise: The Research

Social goals have been identified in the sport and exercise motivation research. Examination of this research reveals two distinct directions for research. That is, research that examined motives for participation and research emphasising a goals focus. In this section the research in these two areas are described and discussed in turn.

Motives for Participation

With regard to research examining motives for participating in sport, consistent results have emerged. Affiliation motives such as wanting to make new friends, be with friends, experience team spirit, and be on a team are frequently reported as important reasons for participating in sport. Passer (1982) summarised the motives children gave for their sport participation, suggesting that six categories of motives existed. These general categories were: skill development; excitement; fitness; energy release; success and status; and affiliation. Both status and affiliation motives reflect social concerns with regard to participation. With only slight variations these six general categories have been supported by subsequent research (see Weiss and Ferrer-Caja, 2002 for a review). Drawing on personal investment theory (Maehr and Braskamp, 1986), Schilling and Hayshi (2001) examined the nature of the personal incentives of high school basketball and cross-country athletes. Task, ego, and social incentives were identified in both groups of athletes, however, social incentives were more salient for the team sport athletes. The social incentives were characterised by positive and negative feelings associated with teamwork, contributing to the team, social support and social approval.

Researchers examining the reasons participants report for withdrawal from sport also highlight social reasons. These reasons included a lower sense of belonging, feeling relatively excluded from the team, less encouragement or support from others for participation, dislike of the coach, parents or friends not wanting me to participate, not meeting new friends, no teamwork, and a desire to spend more time with friends (Gould and Petlichkoff, 1988; Brustad, 1993). Clearly, social aspects of motivation are salient to the participation and attrition processes in sport.

Social reasons for participation in exercise are also commonly reported. Duda and colleagues (Duda and Tappe, 1989; Tappe, Duda, and Menges-Ehrnwald, 1990) employed a personal investment theory framework (Maehr and Braskamp, 1986) to examine exercise behavior in adults and adolescents. In developing a measure of personal incentives for exercise contexts Duda and Tappe (1989) identified a number of diverse incentives including social incentives such as social recognition and affiliation. They found that middle-aged and older males reported engaging in exercise for social recognition reasons more than females of the same age groups. However, for younger adults, females emphasised social recognition more than males. Although not quite reaching significance there was a trend for females to report engaging in exercise for affiliation incentives more than males. In a similar study this time examining predictors of adolescents' exercise behavior, Tappe, et al. (1990) found different predictors of physical activity level for males and females. Incentives such as affiliation, flexibility, and mental benefits were associated with reported level of physical activity. Personal incentives were defined in line with Maehr and Braskamp (1986) as the motivational focus of an activity or the reasons why one engages in a particular activity. This operational definition and the assessment tool developed by Duda and Tappe (1989) provide a broad view of the reasons individuals engage in exercise. Assessed in this way incentives appear similar to motives for participation.

Adopting a self-determination theory (Deci and Ryan, 1985; 2002; Ryan and Deci, 2000) approach Frederick and Ryan (1993) examined the relationship between three motives for participation in physical activity and several indicators of mental well-being including self-esteem, depression, and anxiety. They did not include a social motive, however, in an extension of this study Ryan, et al. (1997) assessed five motives for participation in physical activity and examined the relationship between these motives and adherence, attendance, enjoyment, and challenge. The five motives assessed were competence, enjoyment, appearance, fitness/health, and social (e.g., to be with others in activity). In order to make predictions about the associations between motives and exercise adherence, the motives were classified a priori into either intrinsic motives such as those reasons reflecting qualities inherent in the activity (i.e., enjoyment and competence) and extrinsic motives such as those reflecting gaining something external to the activity itself (i.e., appearance, fitness/health, social). Results indicated that higher ratings of competence, enjoyment, and social motives were predictive of adherence to exercise.

Goals

Early inclusion of social goals in sport motivation research was framed with the theorising of Maehr and Nicholls (1980) and Nicholls (1989). In their theory of motivation, Maehr and Nicholls (1980) were one of the first to highlight the importance of a social goal orientation. They emphasised that in order to understand achievement motivation researchers need to understand the unique meaning of behavior to the individual in a given situation. This unique meaning is inseparably linked to the personal qualities individuals' value, the goals individuals adopt, and how success and failure are construed in the achievement context. Specifically, success and failure are viewed as "psychological states" that are a function of the extent to which the outcomes of goal striving are "perceived to reflect the presence or absence of desirable personal qualities" (p. 228).

Within their framework, they conceptualised goal orientations in terms of views about achievement success. They proposed that there are at least three views of achievement success or goal orientations that are universal across cultures. An ability-orientated motivation emphasised the goal or purpose of behavior being to maximise the probability of attributing high ability to oneself as well as avoiding tasks or situations where failure may imply low ability. A task-mastery-orientated motivation emphasised the goal of behavior being to complete a task, solve a problem, produce a product for its own sake rather than to demonstrate ability. A social approval-orientated motivation emphasised the goal of behavior being to gain approval from significant others and therefore, the behaviours exhibited would depend on what the individual believes is required to gain the desired approval (e.g., effort or ability).

Only limited research has attempted to identify Maehr and Nicholls' social approval universal view of achievement success (goal orientation) in sport (Ewing, 1981; Petlichkoff, 1993a; 1993b; Vealey and Campbell, 1988; Whitehead, 1992; 1995). Ewing (1981) developed the Achievement Orientation Questionnaire (AOQ) for this purpose. Exploratory factor analysis of data from the AOQ revealed three goals (ability, task, and social approval) and one additional factor labelled 'intrinsic' which represented feelings of adventure. Each factor had acceptable internal consistency (alpha coefficients .80 to .91) and the goal orientations discriminated between competitors, dropouts and non-participants in high school sports. Specifically, competitors (i.e., those who persisted longer) were more social approval-oriented and less intrinsic- and ability-oriented than dropouts. An explanation for this finding was that the sport environment provides many opportunities for social-approval oriented individuals to meet their goal with coaches, parents, and peers all providing opportunities to gain social approval. Also even if social approval oriented athletes are not regularly playing in matches their mere presence on the sideline demonstrates loyalty to the team or indicates status and either maybe a sufficient source of satisfaction to encourage them to persist (Roberts, 1984). In contrast, individuals who are ability-oriented want to demonstrate their ability and standing on the sidelines does not give them the opportunity to achieve this goal. Only participation presents the opportunity to demonstrate their ability. However, participation also provides the potential for individuals to expose a lack of ability which would indicate failure and may lead to lower persistence (Roberts, 1984). Roberts' explanation of how a social approval goal orientation is related to persistence in sport has never been empirically examined. Furthermore, what underpins a social approval orientation, why some individuals are more social approval oriented than others and the implications for motivation of adopting a social approval orientation remain unexplored.

Whitehead (1995) attempted to replicate and expand upon Ewing's (1981) findings with a sample of UK children and adolescents. She examined the factor structure of the AOQ and using separate exploratory factor analyses for children and for adolescents revealed four factors similar to those identified in Ewing's original work (i.e., ability, task, social approval, and intrinsic). Furthermore, as Ewing found, the achievement orientations discriminated between competitors, dropouts, and non-participants, although, the major discriminators were different to those found in Ewing's study. In a subsequent study, Whitehead (1992)[5] administered a longer version of the AOQ to 1,198 children aged 9 to 16 years. The modified version included new dimensions based on supplementary responses from the Whitehead (1995) study. Exploratory factor analyses of age and gender sub-groups yielded 13 to 16 factors, but Whitehead determined a six-factor solution was more meaningful. The six factors were considered as three pairs of factors, two pairs reflected mastery and ego orientations while the third reflected social orientations. This social orientation was labelled 'pleasing others' and comprised 'teamwork' and 'social approval' orientations that represented co-operating with others and achievement to gain others' approval. A modified questionnaire based on these six factors was administered to another sample and structural equation modelling techniques used to examine the factor structure of the scale. Confirmatory factor analysis for a six first-order-factor, three second-order-factor model demonstrated acceptable fit (GFI .94, RMSR .055). Vealey and Campbell (1988) also identified a social approval orientation in their research with adolescent figure skaters. These findings, along with those of Ewing, provide preliminary evidence for the existence of Maehr and Nicholls' social approval universal view of success in the physical domain and that it can contribute to explaining participation motivation.

Despite promising initial findings with the AOQ, concern has been expressed over the lack of consistency in research findings examining the psychometric properties of the AOQ, citing failure of subsequent studies to replicate Ewing's findings as a weakness (Weiss and Chaumeton, 1992). For example, Vealey and Campbell (1988) found only two goal orientations. The first was labelled extrinsic and was comprised of items reflecting a focus on gaining social approval by demonstrating ability to others. The second orientation was labelled task and was comprised of items reflecting personal goal attainment and gaining intrinsic satisfaction for accomplishment. Whitehead's research goes some way to address this issue, however, several questions remain regarding the conceptualisation of views of success and the measurement tools developed to assess these orientations. Specifically, in the first of Whitehead's studies, the low internal consistency of the factors, especially for younger children, suggested that the scale needed further refinement. Revisions were made in Whitehead's second study, however, it is not clear how or why the six factor solution was derived from the original 13 to 16 factor solutions. Furthermore, given the variety of solutions produced across gender and age groups the universal nature of these orientations could be questioned.

Maehr and Nicholls (1980) proposed that at least three universal views about success exist in achievement contexts. Researchers in the physical domain have focused on task and ability orientations. The research described above, however, confirms the existence of social, as well as ability, definitions of success in sporting and exercise contexts. Furthermore, it provides empirical evidence supporting the need to conceptualise and explore the role of social goals in motivation in sport and physical activity contexts.

Social views of success have also been identified in exercise research. Hayashi (1996) examined the achievement motivation of adult Anglo-American and Hawaiian exercise

---

5 The Whitehead (1992) study was conducted after the Whitehead (1995) study although it preceded it in publication.

participants. Results from this qualitative study indicated that exercise participants endorsed task, ego, and two socially focused goals which Hayashi termed interdependent perspectives on self and in-group pride and harmony. The interdependent self goal orientation was characterised by the development of positive relationships with others. Exercise participants felt successful when they felt part of the group, experienced camaraderie, and shared experiences with a workout partner. The in-group pride goal orientation was characterised by pride or pleasure gained from the recognition of others and helping others to achieve. Although Hayashi identified social views of success, neither of his social goals were social approval goals and this suggests that other social goals maybe important to exercise participants.

Researchers interested in social goals have identified social goals other than the social approval goal. Grounded within Dweck's (1992) social cognitive theory of motivation, Lewthwaite and Piparo's (1993) identified social acceptance (spend time with friends, be popular) and positive social experience (develop friendships, have fun with others) orientations in their research with gymnasts. Findings from their research suggest that social goals were second only to mastery goals in relative importance for the gymnasts. This finding is similar to that found for male soccer players (Lewthwaite, 1990).

In a study examining early adolescents' sportsmanship Stuntz and Weiss (2003) extended Maehr and Nicholls' (1980) concept of social approval goal orientation to describe three social goals that encompassed different types of social relationships. They proposed and assessed three relationship-focused ways of defining success: group acceptance oriented goal which emphasised gaining liking or approval of peers; friendship-oriented goal which emphasised having a close, supportive relationship with another individual; and coach-praise oriented goal which emphasised gaining approval of the coach. Furthermore, they suggested that these orientations represent extensions of how individuals can show competence. The three social goal orientations were assessed with 15 items which were added to a measure of achievement goals. Initial exploratory factor analysis revealed support for the three social goal factors and each demonstrated acceptable internal consistency. The relationship between these goal orientations and intention to act in an unsportsmanlike manner under a variety of conditions was examined. They found that for girls, when friends or the group did not condone unsportsmanlike play those who were coach-praise oriented were less likely to intend to commit unfair play. For boys, the friendship and group acceptance orientations were important in explaining the relationships among orientation, condition, and intention to act.

Another recent contribution to the social goals literature has been the conceptualisation of the social motivation model (Allen, 2003). This model drew from both achievement goal theory (Maehr and Nicholls, 1980; Nicholls, 1989) and self-determination theory (Deci and Ryan, 1985; 2002; Ryan and Deci, 2000) and defined two general types of social goals. These were a social affiliation orientation where success is construed in terms of developing and maintaining mutual relationships with others in the social context of sport; and a social validation orientation where the emphasis is on reaffirming one's sense of self through gaining social recognition and status from participation in sport. A measure of social motivational orientations in sport (SMOSS) was developed to assess these constructs. Preliminary exploratory research demonstrated that social goals and perceived belonging contributed to the prediction of interest in sport over above that explained by achievement goals and perceived physical ability (Allen, 2003). Further research has demonstrated support for the construct validity of the measurement scale (Allen, 2005). Recently, Sage and Kavussanu (2007) examined the relationships among achievement, social goals and moral behavior in youth soccer participants. They found that endorsement of the social affiliation goal positively predicted prosocial behavior, while endorsement of the social status goal positively predicted antisocial behavior. The social motivation model has also been employed to examine motivational profiles of middle-aged sport participants competing in a Masters Games event (Hodge, Allen, and Smellie, 2008). In this study, a goal profile approach was adopted to examine motivational correlates of both social and achievement goals of sport participants. A goal profile reflecting the endorsement of social goals was associated with the highest levels of enjoyment and perceived belonging, while a goal profile reflecting a focus on achievement goals was associated with the highest levels of intrinsic motivation, commitment and perceived ability.

Summary

Current research demonstrates that participants in sport and exercise endorse social reasons for their involvement. These reasons include to be with friends, make new friends, be part of a group, experience team spirit, gain support, recognition, approval and status. Participants also pursue social goals including approval, social interaction, status, camaraderie, acceptance, recognition, and relationships. Not only are social goals salient to sport and exercise participants they have demonstrated associations with persistence, interest, sportsmanship, enjoyment, and belonging. Despite the interest in social goals, much remains to be explored and clarified if our understanding of the importance and implications of social goal pursuit for the motivation process is to be developed. In the next section two issues central to future development of this area of research are discussed.

Social Goals: The Future?

To further our understanding of social goals in sport and exercise motivation there are at least two areas that warrant clarification. These are how social goals are conceptualised and the meaning of social goal pursuit. Developing a clear conceptual understanding of social goals will assist in addressing issues such as how many and what type of social goals are needed to capture the social focus of motivation; how to assess social goals; and what explanations and predictions can be made about the consequences of social goal pursuit. Research from educational and social psychology is used in conjunction with the research from sport and exercise to illustrate these issues and identify potential pathways for future research examining social goals.

Conceptual Clarity: Motives and Goals

Examination of the literature in sport and exercise psychology relating to social goals revealed that social reasons for participation are prominent in the physical domain and are salient to participants. They have been described as both motives and goals. A useful distinction to make is between motives, discrete goals, and goal orientations and is similar to the distinction that has been suggested for competence goals (Ryan, Sheldon, Kasser, and Deci, 1996; Hall and Kerr, 2001; Duda, 1997; 2001). Motives provide a description of desired outcomes of participation. Similarly, discrete goals focus on what the individual is trying to do. Both motives and discrete goals emphasise the content of the goal. They represent the direction of behavior. In contrast, goals construed as orientations or purposes of activity focus on why the individual is trying to do what they are doing, and how success and failure are defined. Research examining motives and discrete goals has tended to be descriptive and atheoretical, providing researchers with little basis from which to explain findings or predict consequences of pursuing social motives and goals. As a result it has not been well integrated with goal perspectives research and theoretical approaches to understanding motivation. In contrast, research exploring social goals, as goal orientations, have typically been framed in social cognitive theories. This has provided researchers with a theoretical basis for explanation and prediction. Both approaches have potential to contribute to furthering our understanding of social goals in motivation in sport and exercise.

Motives and Discrete Goals

A number of motives for engaging in physical activity, including social motives, have been identified (e.g., Brodkin and Weiss, 1990; Gill, Gross, and Huddleston, 1983, Longhurst and Spink, 1987; Frederick and Ryan, 1993; Ryan et al, 1997). Despite the proliferation of descriptive approaches to motives research, there are two notable exceptions. These are the work in exercise motivation of Frederick and colleagues (Frederick and Ryan, 1993; Ryan et al, 1997, Frederick-Recascino, 2002) and Markland, Ingledew and colleagues (Markland, Ingledew, Hardy, and Grant, 1992; Markland and Ingledew, 1997; Ingledew, Markland and Medley, 1998; Ingledew and Markland, 2007). Both groups of researchers have made links between exercise motives and self-determination theory (Deci and Ryan, 1985; Ryan and Deci , 2000). In doing so they have been able to explain and predict relationships between motives and outcomes such as adherence and well-being. These researchers typically classified motives as either extrinsic if they are typically engaged in as means to some other end or intrinsic if they are likely to satisfy basic psychological needs of competence, autonomy, and relatedness. A similar distinction has been made in research examining life goals (e.g., Kasser and Ryan, 1996). While some exercise motives have been easily classified there has been less agreement over how social motives should be classified.

Ryan et al (1997) classified the social motive as an extrinsic reason for engaging in physical activity. They suggested that engaging in physical activity to be with friends and meet new people is extrinsic, presumably because physical activity is seen as the means of gaining social interaction and that social interaction is considered separable from the activity.

No explanation for this classification was forwarded by the researchers. They went on to suggest that although social motivation was extrinsic it would be associated with the outcome variables such as exercise adherence in a manner similar competence and enjoyment, both of which were viewed as intrinsic motives. The theoretical reasoning for this was unclear. In a more recent discussion of this line of exercise motives research, Frederick-Recascino (2002) did not classify the social motive as either intrinsic or extrinsic but merely stated that it reflected the need for relatedness. In contrast in the research of Markland, Ingledew and colleagues, social recognition motives for exercise were classified as extrinsic (Markland and Ingledew, 1997; Markland et al, 1992) and affiliation motives were classified as intrinsic (Ingledew, Markland and Medley, 1998). Similarly with regard to life goals Kasser and Ryan (1996) classified affiliation and community involvement as intrinsic goals while social recognition and status were classified as extrinsic. Classifying motives as either intrinsic or extrinsic provided researchers with a conceptual basis from which theoretically based explanations and predictions could be made about the consequences of social motives and therefore is a useful step towards integrating motives and motivation theory.

Despite this initial step towards integration, it has been argued that making a priori classifications of motives is limiting (Carver and Baird, 1998; Ingledew and Markland, 2007). Making an assumption about motives, while reasonable, ignores how individuals construe the purpose of their goals. That is, why they aspire to certain ends may be as important as what that end is (Carver and Baird, 1998). Recently, Ingledew and Markland (2007) separated motives and regulatory processes in a general model of exercise participation. They aligned motives with goal content research that examines what individuals are seeking or avoiding in their participation. The behavioural regulation continuum from self-determination theory (Deci and Ryan, 1985; 2002; Ryan and Deci, 2000) was adopted to explain why exercise participants behave as they do. In a study of adult office workers' exercise motivation they found that participants' social engagement motive which was made up of affiliation, challenge, competition, and social recognition was positively related to intrinsic regulation. They argued that this finding supports the notion that social engagement fulfils the needs for competence, autonomy, and relatedness and is therefore intrinsic in nature. This research suggests that, rather than making an assumption about the regulatory processes underpinning motives, to accurately classify motives as either intrinsic or extrinsic the behavioural regulation processes also need to be assessed.

The research of Carver and Baird (1998) examining the behavioural regulation of life aspirations supports the importance of understanding the regulatory processes underpinning motives. They found that endorsing controlling reasons for community involvement were negatively related to self-actualisation while endorsement of identified-intrinsic reasons for community involvement were positively related to self-actualisation. Similar relationships were found for financial success aspiration. This study demonstrates that it is not only the content of the goal pursued that is important in determining outcomes but also whether it is pursued for self-determined or controlled reasons. Furthermore, this study highlights that social motives can be pursued for autonomous or controlled reasons. However, combining multiple social motives with other motives, as Ingledew and Markland (2007) did, does not allow for a detailed examination of the processes underpinning social motives. That is, not all social motives may be intrinsically regulated rather they may vary on a behavioural continuum. To further our understanding of the behavioural regulation of social motives it may be necessary to examine behavioural regulation processes associated with social motives such as affiliation and recognition separately.

Acknowledging that social motives can vary in self-determination and assessing the extent to which they are perceived as controlling and autonomous would enable researchers to describe, explain, and predict the outcomes of the pursuit of multiple social motives. For example, the desire for affiliation, to be with friends and to meet new people is only external to physical activity if one ignores the inherent social nature of most of these activities. Social interaction is as inherent in the majority of physical activities as challenge is and therefore a social motive is no less intrinsic than competence or challenge reasons for engaging in activities. Furthermore, Kasser and Ryan (1996) suggested that life goals that were self-actualising, growth seeking, and likely to satisfy inherent psychological needs are intrinsic. The need for relatedness is likely to be satisfied when socialising during physical activities and therefore behavioural regulation is likely to be self-determined. In contrast, social motives focused on gaining social approval, status, and recognition are likely to lead to more extrinsic behavioural regulations. That is, the person or people from whom recognition or approval is sought may exert some control over the individual's behavior (Urdan and Maehr, 1995). As Ryan and colleagues (1995) suggested "in adapting to the demands of the social world, individuals must at times engage in activities that are not interesting to them but are socially valued or mandated. A central motive that helps to initiate and maintain much of this nonintrinsically motivated action is the need for social connections. Put differently, people often engage in activities that do not interest them, in order to maintain or strengthen their connection with others." (Ryan, et al., 1995, p. 620). Therefore, exploring the behavioural regulation processes associated with different social motives may help to clarify the consequences of social participation motives.

Similar to motives, discrete goals are constructs that focus on what the individual is trying to do. That is, the goal is a discrete, specific objective such as winning a race, mastering a skill, or making friends. Although not as common in sport and exercise research social goals have been examined in education. For example, Wentzel (1989; 1991; 1993; 1996; 1999) has adopted this conception of goals in her research on motivation in the classroom. She has focused specifically on social goals and how they are related to motivation and performance in schools. In her research she has examined the content of students' goals, specifically, what individuals' are trying to achieve. In a study of 9th through 12th graders, Wentzel (1989) assessed how often students reported trying to achieve 12 goals and students' academic achievement. The goals assessed included both academic competence goals and social goals. Wentzel found that students reported trying to achieve social goals (i.e., to make friends, have fun, be dependable and responsible) more often than trying to achieve goals related to learning. In a similar study, this time of 6th and 7th graders, Wentzel (1991) assessed academic achievement, acceptance by peers and teachers and five types of goals including two social responsibility goals and one social interaction goal. Again she found that students reported trying to achieve social interaction goals more often than all other goals and the frequency with which participants reported trying to achieve social interaction goals did not differ as a function of academic achievement. Furthermore, these students reported attempting to achieve social responsibility goals and evaluation goals significantly more often than mastery goals. Wentzel (1993) found that in a group of 6th and 7th graders, students who scored highly on pursuit of both social responsibility and academic goals earned higher grades than students who scored high on pursuit of either type of goal or low on pursuit of both. This research indicates that individuals not only pursue social goals in achievement contexts, they frequently pursue multiple goals, they pursue social goals at least as frequently as academic competence goals, and effective co-ordination of both social and academic goals may enhance performance.

Wentzel's approach may prove useful for researchers in the physical domain. Her approach to the study of goals and motivation does not constrain researchers to the assumption, implicit in other approaches, that individuals desire academic success for task mastery or to prove their ability. Furthermore, it allows for the pursuit of multiple goals, including social goals, and provides a distinction between goals pursued for their own sake and reasons why students try to achieve academically. Parallels for these may be found in the physical domain. Certainly the participation motivation literature in sport and exercise indicates that participants frequently hold multiple motives for their involvement including multiple social motives (Weiss and Ferrera-Caja, 2002). Investigation of the motivational consequences of the pursuit of multiple goals is likely to raise additional questions such as how individuals co-ordinate the pursuit of multiple goals; and the motivational consequences of goal conflict.

Motives and discrete goals typically describe the outcome individuals are seeking when they engage in an activity. Despite the recognition of the importance of social motives to participants, this research does little to explain the mechanisms of action that connect motives to different cognitive, affective, and behavioural consequences. Perhaps the major limitation of these approaches is the same as that of other discrete goal theories of behavior and participation motives research (see Hall and Kerr, 2001; and Ryan, Sheldon, Kasser, and Deci, 1996). That is, theories that hold discrete goals as central lack explanation of the mechanisms underlying goal adoption. Although such theories "examine how one can efficaciously pursue goals, they typically ignore why one pursues particular goals and/or the significance of what specific goals are pursued" (Ryan et al, 1996, p. 7). Examining the extent to which motives (and perhaps discrete goals) are experienced as self-determined or controlling is one way in which motives for participation in physical activities can be theoretically related to motivational outcomes in the physical domain.

Goal Orientations

Much of the research examining social goals in sport and exercise have been grounded in social cognitive theories of motivation. In this research goals are viewed as providing a framework or worldview through which events are interpreted and responded to. Goals are conceptualised as relatively stable (across a variety of achievement situations) orientations that individuals bring with them to situations that are reflected in how success and failure are defined. This conceptualisation of social goals follows closely that of achievement goal orientations common in sport and exercise psychology research (Duda and Whitehead, 1998).

Despite a number of studies examining social goals, there is no consensus on how many social goals are needed to capture the social focus of motivation or how they should be assessed. Early research emphasised a single social approval goal orientation (e.g., Ewing, 1981; Whitehead, 1995). However, it has not always been clear what approval was for. Roberts (1984) suggested several ways in which approval might be gained including performance, loyalty to the team, and status. Whitehead (1992; 1995) emphasised achievement to gain approval. Vealey and Campbell (1988) focused on demonstrating ability to others to gain approval. The coach praise orientation of Stuntz and Weiss (2003) reflects an approval goal, however, what approval is for is not specified. Several measurement items suggest gaining approval for performance but others are more general. Maehr and Nicholls (1980) suggested that what approval was for would be determined by the significant others from whom approval was sought. While Urdan and Maehr (1995) suggested that both the target person and target behavior would influence the actual behavioural consequences of approval oriented individuals. Therefore, to better understand the motivational implications of the social approval goal, future research should explore the range of target people (e.g., peers, coaches, parents) and target behaviours (e.g., ability, effort, improvement, support for others, helping) for which participants might gain approval.

The social approval goal is not the only social goal identified in the research. Other researchers have identified or proposed multiple social goals. For example, Lewthwaite and Piparo (1993) described a social acceptance/affiliation goal and a positive social experience goal, Stuntz and Weiss (2003) proposed and assessed three relationship focused goals: coach praise, friendship, group acceptance. Allen (2003) included affiliation, social recognition, and social status goal orientations. Research in education has described at least 3 types of social goals (Anderman, 1999; Anderman and Anderman, 1999; Patrick et al, 1997; Ryan, Hicks, and Midgley, 1997). A social responsibility goal emphasised adherence to social rules and role expectations as the primary concern. An intimate peer relationship goal focused on forming and maintaining intimate social relationships with peers. A social status goal emphasised social visibility and prestige within the larger peer group and being part of the 'popular' group. Urdan and Maehr (1995) described four types of social goals relating to why students try to do well academically at school. These were trying to achieve academically to: gain or keep the approval others (social approval); raise the esteem or status of their in-group (social solidarity); be viewed as a good girl or boy (social compliance); and benefit the larger society by becoming a productive member (social welfare).

Despite the variety of social goals described in the research, they tend to fall into three broad categories: approval, affiliation, and prosocial goals (Allen, 2005b). The approval goal orientation emphasises recognition, status, pleasing others, and acceptance. The affiliation goal emphasises positive social experiences, solidarity, friendship, in-group-pride, and relationships. The prosocial orientation emphasises welfare, responsibility, helping, and contribution to others (Allen, 2005b). Research is needed to empirically test this categorisation of social goals and examine whether these three goals provide a meaningful contribution to our understanding of socially focused motivation. In doing so, it will be important to clarify the theoretical basis of these goals and the meaning of social goal pursuit to participants (see discussion in next section).

In addition to clarifying the focus of social goals it is important to recognise that all the goals described in the research here are approach focused goals. That is, they focus on the desired end state rather than the avoidance of undesired outcomes. Recently, Gable and colleagues (Gable, 2006; Elliot, Gable, Mapes, 2006; Strachman and Gable, 2006) proposed a model of general social goals in social psychology that emphasises approach *and* avoidance social goals. Although not developed in the physical domain, whether similar avoidance social goals are relevant to understanding sport and exercise motivation remains to be explored.

Establishing how many and what type of social goals will be useful, however, assessment tools may need to be developed or adapted to measure these social goals. As already discussed there has been concern over Ewing's (1981) AOQ developed to assess the social approval orientation. Whitehead's research goes some way to addressing this but further research is needed to demonstrate the reliability and validity of this measure. Furthermore, as researchers clarify the target people and behaviours relevant to the social approval orientation, these scales will need to be modified to reflect these newer conceptualisations of social approval. With regard to other social goals, several studies have been qualitative (e.g., Hayashi, 1996; Schilling and Hayashi, 2001) and although providing useful insight their small sample sizes limits the generalizability of findings to other populations. However, the themes developed in these studies may provide useful direction for subscale and item development. Other quantitative measures developed to assess social goal orientations have received only limited psychometric evaluation and have frequently been used on only one occasion. Some have employed exploratory factor analyses to establish subscales (Lewthwaite and Piparo, 1993; Stuntz and Weiss, 2003) and additional research is needed to provide further evidence of validity and reliability. Research employing the Social Motivational Orientations in Sport Scale (SMOSS) (Allen, 2003; 2005; Hodge, et al, 2008; Sage and Kavussanu, 2007) has demonstrated the scale's adequate factorial validity through confirmatory factor analysis as well as evidence of convergent, discriminant and predictive validity in adolescent and adult populations. This scale is, however, not without limitations and there is room for future development. For example, it does not include a prosocial goal and the recognition goal focuses on recognition for ability only. Recognition could be given for effort or improvement or other non-physically-based behaviours such as support for teammates. Therefore, modification of this scale is likely to be necessary if it is to adequately capture social goals in sport.

Another important issue related to social goal orientations and their measurement is related to the hypothesised relative stability of orientations. Although conceptualised at the orientation level there is limited evidence that all the social goals proposed and assessed reflect a relatively stable general disposition. For example, in education research, A. Ryan et al's (1997) conceptualisation of social goals emphasised the meaning assigned to *a given act* which suggests a situation-specific goal rather than a relatively stable orientation. In addition, with regard to the definition of the social responsibility goal Patrick et al, (1997), Anderman (1999), and Anderman and Anderman (1999) all employed Wentzel's (1991) conceptualisation of this goal. Wentzel focused on the *content* of goals viewing them as *what* the individual is trying to do not as a relatively stable general disposition or worldview through which events are interpreted and responded to. Furthermore, the psychometric properties of the instruments developed to assess these social goals have not been documented. At least one of the sub scales has exhibited questionable reliability and for this reason further research to validate these scales would be valuable. In sport and exercise research there are no published studies assessing the relative stability of social goal orientations. An unpublished study employing the SMOSS has demonstrated some support for the cross domain stability of the three social orientations contained within this scale (Allen, 2001). Future research should continue to clarify the level at which social goals are conceptualised and examine the general nature, including stability across domains, of social goal orientations.

Summary

The research to date on social goals provides a useful beginning to social motivation research, however, as a body of literature it demonstrates a lack of conceptual clarity with regard to nature of social goals. To move beyond describing social reasons for engaging in sport and exercise the integration with theory is critical. The work of Ingledew and Markland (2007) in exercise provides an avenue for conceptualising motives within self-determination theory (Deci and Ryan, 1985; 2002; Ryan and Deci, 2000). This could be expanded to examine social motives in sport participation. Social cognitive theories of motivation have also proven useful in providing explanations and predictions about social goal pursuit. However, questions remain regarding how many and what type of social goals adequately express the social focus on motivation in sport and exercise and whether goals are discrete objectives or relatively stable general dispositions. On their own participation motives and discrete goals are only partial theories of motivation in that they only describe what a person is striving for. In contrast, goal orientations explain why the behavior is important. Furthermore, much remains to be explored and demonstrated with regard to the psychometric properties of measurement tools developed to assess social goals. As Brewer (2000) indicated "validity is never the achievement of a single research project but the product of cumulative theory-testing and application." (p. 15).

Meaning of Social Goal Pursuit: Psychological Needs

In addition to clarifying how many and what type of social goals are necessary to adequately capture the social focus of motivation in sport and exercise, the meaning of social goal pursuit also warrants clarification. Researchers in sport and exercise psychology have described social motives, goals, and orientations. This work indicates the salience of social goals to individuals engaging in physical activities. However, an explanation of why social goals are salient and how they influence the motivation process is limited. The concept of psychological needs may provide insight and enable researchers to further integrate social goal research within motivation theory. Deci and Ryan (1985; 2002) proposed that three needs, autonomy, competence, and relatedness, were essential for and could parsimoniously account for psychological growth and development. As already discussed researchers examining exercise motives have suggested that motives can vary in self-determination and also that there is an association between social motives and the need for relatedness (Ingledew and Markland, 2007; Frederick-Recascino, 2002). However, the exact nature of these associations has received little attention. Furthermore, the relative importance of the need for relatedness, social motives, and perceived relatedness compared with the needs for competence and autonomy, their associated motives and perceptions has yet to be examined. This provides an avenue for future development of our understanding of the meaning of social motives.

In research examining social goals, a limiting factor appears to be a narrow focus on achievement goals and the underlying assumption that the meaning associated with these goals comes from the extent to which they satisfy the need for competence. Nicholls (1984) proposed that in achievement contexts individuals' primary concern was to develop or demonstrate ability and avoid demonstrating low ability. As a result, success and failure where physical ability is salient says something about one's physical competence which in turn may contribute to one's self-definition and sense of personal worth. As Maehr and Nicholls (1980) stated "people do not strive for goals because the goals are there, rather a goal is only there when reaching it implies something desirable about the person, such as that they are competent, courageous, or tenacious" (Maehr and Nicholls, 1980, p. 235). Therefore, the question can be raised as to whether the need for competence is the only relevant need. If the need for physical competence underpins and gives meaning to competence-based goals then could other needs such as relatedness give meaning to socially focused goals?

Achievement motivation theories (Dweck, 1999; Maehr and Nicholls, 1980; Nicholls, 1984; 1989) are perhaps the most commonly adopted theory for the examination of social goals in sport and exercise (e.g., Ewing, 1981; Hayashi, 1996; Lewthwaite and Piparo, 1993; Stuntz and Weiss, 2003; Whitehead, 1995). Researchers, however, have not explicitly described or explained the connection between social goals and competence. As has been discussed already the social approval goal orientation could be related to the achievement of physical competence. That is, approval can be gained through the development and/or demonstration of physical ability. However, it is not clear whether competence is seen to mediate or moderate the relationship between social goals and motivated behavior as has been proposed for physical achievement goals. Furthermore, it is not clear whether the development or demonstration of competence is even conceived as the energizer of social goal-directed behavior. Nor is it clear whether researchers are emphasising physical or social competence. Rather it appears that the goal concept from achievement motivation theories has been adopted without consideration for the other propositions of the theories. This also raises the question as to whether achievement goal theories are the most appropriate for examining social goals and understanding the antecedents and consequences social goal pursuit. In fact Nicholls, Cheung, Lauer, and Patashnick (1989) stated that "the nature of social goal orientations is a topic in its own right" (p. 70) and suggested that it had been poorly dealt with in the research.

In education, Dweck (Dweck, 1999; Dweck and Elliot, 1983; Dweck and Leggett, 1988) proposed two classes of goals could be used to describe the focus or concerns individuals had in achievement contexts. Specifically, performance goals are goals where the purpose of activity was to demonstrate ability or to document the adequacy of one's ability. The second class of goals was termed learning goals and represented the purpose of developing one's ability. Much of the research by Dweck and her colleagues has focused on academic competence goals (i.e., the development and demonstration of competence) as central to understanding achievement motivation in the classroom (see Dweck, 1999 for a review). Despite this focus on academic competence, however, there is also empirical support for aspects of Dweck's theory in the social domain. Specifically, when children focused on practicing and improving their social skills (i.e., a learning goal) they displayed a more adaptive, mastery-oriented response to rejection than when the focus was on evaluating their social skills (i.e., performance goal) (Erdley, Loomis, Dumas-Hines, and Dweck, 1997; Goetz and Dweck, 1980).

In an alternative approach, but one that still focused on competence as the energizer of motivated behavior, Klint and Weiss (1987) adopted Harter's (1978) competence motivation theory in their examination of the relationship between participation motives and perceptions of physical and social competence. They found that children high in perceived social competence were more motivated by affiliation aspects of sport compared with individuals lower in perceived social competence. A similar relationship was found between perceived physical competence and skill development motives. Despite demonstrating that different competencies may be related to different participation motives, specifically that social competence was associated with social motives, researchers in sport and exercise psychology have continued to emphasise physical competence (see Weiss and Ferrer-Caja, 2002 for a review). Whether, Dweck's or Harter's theories and social competence can provide further insight into socially focused motivation and consequences of social goal pursuit remains to be explored. However, the research of Klint and Weiss (1987) and Dweck and colleagues (Erdley, et al, 1997; Goetz and Dweck, 1980) suggests future research examining the connection between social goals and social competence rather than physical or academic competence may prove useful to further our understanding of the meaning and consequences of social goal pursuit.

In the model of social motivation Allen (2001; 2003) proposed that, rather than viewing competence as the energizer of behavior in social contexts such as sport and exercise, researchers consider a social need as the energizer. Drawing from theorists such as Baumeister and Leary (1995) and Deci and Ryan (1985; 2002; Ryan and Deci, 2000) it was proposed that the need for belonging gave meaning to the pursuit of social goals. That is, the fundamental psychological need to feel connected with others would stimulate goal-directed behavior designed to satisfy it (Baumeister and Leary, 1995). Individuals should show tendencies to seek out interpersonal contacts and cultivate relationships. Their thoughts should reflect a pervasive concern with forming and maintaining relationships. They should experience positive affect from forming and solidifying social bonds and negative affect when relationships are broken, threatened, or refused (Baumeister and Leary, 1995). Allen proposed that belonging not only provides the impetus for social behaviours but also provides the basis for two qualitatively different forms of motivation or motivational orientations: affiliation and validation. In several studies, perceived belonging and social goals have been associated with interest/enjoyment, and adaptive motivational profiles (Allen, 2003; 2006; Hodge, et al, 2008).

The concept of psychological needs provides a useful avenue for researchers to further explore and develop an understanding of the meaning and consequences of social goal pursuit. At least three directions show potential for future research. First, the integration of participation motives within self-determination theory. For example, researchers might examine the extent to which motives, particularly social motives, are experienced as autonomous or controlling and the related thoughts, feelings, and actions. Research along this line has begun with regard to exercise motivation, however, the types of social motives and their behavioural regulation warrant further investigation as does the connection between social motives and the need for relatedness. Sport participation motivation research could also be developed further by adopting a similar theoretical approach. Second, within achievement motivation approaches clarifying the target people and behaviours of the social approval orientation and the examination of the relationship between social goals and social competence rather than physical competence may assist in clarifying the meaning and consequences of social goal pursuit. Third, the social motivation model (Allen, 2003) provides testable propositions about the relationship between social goals, belonging, and motivational consequences. Future research within this framework would also be useful to further develop the model.

Conclusion

As long as there has been interest in motivation there has been acknowledgement of a social focus to motivation. Social motives, goals, and orientations for physical activity have been described by sport and exercise psychology researchers. Unfortunately, the research has been somewhat piecemeal and lacking clear conceptual frameworks. There are a number of avenues that show promise for future development of the social goal research. With greater attention to the theoretical basis of social goals prominent issues can be addressed. These include the number and content or focus of social goals needed to adequately represent socially focused motivation and the meaning and consequences of social goal pursuit.

References

Allen, J. B. (2001). *Social motivation in youth sport*. Unpublished PhD, DeMontfort University, Bedford, UK.

Allen, J. B. (2003). Social motivation in youth sport. *Journal of Sport and Exercise Psychology, 25*(4), 551-567.

Allen, J. B. (2005). Measuring social motivational orientations in sport: An examination of the construct validity of the SMOSS. *International Journal of Sport and Exercise Psychology, 3*(2), 147-162.

Allen, J. B. (2005b). *Pursuing social goals in sport and exercise: Beyond social approval.* Paper presented at the International Society for Sport Psychology Congress, Sydney, Australia, August 15 -19.

Allen, J. B. (2006). The perceived belonging in sport scale: Examining validity. *Psychology of Sport and Exercise, 7*, 387-405.

Anderman, L. H. (1999). Classroom goal orientation, school belonging and social goals as predictors of students' positive and negative affect following the transition to middle school. *Journal of Research and Development in Education, 32*(2), 89-103.

Anderman, L. H., and Anderman, E. M. (1999). Social predictors of changes in students' achievement goal orientations. *Contemporary Educational Psychology, 25*, 21-37.

Baumeister, R. F., and Leary, M. R. (1995). The need to belong: Desire for interpersonal attachments as a fundamental human motivation. *Psychological Bulletin, 117*(3), 497-529.

Brewer, M. B. (2000). Research design and issues of validity. In H. T. Reis and C. M. Judd (Eds.), *Handbook of research methods in social and personality psychology* (pp. 3-16). Cambridge: Cambridge University Press.

Brodkin, P., and Weiss, M. R. (1990). Developmental differences in motivation for participating in competitive swimming. *Journal of Sport and Exercise Psychology, 12*, 248-263.

Brustad, R. J. (1993). Youth in sport: Psychological considerations. In R. N. Singer, M. Murphey and L. K. Tennant (Eds.), *Handbook of research on sport psychology* (pp. 695-717). New York: Macmillan.

Carver, C. S., and Baird, E. (1998). The American dream revisited: Is it what you want or why you want it that matters? *Psychological Science, 9*(4), 289-292.

Deci, E., and Ryan, R. M. (2002). *Handbook of self-determination research*. Rochester, NY: University of Rochester Press.

Deci, E. L., and Ryan, R. M. (1985). *Intrinsic motivation and self-determination in human behavior*. New York: Plenum.

Duda, J., and Nicholls, J. (1992). Dimensions of achievement motivation in schoolwork and sport. *Journal of Educational Psychology, 84*(3), 290-299.

Duda, J., and Whitehead, J. (1998). Measurement of goal perspectives in the physical domain. In J. Duda (Ed.), *Advances in sport and exercise psychology measurement* (pp. 21-48). Morgantown: Fitness Information Technology.

Duda, J. L. (1997). Perpetuating myths: A response to Hardy's 1996 Coleman Griffith address. *Journal of Applied Sport Psychology, 9*(2), 303-309.

Duda, J. L. (2001). Achievement goal research in sport: Pushing the boundaries and clarifying some misunderstandings. In G. Roberts (Ed.), *Advances in motivation in sport and exercise* (pp. 129-182). Champaign, IL: Human Kinetics.

Duda, J. L., and Hall, H. K. (2001). Achievement goal theory in sport: Recent extensions and future directions. In R. Singer, C. Janelle and H. Hausenblas (Eds.), *Handbook of Research in Sport Psychology* (2nd ed., pp. 417-443). New York: John Wiley and Sons.

Duda, J. L., and Tappe, M. K. (1989). Personal investment in exercise among adults: The examination of age and gender-related differences in motivational orientation. In A. Ostrow (Ed.), *Motor behavior and aging* (pp. 239-256). Indianapolis: Benchmark.

Dweck, C., and Leggett, E. (1988). A social-cognitive approach to motivation and personality. *Psychological Review, 95*(2), 256-273.

Dweck, C. S. (1992). The study of goals in psychology. *Psychological Science, 3*(3), 165-167.

Dweck, C. S. (1999). *Self-theories: Their role in motivation, personality, and development.* Philadelphia, PA: Psychology Press.

Dweck, C. S., and Elliott, E. S. (1983). Achievement motivation. In P. Mussen (Ed.), *Handbook of child psychology* (Vol. 4, pp. 643-691). New York: Wiley.

Eccles, J. S., Wigfield, A., and Schiefele, U. (1998). Motivation to succeed. In W. Damon (Ed.), *Handbook of child psychology* (5 ed., Vol. 3, pp. 1017-1095). New York: John Wiley and Sons.

Elliot, A. J., Gable, S. L., and Mapes, R. R. (2006). Approach and avoidance motivation in the social domain. *Personality and Social Psychology Bulletin, 32*(3), 378-391.

Erdley, C., Cain, K., Loomis, C., Dumas-Hines, F., and Dweck, C. S. (1997). The relations among children's social goals, implicit personality theories and response to social failure. *Developmental psychology, 33*, 263-272.

Ewing, M. E. (1981). *Achievement orientations and sport behavior of males and females.* University of Illinois at Urbana-Champaign, Champaign, IL.

Frederick, C. M., and Ryan, R. M. (1993). Differences in motivation for sport and exercise and their relations with participation and mental health. *Journal of Sport Behavior, 16*, 124-146.

Frederick-Recascino, C. M. (2002). Self-determination theory and participation motivation research in the sport and exercise domain. In E. Deci and R. M. Ryan (Eds.), *Handbook of self-determination research* (pp. 277-296). Rochester, NY: University of Rochester.

Gable, S. L. (2006). Approach and avoidance social motives and goals. *Journal of Personality, 74*(1), 175-222.

Gill, D. L., Gross, J. B., and Huddleston, S. (1983). Participation motivation in youth sports. *International Journal of Sport Psychology, 14*, 1-14.

Goetz, T. E., and Dweck, C. S. (1980). Learned helplessness in social situations. *Journal of Personality and Social Psychology, 39*, 246-255.

Gould, D., and Petlichkoff, L. (1988). Psychological stress and the age-group wrestler. In E. W. Brown and C. F. Branta (Eds.), *Competitive sports for children and youth* (pp. 63-74). Champaign, IL: Human Kinetics.

Hall, H. K., and Kerr, A. W. (2001). Goal setting in sport and physical activity: Tracing empirical developments and establishing conceptual direction. In G. C. Roberts (Ed.), *Motivation in sport and exercise* (pp. 183-234). Champaign, IL: Human Kinetics.

Harter, S. (1978). Effectance motivation reconsidered: Toward a developmental model. *Human Development, 21*, 34-64.

Hayashi, C. T. (1996). Achievement motivation among Anglo-American and Hawaiian male physical activity participants: Individual differences and social contextual factors. *Journal of Sport and Exercise Psychology, 18*(2), 194-215.

Hodge, K., Allen, J. B., and Smellie, L. (2007). Motivation in masters sport: Achievement and social goals. *Psychology of Sport and Exercise*, 9, 157-176.

Ingledew, D. K., and Markland, D. (2007). The role of motives in exercise participation. *Psychology and Health*, 1-22.

Ingledew, D. K., Markland, D., and Medley, A. (1998). Exercise motives and stages of change. *Journal of Health Psychology., 3*, 477-489.

Kasser, T., and Ryan, R. M. (1996). Further examining the American dream: Differential correlates of intrinsic and extrinsic goals. *Personality and Social Psychology Bulletin, 22*(3), 280-287.

Klint, K. A., and Weiss, M. R. (1987). Perceived competence and motives for participating in youth sports: A test of Harter's competence motivation theory. *Journal of Sport Psychology, 9*, 55-65.

Lewthwaite, R. (1990). Threat perception in competitive trait anxiety: The endangerment of important goals. *Journal of Sport and Exercise Psychology, 12*, 280-300.

Lewthwaite, R., and Piparo, A. J. (1993). Goal orientations in young competitive athletes: Physical achievement, social-relational, and experiential concerns. *Journal of Research in Personality, 27*, 103-117.

Longhurst, K., and Spink, K. S. (1987). Participation motivation of Australian children involved in organized sport. *Canadian Journal of Applied Sport Sciences, 12*, 24-30.

Maehr, M. (1984). Meaning and motivation: Toward a theory of personal investment. In R. Ames and C. Ames (Eds.), *Research on motivation in education: Student motivation* (Vol. 1, pp. 115-207). Orlando, FL: Academic Press.

Maehr, M. L., and Braskamp, L. A. (1986). *The motivation factor: A theory of personal investment*. Lexington, MA: Lexington Books.

Maehr, M. L., and Nicholls, J. G. (1980). Culture and achievement motivation: A second look. In N. Warren (Ed.), *Studies in cross-cultural psychology, Vol. 3* (pp. 221-267). New York: Academic Press.

Markland, D., and Hardy, L. (1993). The Exercise Motivations Inventory: Preliminary development and validity of a measure of individuals' reasons for participation in regular physical exercise. *Personality and Individual Differences, 15*, 289-296.

Markland, D., and Ingledew, D. K. (1997). The measurement of exercise motives: Factorial validity and invariance across gender of a revised Exercise Motivations Inventory. *British Journal of Health Psychology, 2*, 361-376.

Markland, D., Ingledew, D. K., Hardy, L., and Grant, L. (1992). A comparison of the exercise motivations of aerobics participants and weight-watcher exercisers. *Journal of Sport Sciences, 10*, 60.

Maslow, A. (1954). *Motivation and personality*. New York: Harper and Row.

McClelland, D. C. (1987). *Human Motivation*. Cambridge, UK: Cambridge University.

Murray, H. A. (1938). *Explorations in personality: A clinical and experimental study of fifty men of college age*. New York: Oxford University.

Nicholls, J. G. (1984). Achievement motivation: Conceptions of ability, subjective experience, task choice, and performance. *Psychological Review, 91*, 328-346.

Nicholls, J. G. (1989). *The competitive ethos and democratic education*. Cambridge, MA: Harvard University Press.

Nicholls, J. G., Cheung, P. C., Lauer, J., and Patashnick, M. (1989). Individual differences in academic motivation: Perceived ability, goals, beliefs and values. *Learning and individual differences, 1*, 63-84.

Passer, M. W. (1982). Children in sport: Participation motives and psychological stress. *Quest, 33*, 231-244.

Patrick, H., Hicks, L., and Ryan, A. M. (1997). Relations of perceived social efficacy and social goal pursuit to self-efficacy for academic work. *Journal of Early Adolescence, 17*(2), 109-128.

Petlichkoff, L. M. (1993). Group differences on achievement goal orientations, perceived ability, and level of satisfaction during an athletic season. *Pediatric Exercise Science, 5*, 12-24.

Petlichkoff, L. M. (1993). Relationship of player status and time of season to achievement goals and perceived ability in interscholastic athletes. *Pediatric Exercise Science, 5*, 242-252.

Roberts, G. C. (1984). Toward a new theory of motivation in sport: The role of perceived ability. In J. M. Silva and R. S. Weinberg (Eds.), *Psychological foundations in sport* (pp. 214-228). Champaign, IL: Human Kinetics.

Roberts, G. C. (2001). Understanding the dynamics of motivation in physical activity: The influence of achievement goals on motivational processes. In G. C. Roberts (Ed.), *Advances in motivation in sport and exercise* (pp. 1-50). Champaign, IL: Human Kinetics.

Rogers, C. R. (1951). *Client-centered therapy: Its current practice, implications, and theory.* Boston: Houghton Mifflin.

Ryan, A. M., Hicks, L., and Midgley, C. (1997). Social goals, academic goals, and avoiding seeking help in the classroom. *Journal of Early Adolescence, 17*(2), 152-171.

Ryan, R., Frederick, C. M., D., L., Rubio, N., and Sheldon, K. M. (1997). Intrinsic motivation and exercise adherence. *International Journal of Sport Psychology, 28*, 335-354.

Ryan, R. M. (1993). Agency and organization: Intrinsic motivation, autonomy and the self in psychological development. In J. E. Jacobs (Ed.), *Nebraska symposium on motivation: Developmental perspectives on motivation* (Vol. 40, pp. 1-56). Lincoln, NE: University of Nebraska.

Ryan, R. M., and Deci, E. L. (2000). Self-determination theory and the facilitation of intrinsic motivation, social development, and well-being. *American Psychologist, 55*(1), 68-78.

Ryan, R. M., Sheldon, K. M., Kasser, T., and Deci, E. L. (1996). All goals are not created equal: An organismic perspective on the nature of goals and their regulation. In P. M. Gollwitzer and J. A. Bargh (Eds.), *The Psychology of Action: Linking cognition and motivation to behavior* (pp. 7-26). New York: The Guilford Press.

Sage, L., & Kavussanu, M. (2007). Multiple goal orientations as predictors of moral behaviour in youth soccer. *The Sport Psychologist, 21*(4), 417-437.

Schilling, T. A., and Hayashi, C. T. (2001). Achievement motivation among high school basketball and cross-country athletes: A personal investment perspective. *Journal of Applied Sport Psychology, 13*(1), 103-128.

Strachman, A., and Gable, S. L. (2006). What you want (and do not want) affects what you see (and do not see): Avoidance social goals and social events. *Personality and Social Psychology Bulletin, 32*(11), 1446-1458.

Stuntz, C. P., and Weiss, M. R. (2003). Influence of social goal orientations and peers on unsportsmanlike play. *Research Quarterly for Exercise and Sport, 74*(4), 421-435.

Tappe, M. K., Duda, J. L., and Menges-Ehrnwald, P. (1990). Personal investment predictors of adolescent motivational orientation toward exercise. *Canadian Journal of Sport Sciences, 15*(3), 185-192.

Urdan, T. C., and Maehr, M. L. (1995). Beyond a two-goal theory of motivation and achievement: A case for social goals. *Review of Educational Research, 65*(3), 213-243.

Vallerand, R. J. (1997). Toward a hierarchical model of intrinsic motivation. *Advances in Experimental Social Psychology, 29*, 271-360.

Vealey, R. S., and Campbell, J. L. (1988). Achievement goals of adolescent figure skaters: Impact on self-confidence, anxiety, and performance. *Journal of Adolescent Research, 3*(2), 227-243.

Weiner, B. (1996). Foreword. In J. Juvonen and K. R. Wentzel (Eds.), *Social motivation: Understanding children's school adjustment* (pp. xiii-xv). New York: Cambridge.

Weiss, M. R., and Chaumeton, N. (1992). Motivational orientations in sport. In T. S. Horn (Ed.), *Advances in sport psychology* (pp. 61-99). Champaign, IL: Human Kinetics.

Weiss, M. R., and Ferrer-Caja, E. (2002). Motivational orientations and sport behavior. In T. Horn (Ed.), *Advances in sport psychology* (pp. 101-184). Champaign, IL: Human Kinetics.

Wentzel, K. R. (1989). Adolescent classroom goals, standards of performance, and academic achievement: An interactionist perspective. *Journal of Educational Psychology, 81*, 131-142.

Wentzel, K. R. (1991). Social competence at school: The relation between social responsibility and academic achievement. *Review of Educational Research, 61*, 1-24.

Wentzel, K. R. (1993). Social and academic goals at school: Motivation and achievement in early adolescence. *Journal of early adolescence, 13*, 4-20.

Wentzel, K. R. (1996). Social goals and social relationships as motivators of school adjustment. In J. Juvonen and K. R. Wentzel (Eds.), *Social motivation: Understanding children's school adjustment* (pp. 226-247). New York: Cambridge.

Wentzel, K. R. (1999). Social-motivational processes and interpersonal relationships: Implications for understanding motivation at school. *Journal of Educational Psychology, 91*(1), 76-97.

White, R. (1959). Motivation reconsidered: The concept of competence. *Psychological Review,, 66*, 297-333.

Whitehead, J. (1992). Toward the assessment of multiple goal perspectives in children's sport. *Olympic Scientific Congress, Malaga, Spain, Abstracts, 2*, PSY14.

Whitehead, J. (1995). Multiple achievement orientations and participation in youth sport: A cultural and developmental perspective. *International Journal of Sport Psychology, 26*, 431-452.

Wigfield, A., and Eccles, J. S. (1992). The development of achievement task values: A theoretical analysis. *Developmental Review, 12*, 265-310.

Wylleman, P. (2000). Interpersonal relationships in sport: Uncharted territory in sport psychology research. *International Journal of Sport Psychology, 31*(4), 555-572.

In: Sport and Exercise Psychology Research Advances   ISBN: 978-1-60456-157-9
Editors: M. P. Simmons, L. A. Foster, pp. 111-133   © 2008 Nova Science Publishers, Inc.

Chapter IV

The Explicit Consequences of Error in Motor Learning

J.P. Maxwell[6] and R.S.W. Masters

Institute of Human Performance, University of Hong Kong, China

Abstract

There has been an ongoing debate in the motor learning literature regarding the role of performance error (Holding, 1970a, 1970b; Ohlsson, 1996; Prather, 1971; Singer, 1977). Some practices assume that errors promote learning (i.e., learning from mistakes; Schmidt, 1975) whereas others consider the elimination of error as necessary because repeated errors may interfere with correct performance (e.g., Kay, 1951; Von Wright, 1957; Wulf, Shea, and Whitacre, 1998). A second debate has revolved around considerations of the extent to which individuals' motor learning should be reliant upon processes that are explicit/declarative (readily verbalisable and attention demanding) or implicit/procedural (difficult to verbalise and minimally attention demanding; e.g., Masters and Maxwell, 2004; Willingham, 1998). In this chapter we review recent research, which suggests that errors in performance have important implications for the involvement of implicit and explicit processes in movement control, and discuss the implications for sports performance and rehabilitation.

Keywords: Implicit, Lifespan Development, Rehabilitation, Sport

---

6 Address all correspondence to: J.P. Maxwell Institute of Human Performance The University of Hong Kong, 111-113 Pokfulam Road, Hong Kong SAR, China, Email: maxwellj@hku.hk, Tel: +852 2589 0583, Fax: +852 2855 1712.

The Process of Acquiring Motor Skills

Motor skill is the ability to coordinate the action of muscles, attached to a variety of bones, and spanning various joints to produce a specialised movement that is finely tuned to accomplish a certain goal (Bernstein, 1967; Kelso, 1995; Newell, 1996; Schmidt and Lee, 2005; Thach, 1998). Motor learning is the process of acquiring motor skills. A movement error describes occasions when the motor skill fails to achieve the goal or purpose for which it was intended for reasons that are intrinsic (e.g., selection of incorrect movement parameters), rather than external (e.g., an unexpected perturbation), to the performer. Thus, motor learning can also be viewed as the process of reducing movement error. However, it should be noted that more than one pattern of movement can result in successful goal attainment; therefore, motor skill does not imply a single invariant movement pattern. Rather, a single motor skill is represented by a range of movements that are capable of achieving the same goal and can be modified to accommodate relatively minor changes in task conditions.

Without external intervention (e.g., instructions from a coach), new motor skills can be acquired through a process of trial-and-error[7] that is typically referred to as discovery learning. Discovery learning involves overcoming a movement problem by somehow generating an adequate motor response, often based on successful movements applied previously to similar problems, and then refining the movement based on feedback. In other words, the learner generates a hypothesis (e.g., "If I throw the stone harder it will be more likely to reach the target") and uses outcome feedback to evaluate its effectiveness (Frese and Altmann, 1989; Guadagnoli and Kohl, 2001; Masters and Maxwell, 2004). The testing of hypotheses generates a set of action rules that can then be used to inform current task performance and to generate modified responses to novel task variations (Gick and McGarry, 1992; Ohlsson, 1996; Schank, 1982). Discovery learning is normally a purposeful process, rather than incidental, because the learner intentionally acts in order to obtain a conscious goal and can often describe the techniques used to accomplish the task to other individuals (Hodges and Franks, 2002; Hodges and Lee, 1999; Raab et al., in press; Smeeton, Williams, Hodges, and Ward, 2005).

Discovery learning suffers from the availability of an almost unlimited number of possible movement combinations that could be adopted for the performance of a particular task compared with the relatively small number of effective movement combinations. Discovery learning is likely to be slow and inefficient, particularly for truly novel tasks. An alternative to discovery learning involves guiding the learner to the correct movement parameters.[8] The imposition of constraints on the learner's selection of appropriate movements is designed to reduce or even eliminate error (Schmidt, 1991; Wulf, et al., 1998). Guidance may take many forms that differ in the severity of the constraints imposed on the

---

[7] Discovery learning and trial-and-error are used interchangeably throughout this chapter, consistent with the original conception of the trial-and-error process as deterministic and intentional. More recent interpretations of trial-and-error have emphasized the role of randomness in the process to such an extent that even 'trial' generation may be stochastic rather than deterministic or intentional (Thorndike, 1898/2000).

[8] It is not implied here that all learning methods fall under the heading of either discovery or guidance, they are simply used as examples of the dominant methods employed to date. Learning from subliminally presented information, for example, may be an entirely unique process (Masters, Eves, & Maxwell, 2007).

learner. At one extreme, the learner may be physically constrained so that only correct actions can be performed (e.g., Lippman and Rees, 1997; Masters, MacMahon, and Pall, 2004). For example, a contraption might be designed that physically constrains the dynamics of a golfer's swing such that the optimal movement is produced. At the other extreme, verbal instructions may be provided that suggest the correct course of action (e.g., Hodges and Lee, 1999). The latter guidance technique is probably the most dominant within the sport coaching/motor learning context.

Implicit and Explicit Motor Learning

Masters and Maxwell (2004) argued that the acquisition of motor skills, and their subsequent performance, is subsumed by two cognitive processes, one explicit and the other implicit. According to Masters and Maxwell, explicit motor learning refers to increases in performance that are accompanied by an awareness of and ability to verbally communicate to others the intricate details of the movement dynamics underlying performance. The learning process is characterised by a hypothesis testing approach; the learner formulates a hypothesis about how to accomplish the task and then uses naturally occurring feedback to assess the validity of the hypothesis. Incorrect hypotheses are abandoned (eventually) and correct hypotheses are pursued further. This process leads to the development of a 'do and do not' list of instructions that can be applied to future performance and informs strategies for coping with novel task variations. Maxwell and Masters have argued that explicit motor learning places a heavy load on working memory resources (Baddeley, 1986; 1997; Baddeley and Logie, 1999). They also argue that the learner becomes reliant on the availability of working memory resources due to their habitual use during learning. Considerable evidence has been produced to support this contention (e.g., Maxwell, Masters, and Eves, 2003). Typically, explicit learners are asked to perform a primary motor skill whilst concurrently performing a secondary task that loads working memory (e.g., random letter generation; Baddeley, 1966). Performance of the primary motor skill typically deteriorates under these conditions, demonstrating reliance on the availability of working memory.

Implicit motor learning is the acquisition of a movement skill without the concomitant accrual of explicit or declarative knowledge. Whilst implicit learners are aware of the fact that they are learning, they are much less aware of the underlying processes or mechanisms that characterise improved performance. Importantly, the motor performance of implicit learners places a lower load on working memory or attentional resources and is less susceptible to disruption from secondary tasks (e.g. Liao and Masters, 2001; Maxwell, et al., 2003). That is, when performing a secondary task, such as random letter generation, performance of the primary motor skill is unaffected.

'Errorless' Learning

As part of an extensive research program, Masters, Maxwell, and colleagues have sought to develop learning protocols that maximise performance whilst concurrently limiting the accrual of explicit knowledge by minimising hypothesis testing behaviours. One method of maximising performance may be to guide the learner through the learning process, such that the probability of performing only correct movements is increased. This might be accomplished via the imposition of constraints on the learner's selection of appropriate actions so that error rates are reduced or eliminated (Schmidt, 1991; Wulf, et al., 1998). For example, a simple push button response may be cued in advance such that timing error is avoided (Prather, 1971) or the learner may be physically constrained so that only correct actions can be performed (e.g., Lippman and Rees, 1997; Masters, et al., 2004). In other words, the learner is "guided" to the correct movement solution for a particular task.

Whilst some researchers argue that errors impede the formation of the correct motor program and must be either 'unlearned' or 'washed out' by subsequent correct movements (e.g., Hebb, 1961; McClelland, Thomas, McCandliss, and Fiez, 1999) others argue that errors are beneficial for learning (i.e., learning from our mistakes; Ivancic and Hesketh, 1996; Neisser, 1976; Ohlsson, 1996). The former argument favours guided learning, whilst the latter favours discovery learning. Unfortunately, the empirical evidence is not as straightforward as the logical argument. Performance is generally higher following guided learning, when compared to discovery, partly because the learner has multiple experiences of executing the correct movement (e.g., Maxwell, Masters, Kerr, and Weedon, 2001). However, transfer to novel task variations is generally superior following discovery learning (e.g., Prather, 1971; Prather and Berry, 1970; Singer and Gaines, 1975; Singer and Pease, 1976).

In his review of the early evidence, Singer (1977) concluded that guided learning should be adopted when time efficiency and performance maximisation are crucial; conversely, when generalisability to novel task variations is crucial, discovery or trial-and-error learning should be the paradigm of choice. However, more recent experimental evidence (e.g., Wulf, et al., 1998) and reviews of guidance learning's use within special populations (e.g., Evans et al., 2000; Fillingham, Hodgson, Sage, and Lambon Ralph, 2003) indicate that additional factors need to be considered.

Wulf et al. (1998), for instance, pointed out that task complexity may be an important issue, with complex tasks more amenable to the positive effects of guidance. Wulf, et al. (1998) had participants learn to perform a ski-simulation task with or without physical guidance (with or without ski poles, respectively). They reported benefits of guided learning (where errors are reduced) for movement amplitude during learning but not when the task was performed under non-guided conditions. However, guided learners adopted a more efficient movement pattern than non-guided learners suggesting that physically guided practice was superior to non-guided practice for skill acquisition. Wulf, et al. proposed that guided practice allowed the performer to experience the target movement pattern at an earlier stage in learning than would normally be the case during non-guided practice. Their results also highlight the problem that discovery learning is unlikely to be efficient for complex tasks for which the correct movement is difficult to generate.

Depending on the constraints imposed and the motivation of the performer, guided learning may be incidental (or implicit), intentional (or explicit), or a complex mixture of the two. Prather (1971), for example, observed that participants in his cued response experiment tended to learn in a passive or incidental manner, suggesting a low level of intentionality that is consistent with implicit learning (Berry, 1997). Providing verbal instructions as guidance, on the other hand, is clearly explicit in nature and relies on the learner consciously and intentionally applying the rules to the task at hand.

The 'errorless' learning paradigm has been promoted as a method that maximises motor skill whilst reducing the build up of explicit knowledge (Maxwell, et al, 2001). Maxwell et al. (2001) and others (e.g. Winstein, Pohl, and Lethwaite, 1994) reasoned that guidance should reduce errors and promote learning without allowing the learner to become reliant on its presence. Maxwell et al. claimed that this could be achieved by gradually increasing the difficulty of task variations until the required difficulty level is reached. At each level of difficulty no extraneous constraints are imposed; therefore, learners must generate, initiate, and control their own movements. This simple process should reduce errors but, critically, maintain a certain amount of variability during the learning experience and leave the performer in control of skill execution. Thus, performance should be maximised without a concomitant loss in generalisability. Similar procedures, labelled adaptive training, used in previous research have produced mixed results (Cote, Williges, and Williges, 1981; Lintern and Gopher, 1978; Mané, Adams, and Donchin, 1989); however, adaptive training usually adopts a criterion performance level before increases in task difficulty are implemented. This may confound learning with amount of practice. Maxwell et al. implemented a fixed schedule of difficulty manipulations to avoid this potential problem.

In the Maxwell et al. (2001) study, novice golfers were assigned to one of three groups with differential practice schedules. The first group (Errorless) performed 400 learning trials from distances to the hole that were increased by 25cm after each 50 trials (i.e. first 50 from 25cm, second 50 from 50cm and so on until 200cm). The second group (Errorful) practiced from the same distances, but in reverse order. The final group (Random Errorful) practiced at each of the eight distances in a pseudorandom order. No physical constraints, verbal instructions, or augmented feedback were used; thus, learners were constrained only by the objective difficulty of the task at hand. During the learning phase, the Errorless group consistently outperformed the other two groups, which did not differ from each other. Following learning, all groups performed a 50 trial retention test at a distance of 200cm from the target and a 50 trial transfer test from 300cm. Again the Errorless group's performance was superior despite performance decrements at the longer distance. Maxwell et al.'s results suggest that the generation, selection, and execution of movement parameters by the learner may be crucial during guided learning.

In addition to the performance and novel distance transfer benefits associated with errorless (or guided) learning, Maxwell et al. (2001) suggested that the reduction of errors during learning would have further benefits related to the allocation of attentional resources, particularly the role of working memory (Baddeley, 1986). Working memory has been implicated in the identification, correction, and recall of performance errors (Baddeley and Wilson, 1994). As noted earlier, in a typical discovery learning situation, the learner formulates a hypothesis (in working memory) about the correct action to achieve a goal, assesses the outcome (again possibly involving working memory) and integrates this information with the original hypothesis to inform future attempts. Therefore, working memory is likely to be most active when errors are frequent and, eventually, the performer comes to rely on its availability (Masters and Maxwell, 2004; Maxwell, et al., 2003).

Working memory is a predominantly verbal system, therefore, learning that is accompanied by high levels of working memory involvement is likely to be explicit; but, when errors are infrequent, the participation of working memory is likely to be reduced or minimal and learning is more likely to be implicit.

To test their 'error-induced working memory dependence' argument, Maxwell et al. (2001) inserted a secondary task transfer test between their retention and novel distance tests. It was predicted that dependence on working memory for performance of the putting task would be demonstrated by performance breakdown when working memory was diverted to a secondary task, in this case counting tones. The use of secondary tasks to estimate working memory involvement in motor tasks is a well established technique (e.g., Abernethy, 1988; Li and Wright, 2000; MacMahon and Masters, 2002; Marsh and Geel, 2000; Maxwell et al., 2003; Wulf, McNevin and Shea, 2001). The putting performances of both the Errorful and Errorful Random groups deteriorated when working memory was occupied by the secondary tone counting task, suggesting that both groups relied on its availability to perform the primary task. The Errorless group was unaffected by the imposition of the secondary task load, suggesting that this group was less reliant on the availability of working memory resources for primary task performance. These results were interpreted as providing evidence that errorful learning is explicit whereas errorless learning is implicit.

However, verbal protocols revealed that all groups had accumulated a moderate amount of verbal knowledge about how to perform the putting task, suggesting working memory activity during learning. This result presented a potential paradox; one measure suggested working memory independence for the errorless group but another suggested dependence. Maxwell et al. noted that the performance of their errorless group was not completely error free. At longer distances, a large number of errors were made. Maxwell et al. speculated that verbal rules had been accumulated during these later trials, but that the initial period of errorless learning had somehow inoculated the learner against the negative influence of the later accumulation of explicit knowledge. A second experiment confirmed these speculations by providing evidence that the Errorless group tested fewer hypotheses about their movements and made fewer adjustments to their technique at the shorter distance.

Maxwell et al's second experiment also eliminated a possible confound in the first experiment (see also Poolton, Masters, and Maxwell, 2007). Errorless learners in the first experiment had recently experienced putting at the retention and transfer distances, but the other two groups had not. This recency effect may have accounted for test phase performance. In the second experiment, errorless and errorful groups converged on an intermediate distance that neither experienced during practice, thereby eliminating this problem. Errorless learners were unaffected by secondary task load relative to a control group who performed only the putting task, but the performance level of errorful learners once again dropped relative to controls, suggesting that transfer distance relative to final practice distance did not account for the effects seen in the test phase. Crucially, errorless learners also report fewer rules pertaining to their motor skill than did the errorful group. Errorful learners were also witnessed making more adjustments to their putting technique during the learning and transfer phases than did errorless learners, again suggesting the involvement of explicit, working memory processes in the former, but not the latter, group.

The results of Maxwell et al's (2001) experiments imply that only the initial trials of practice need be error-free and devoid of explicit knowledge for benefits associated with implicit learning (or low working memory involvement) to take effect. In a direct test of this implication, Poolton, Masters, and Maxwell (2005) had two groups of novice golfers follow Maxwell et al's errorless learning procedure. One group (Explicit) were provided with a set of six instructions about the movements required to putt successfully (e.g., "Place your right hand below your left when gripping the handle"); the other group (Implicit-Explicit) received the same instructions after they had completed the first 150 trials at the shortest distances from the hole (i.e. 25, 50, and 75cm). Following completion of the learning trials, all participants completed a three block (150 trials in total) test phase consisting of a secondary task transfer test sandwiched between two retention tests. It was predicted that the Explicit group's putting performance would deteriorate during the transfer test, but the performance of the Implicit-Explicit group would be unaffected. These predictions were supported by the performance data; however, the mechanism for this effect remains unclear. It is possible that the interaction of implicit and explicit processes is more efficient when implicit learning is experienced before the introduction of explicit knowledge.

Transfer to Novel Task Variations

Singer (1977) suggested that trial-and-error learning was superior to errorless learning when transfer to novel task variations is required. In addition, it has been claimed that implicit processes are poor for adapting to novel task constraints, the latter quality being better served by explicit processes (Beek, 2000). Maxwell et al. (2001) pointed out several flaws with previous research examining the effects of errorless learning on transfer. Typically, guidance is provided throughout the learning experience then removed for retention and transfer tests, critically altering task parameters (Ivens and Marteniuk, 1997) and leading to poorer performance. In the most extreme cases, the performer may not even be required to generate solutions to task problems during the learning experience because guidance constraints are so severe (e.g., Holding and Macrae, 1964; Prather, 1971). Maxwell et al. argued that the learner becomes reliant on the availability of guidance, such that when guidance is removed in transfer tests, performance drops significantly. A similar suggestion, ironically dubbed the guidance hypothesis, has been reported for the effects of augmented feedback on learning and subsequent performance (Schmidt, 1991; Schmidt, Young, Swinnen, and Shapiro, 1989; Swinnen, Schmidt, Nicholson, and Shapiro, 1990; Winstein, et al., 1994). Again, performance level drops when augmented feedback is removed. These results highlight the importance of requiring the learner to actively generate movements rather than passively conform to external constraints.

In their original errorless learning experiment, Maxwell et al., (2001) examined transfer to a novel performance distance (300cm) compared with performance during retention tests (200cm). Performance at the transfer distance was worse than at the retention distance for both errorless and errorful groups, but the errorless group maintained their performance superiority. Further evidence to suggest that implicit processes are capable of adapting to novel task variations was slow in arriving.

In a recent examination of the transfer issue, we conducted a direct test of the relative efficacy of errorless and errorful learning protocols (Maxwell and Masters, 2007a; Maxwell, Masters, and Lam, 2006a). We found that transfer to a sloped putting surface following practice on a flat surface was equivalent for errorless and errorful learners, but that errorless learners maintained an overall performance advantage. However, verbal protocols suggested that the errorless and errorful groups developed an equivalent amount of verbalisable knowledge, suggesting that both had learned explicitly. Thus, the requirement that transfer be supported by explicit knowledge could not be refuted.

In a follow-up experiment, probe reaction times were used to identify changes in attentional allocation (and by implication explicit processing) for errorless and errorful learners during practice and novel task (altered putter characteristics) transfer trials (Lam, Maxwell, and Masters, 2007; Maxwell, Masters, and Lam, 2006b; Poolton, Maxwell, Lam, and Masters, 2007). Again, transfer performance was identical for both groups. Prior to movement execution both groups had equivalent (slow) reaction times to auditory probes; however, reaction time was significantly quicker for the errorless group, relative to the errorful group, during movement execution. Lam et al. argued that both groups used explicit knowledge to plan their movements but that errorless learners relinquished online conscious control for movement execution. This argument fits neatly with Shiffrin and Schneider's (1977) contention that automatic processes can be initiated 'consciously', for example by an explicit decision (or plan) in working memory, then run to completion without further contributions from controlled processes. Thus, errorless learning may promote the automaticity of movement execution, but does not prevent the use of explicit knowledge during movement planning. It has yet to be demonstrated whether this interaction between explicit and implicit processes is optimal, but the evidence to date suggests that it may be.

Psychological and Physiological Stress

One of the first experimental investigations of implicit motor learning suggested that motor skills learnt implicitly might be less susceptible to the effects of psychological stress than are explicitly acquired motor skills (Masters, 1992). Masters argued that explicit learners would attempt to control their movements using explicit knowledge when placed under pressure. Crucially, Masters argued that implicit learners would be unable to utilise explicit knowledge because it would, as a consequence of learning implicitly, be unavailable. Further, Masters argued that attempting to control movements using explicit knowledge would prove ineffective as evidenced by a significant breakdown in performance under pressure. Masters' results supported these arguments, with implicit learners demonstrating continuing performance improvement under pressure (induced by expert evaluation and financial penalties for poor performance) and the explicit learners demonstrated a relative inability to cope with performance pressure. These results have since been independently replicated and extended (Hardy, Mullen, and Jones, 1996; Mullen, Hardy, and Oldham, 2007), adding support to the contention that implicitly learnt motor skills are resistant to the effects of psychological pressure.

In Masters' (1992) study and its subsequent replications (Hardy et al., 1996, Mullen, et al., 2007), implicit learning was induced by having learners perform a secondary random letter generation task (Baddeley, 1966) continuously and concurrently whilst practicing the primary motor task (golf putting). Whilst secondary tasks have been found to suppress the accumulation of explicit knowledge over at least 3000 trials (Maxwell, Masters, and Eves, 2000), they also suppress performance. Thus, the effects of psychological pressure on errorless (implicit) and errorful (explicit) learners was investigated because these protocols do not suffer from the negative effects of secondary tasks on practice performance (Maxwell and Masters, 2007b).

In a first experiment, novice golfers followed the standard 400 trial errorless and errorful learning protocols established by Maxwell et al. (2001). Following the learning phase and a short rest of 15 minutes, participants completed a test phase consisting of three blocks of 50 trials. The first and third blocks were performed at 200cm from the hole on a flat artificial grass surface and acted as retention tests. The second block acted as the stressed transfer test (stress test) and was performed at the same distance from the hole as the two retention tests. During the stress test, participants were evaluated by a single 'golf expert' and were informed that if their performance did not meet expectations they would lose part of the fee that they had been promised for participating in the experiment. Degree of anxiety was measured using the state portion of the State-Trait Anxiety Inventory (STAI; Speilberger, Gorsuch, and Lushene, 1970) and heart rate. It was predicted that the errorless group's performance would be unaffected by pressure during the stress test, but that the performance of the errorful group would deteriorate. Although both STAI score and heart rate increased (mean increase was approximately five points and ten beats per minute, respectively), neither group demonstrated breakdown under pressure; in fact, the performance of both groups increased significantly. It was concluded that the small increase in stress was more likely to have motivated participants to perform better, rather than causing performance breakdown. Typically, mild to moderate anxiety facilitates performance up to an individualized optimal level after which performance catastrophically declines as anxiety increases (e.g., Burton, 1988; Fazey and Hardy, 1988; Hardy and Parfitt, 1991; Hardy, Parfitt, and Pates, 1994; Yerkes and Dodson, 1908).

In order to examine the possibility that the mild increase in anxiety was responsible for the lack of performance decrement in the errorful (explicit) group, the experiment was repeated with the addition of a small group of evaluators during the stress test, rather than a single evaluator. The performance of the errorless group once again improved during the stress test; however, the performance of the errorful group did not, suggesting that the latter group's performance may have been adversely affected by the anxiety manipulation. In addition, the changes in STAI score and heart rate from baseline to stress test was approximately double that found in the first experiment; confirming the efficacy of the stress manipulation. It must be noted that previous studies examining the effects of anxiety on explicit and implicit learning have also failed to demonstrate performance breakdown in the explicit group, but have consistently demonstrated increased performance in the implicit groups (Hardy et al., 1996; Masters, 1992; Mullen, et al., 2007). If it is assumed that the stress manipulation increased motivation to succeed in both groups equally, then failure to improve performance can be viewed as evidence of the negative consequences of increased anxiety.

The mounting evidence seems to indicate that implicit learners may actually benefit from mild to moderate levels of psychological stress whilst performing. It is plausible that other types of stress might also enhance the performance of implicit learners relative to explicit learners. Poolton, Masters, et al. (2007) examined the effect of physiological fatigue on performance of a rugby passing task learnt under either errorless (implicit) or errorful (explicit) conditions. Physiological fatigue is generally associated with performance decrements (e.g., Davey, Thorpe, and Williams, 2002; McGregor, Nicholas, Lakomy and Williams, 1999; Sullivan and Hooper, 2005); however, it can be reasonably argued that participants in previous studies had acquired their movement skills explicitly (Poolton, Masters, et al. 2007); therefore, a differential response to physiological fatigue may be witnessed in implicit learners.

Poolton, Masters, et al. (2007) utilised errorless and errorful learning paradigms to encourage implicit or explicit motor learning, respectively. The motor skill acquired was a modified two-handed rugby passing task with performance measured as distance from the centre of a wall mounted target. Following a 100 trial practice phase, participants were tested over five blocks of 10 passes under various conditions. During the first and third test blocks (Retention 1 and Retention 2), participants performed the passing task over a distance of 350cm; the retention tests were used as baseline measures to judge the relative impact of manipulations in the remaining three transfer test blocks. During the second test block (Secondary Transfer) all participants performed ten passing trials whilst concurrently performing the random letter generation task. During the fourth and fifth test blocks, participants performed the passing task whilst physically fatigued (Fatigue Transfer). Physiological fatigue was induced using a double Wingate protocol (Inbar, Bar-Or, and Skinner, 1996) immediately prior to commencement of the final two blocks.

Results of the Secondary Transfer test replicated previous findings; the performance of the errorful group deteriorated whereas the performance of the errorless group was unaffected. These results were replicated during the fatigue Transfer test; again, the errorful group's performance worsened but the errorless group's performance was unchanged. These results reinforce the notion that errorless learning produces motor skills that are less reliant on working memory resources, consistent with previous research (e.g., Maxwell et al., 2001), and extend previous work by demonstrating that errorless learning also promotes resistance to physiological fatigue. A replication of the Poolton, Masters, et al., (2007) study, using a more aerobic physiological stressor (running VO_2 max test), produced identical results (Masters, Poolton, and Maxwell, in press), reinforcing the evidence that suggests that motor skills acquired implicitly are resistant to both psychological and physiological stress.

Errorless Learning in Young Children

All of the experiments discussed thus far used adult participants who would have brought a considerable amount of 'movement experience' to the lab. The utility of the errorless learning paradigm when adapted for other healthy populations has received much less attention. It is possible that individuals with underdeveloped cognitive resources (e.g., young children) may particularly benefit from learning paradigms that reduce the committal of errors and, as a consequence, reduce the cognitive demands of learning movement skills. It is also likely that errorless learning will be most beneficial for individuals with poor natural coordination, because it limits the initial difficulty of the task and is likely to enhance self-efficacy through the experience of success (Bandura, 1977).

To test these possibilities, we asked young children (aged 9-12) to learn a golf putting task via our errorless or errorful procedures (Maxwell, Masters, and Hammond, 2007). Prior to learning the putting skill, 261 children were categorised as either low or high motor ability based on their performance of a battery of four fundamental movement skills (running, balancing on one leg, hopping, and bouncing a ball; *adapted from* Larkin and Revie, 1994) and their score on the Fundamental Movement Skills Rating scale (Revie and Larkin, 1993). Children scoring in the top 20% were labelled "high ability" and children scoring in the bottom 20% were labelled "low ability". Of those eligible for participation, 45 subsequently completed the golf-putting experiment.

Children were assigned, pseudo-randomly, to one of four groups: Errorless High Ability, Errorless Low Ability, Errorful High Ability, and Errorful Low Ability. All participants completed 300 practice trials at six distances ranging from 25cm to 150cm from the hole. Order of practice for the errorless and errorful conditions was consistent with previous studies. Following the practice phase, all children performed three blocks of 50 trials from 150cm. During the first and third blocks (Retention 1 and Retention 2), only the putting task was performed; during the second block, the children also performed a secondary tone counting task (Secondary Transfer). The tone counting task required the children to monitor a random sequence of high and low pitched tones and, following completion of the transfer test, report the number of high pitched tones they had heard. Following the test phase, all children completed the traditional verbal protocol.

It was predicted that performance during the secondary task transfer test, relative to baseline performance in the two retention tests, would be a function of ability and learning condition. We also expected differences between high and low ability groups in the errorful condition, but not the errorless condition. The results were largely consistent with this prediction. Errorless learners, regardless of ability, were unaffected by the imposition of a secondary task load. Errorful learners of high ability were also unaffected by the secondary task; however, the performance of low ability errorful learners deteriorated significantly under secondary task load. Although there was an overall effect of ability favouring the high ability group, post-hoc tests found significant performance differences between the errorful high and low ability groups only during the secondary task transfer test. In addition, the errorless groups reported significantly fewer task relevant rules than the errorful groups, supporting the contention that errorless learning is largely implicit.

The pattern of results suggests that by initially reducing the difficulty of a task and then gradually increasing its difficulty to normal levels, children who are naturally low in ability will perform at a standard that is equivalent to that of high ability children, even when required to perform two tasks simultaneously. The results also suggest that the mechanism underlying this effect is a lowering of attentional demands from movement control. In other words, errorless learners acquire their skills implicitly with less contribution from explicit working memory resources. Promoting error early in learning has a negative effect for low ability children, particularly when required to perform a secondary task. The fact that high ability children in the errorful condition seemed to improve slightly under secondary task load suggests that they may have more working memory resources available to devote to task performance (i.e., higher capacity). This suggestion is speculative and requires validation; however, the positive correlation found between academic, particularly reading, and motor abilities in youg children (e.g., Kaplan, Wilson, Dewey, & Crawford, 1998; Smits-Engelsman, Wilson, Westenberg, & Duysens, 2003; Sugden & Wann, 1987; Waber et al., 2000) would tend to support the idea.

Errorless Learning in Healthy Older Adults

The functional ability of working memory to control actions declines with age (Park, O'Connell, and Thomson, 2003; West, 1996) leading to, among other things, forgetfulness, a reduced ability to acquire new information, and difficulty with processing multiple sources of information simultaneously. There is also a notable decrease in motor functioning with increased age (Seidler and Stelmach, 1995; Tunney et al., 2003), with the critical age of deficit onset, for both cognitive and motor skills, estimated at about 60 years (Smith et al., 1999). However, research suggests that slowing of cognitive processes may be responsible for the majority of deficits in movement control and learning (e.g., Chaput and Proteau, 1996; Contreras-Vidal, Teulings, and Stelmach, 1998).

Despite decreasing working memory ability, when faced with uncertainty or low confidence, as is typical of older adults engaging in fine motor tasks, there is a paradoxical tendency to assume explicit control over movements (Heuninckx, Wenderoth, Debaere, Peeters, and Swinnen, 2005). The idea of increased reliance on explicit processes with increasing age has received support from neuroimaging studies that show increased utilization of prefrontal areas by the elderly during externally- and self-paced motor control and learning tasks (Heuninckx, et al., 2005; Mattay et al., 2002; Ward and Frachowiak, 2003). Using a hand-foot coordination task Heuninckx et al., found activity of the superior frontal gyrus and precentral gyrus, areas that are more closely related to cognitive than motor processes. However, it must be noted that the motor tasks used in these experiments were extremely simple (e.g. tapping hands and feet alternately) and cannot be easily generalized to more complex tasks.

Whilst working memory based explicit learning seems to be impaired in older age, learning that is not based on the availability of working memory (i.e., as in our conception of implicit motor learning) appears to be intact (see Howard, 1988; Reber, 1993; Toates, 2006). Assuming these assertions are true, it would follow that errorless (implicit) motor learning in older adults should be superior to errorful (explicit) motor learning and that the disparity between the two methods should increase as working memory declines with increasing age. To test this possibility, Chauvel, Maquestiaux, Joubert, Benguigui, and Bertsch (2007) had young and healthy older adults (mean age 23.59 and 65.00 years, respectively) learn a golf putting task under errorless or errorful conditions in a protocol that was similar to Maxwell et al's (2001) Experiment 2. Errorless learners practiced for 160 trials at distances that were close to the hole (25cm, 50cm, 75cm, and 100cm) and then transferred to a distance of 125cm for a transfer test. The errorful group practiced at longer distances (225cm, 200cm, 175cm, and 150cm) before also completing a transfer test (125cm). During the transfer test, half the participants performed only the primary putting task, whereas, the remaining participants performed the putting task and a secondary tone counting task concurrently.

Working memory ability in younger adults was significantly better than the older adults on a digit-number sequence test (mean = 12.56 and 9.22 for young and older adults, respectively). During learning, errorless learners made significantly fewer errors than errorful learners, as expected from the unique practice protocols. Crucially, for the errorless learning condition, no differences were found between young and older adults for number of errors made, but significant differences were found between the two age groups in the errorful condition. Older adults made significantly more errors during learning suggesting that their poorer working memory was in some way disruptive to performance. The results of the transfer test showed that the putting performance of the errorless group was unaffected by the imposition of a secondary task load. No age difference was observed in this condition. The motor performance of the errorful group, however, was impaired by the imposition of a secondary cognitive task. This impairment was more pronounced in older adults than in younger adults, supporting the idea that errorful learning had promoted a reliance on the availability of working memory resources. The secondary task probably placed identical limitations on the young and older adults, but consumed a larger relative proportion in the older adults leaving them with fewer resources to complete the primary putting task.

Chauvel et al's (2007) results support the idea that implicit motor learning is less affected by the cognitive deterioration associated with aging than is explicit motor learning. They also suggest that the errorless learning technique may be useful in the rehabilitation of elderly adults who may have to learn new skills or relearn old ones, perhaps following a fall or a stroke. As we age, from infancy to death, we are constantly relearning and re-calibrating our movement control systems as body proportions and muscular capabilities change. Normally, compensatory adjustments are made gradually and we are largely unaware of them (growth spurts in adolescence are perhaps the most obvious example of rapid changes causing clumsiness of which we may be very aware). Because the 60+ individual is starting to experience rapid changes in multiple capabilities, healthy ageing means re-adjusting and re-learning old tasks. The individual who knocks over objects or falls may often be the one who attempts a task in the same way that they did when younger, without re-adjustment to their new capabilities (cognitive and motor). Using a walking stick or manipulating objects with an arthritic hand are new skills that must be (re)mastered. It is important, therefore, to analyse how effectively older adults cope with these changes and determine conditions that optimise adaptation; errorless learning may be a technique that fulfils this function. If more golf instructors adopted the errorless method might we see more silver swingers on the golf course? Throw into this recipe the increased health benefits of regular exercise and the implications begin to broaden.

Errorless Learning and Neuropsychological Impairment

The success of errorless learning for motor skill acquisition by healthy adults and young children suggests that it may also be useful for individuals who are movement impaired. For example, it may be appropriate to rehabilitate patients recovering from stroke using techniques that reduce errors and, for example, risk of injury, rather than techniques that promote error. Within the cognitive domain, errorless learning techniques have proved extremely successful for the promotion of learning in memory disordered patients (for reviews of errorless learning in the treatment of various neurological disorders see Evans, Levine, and Bateman, 2004; Fillingham, et al., 2003; Fillingham, Sage, and Lambon Ralph, 2006); however, there is a scarcity of work examining errorless motor learning in movement disordered patients.

In one of the few studies using motor skills, Masters et al. (2003) used a guided hammering task to examine the effects of errors during learning on the subsequent performance of Parkinson patients under single and dual task conditions. During a 120 trial learning phase, errorless learners performed a hammering task that was physically constrained by a manipulandum whereas errorful learners performed the hammering task without constraint. Whilst no differences were found during single task (hammering alone) retention tests, the errorless learners were significantly better than the errorful group during dual task transfer trials (hammering and counting backwards). In addition, patients in the errorless condition were able to verbally report significantly more task relevant knowledge that the errorless group. Masters et al interpreted these results as evidence for implicit learning in the errorless group (i.e., working memory independence and poor conscious access to knowledge). They argued that implicit learning techniques should be adopted during rehabilitation because everyday tasks often require attention to, and integration of multiple sources of information in working memory.

The Masters et al's (2003) study suffered from a number of limitations that require further study. Firstly, as the authors noted, there was minimal evidence of learning in the errorless or errorful groups; whilst accuracy did not change over blocks, variability decreased significantly. Masters et al. suggested analysis of the kinematic properties of the movement as a possible solution to this problem. Parkinson patients tend to have a prolonged deceleration phase for ballistic movements, rather than the typical symmetrical, bell-shaped, acceleration curve seen in healthy individuals (Inzelberg, Flash, and Korczyn, 1990). In addition, Master et al's errorless condition involved a physical constraint to prevent errors. Previous studies using cognitive tasks have found that self-generation of responses is a crucial factor in the rehabilitation of memory impaired patients (Tailby and Haslam, 2003). Similar arguments were put forward by Maxwell et al., (2001) for the generation of movement during the acquisition of motor skills. It might be predicted that stronger effects may be apparent when Parkinson patients are required to generate their own movements (i.e. without physical guidance) but still with minimal error. Masters et al. suggested gradually increasing task difficulty (similar to the protocol used in the errorless golf-putting studies, Maxwell et al., 2001) as a possible alternative; however, this possibility has yet to be examined. Finally, the durability of the effects seen in the Masters et al. study (and in many other errorless learning paradigms; for an exception see Poolton, Masters, et al., 2007) is not known because their retention test was conducted almost immediately after their acquisition trials. A delayed retention test of at least 24 hours would help to resolve this issue. Thus, whilst it appears promising for the use of errorless learning in the rehabilitation of patients with movement impairment, significantly more experimental work is required.

Can Errors be Beneficial?

Some authors have argued that human performance is inevitably error strewn and that to utilise learning conditions that are free from error ignores this basic quality. It is argued that errorless learners will be devoid of the relevant abilities to cope with error when it is eventually encountered. In response to these assertions, error management training (EMT) has been proposed as a possible alternative to errorless (and errorful or trial-and-error) learning (Chillarege, Nordstrom, and Williams, 2003; Frese et al., 1988, 1991; Nordstrom, Wendland, and Williams, 1998). In EMT the learner is encouraged to reframe the negative connotations normally associated with making a mistake into a positive experience. The EMT protocol also leads the learner to believe that errors actually increase rate of learning. Chillarege et al. (2003) found that EMT resulted in better learning of a word processing package than did error avoidant training (which emphasised the negative aspects of error committal). These results would suggest that errors may be either beneficial or detrimental, depending on how they are construed by the learner. This approach has yet to be applied to movement skills.

In a similar vein, some research has demonstrated that estimating performance error following movement appears to enhance learning (e.g., Adams and Goetz, 1973; Guadagnoli and Kohl, 2001; Swinnen, 1990; Swinnen, et al., 1990). Guadagnoli and Kohl argued that estimation of outcome error may serve to enhance the functionality of hypothesis testing behaviours, thereby improving performance. If this assertion is true, it could be argued that this form of learning is highly explicit, leading to a heightened awareness of body movements. Performers who adopt the error-estimation technique are likely to be susceptible to the effects of secondary task loading and psychological/physiological stress described earlier. This possibility could be easily investigated using the protocols typically adopted by researchers investigating implicit motor learning (e.g., Masters, 1992; Maxwell et al., 2001; Poolton, Masters, et al., 2007).

Conceding that it is a possibility that errors may be beneficial under some conditions, it remains obvious that the errorless learning technique is not completely void of error. Typically, only the early experiences are truly error free with later attempts at longer distances or with novel task constraints (e.g., the adapted putter used by Lam et al., 2007) characterised by increasing error. Nevertheless, errorless learners are no less able to cope with the appearance of error than errorful learners. Rather than indefinitely protect the performer from error, it has been argued that only the initial learning trials be error free so that a concrete platform is established that can be used to support later performance. If initial performance is ridden with error, a stable motor program is unlikely to be established and subsequent performances will be built upon shaky foundations.

Conclusion

Based on the research reviewed in this chapter, it appears that the practice of reducing the committal of errors during the very early stages of acquiring a new motor skill may have several distinct advantages over practice that is plagued with error. Movement errors appear to cause superfluous cognitive processing. Increased cognitive processing becomes habitual (over analysis), triggering a reliance on the availability of working memory processes, and leads to further errors when pressure is high or the performer is required to process additional information whilst performing the motor skill. When errors are frequent during the early stages of learning, the formation of a stable movement pattern may be difficult due to the high variability associated with making frequent changes to technique.

Skills that have been learnt with errors minimised during the early stages of learning appear to be resistant to the negative effects of psychological and physiological fatigue, robust to secondary task loads, are independent of age and natural ability, and transfer well to other task variations. These benefits appear to be associated with reductions in conscious processing during the movement execution phase of skill execution rather than the movement planning stage. Of considerable importance, is the possibility that benefits may be experienced by individuals with impaired movement control following an errorless motor learning paradigm. Not only will injury be prevented, but repeated success is likely to increase self-efficacy and aid the recovery process. However, considerable work is required before definitive conclusions can be made and the debate about the relevant importance of learning from errors versus error elimination is likely to continue.

Acknowledgments

The production of this chapter was supported by a Competitive Earmarked Research Grant (HKU 7231/04H) awarded by the Hong Kong Research Grants Council.

References

Abernethy, B. (1988). Dual-task methodology and motor skills research: Some applications and methodological constraints. *Journal of Human Movement Studies, 14,* 101-132.

Adams, J. A., and Goetz, E. T. (1973). Feedback and practice as variables in error detection and correction. *Journal of Motor Behavior, 5,* 217-224.

Baddeley, A. D. (1966). The capacity for generating information by randomization. *Quarterly Journal of Experimental Psychology, 18,* 119-129.

Baddeley, A. D. (1986). *Working memory.* New York: Oxford University Press.

Baddeley, A. D. (1986). *Human memory: Theory and practice* (revised edition). Hove, UK: Psychology Press.

Baddeley, A. D., and Logie, R. H. (1999) Working Memory: The Multiple-Component Model. In A. Miyake and P. Shah (Eds.), *Models of working memory: Mechanisms of active maintenance and executive control* (pp. 28-61). Cambridge, UK: Cambridge University Press.

Baddeley, A. D., and Wilson, B. A. (1994). When implicit learning fails: Amnesia and the problem of error elimination. *Neuropsychologia, 32,* 53-68.

Bandura, A. (1977). Self-efficacy: Toward a unifying theory of personality change. *Psychological Review, 84,* 191-215.

Inbar, O., Bar-Or, O., and Skinner, J. S. (1996). *The Wingate anaerobic test.* Champaign, IL: Human Kinetics.

Beek, P. J. (2000). Toward a theory of implicit learning in the perceptual-motor domain. *International Journal of Sport Psychology, 31,* 547-554.

Bernstein, N. A. (1967). *The control and regulation of movements.* London: Pergamon Press.

Berry, D. C. (1997). *How implicit is implicit learning?* New York: Oxford University Press.

Burton, D. (1988). Do anxious swimmers swim slower? Re-examining the elusive anxiety-performance relationship. *Journal of Sport and Exercise Psychology, 10,* 45-61.

Chaput, S. and Proteau, L. (1996). Aging and motor control. *Journal of Gerontology: Psychological Sciences, 51B,* 346-355.

Chauvel, G., Maquestiaux, F., Joubert, S., Benguigui, N., and Bertsch, J. (2007). Can older adults acquire a novel motor skill independently of working memory load? *12th European Congress of Sport Psychology, Halkidiki, Greece.*

Chillarege, K. A., Nordstrom, C. R., and Williams, K. B. (2003). Learning from our mistakes: Error management training for mature learners. *Journal of Business and Psychology, 17,* 369-385.

Contreras-Vidal, J. L., Teulings, H. L., and Stelmach, G. E. (1998). Elderly subjects are impaired in spatial coordination in fine motor control. *Acta Psychologica, 100,* 25-35.

Cote, D. O., Williges, B. H. and Williges, R. C. (1981). Augmented feedback in adaptive motor skill training. *Human Factors, 23,* 505-508.

Davey, P. R., Thorpe, R. D., and Williams, C. (2002). Fatigue decreases skilled tennis performance. *Journal of Sport Sciences, 20,* 311-318.

Evans, J. J., Levine, B., and Bateman, A. (2004). Research digest. *Neuropsychological Rehabilitation, 14,* 467-476.

Evans, J. J., Wilson, B. A., Schuri, U., Andrade, J., Baddeley, A., Bruna, O., Canavan, T., Della Sala, S., Green, R., Laaksonen, R., Lorenzi, L., and Taussik, I. (2000). A comparison of 'errorless' and 'trial-and-error' learning methods for teaching individuals with acquired memory deficit. *Neuropsychological Rehabilitation, 10,* 67-101.

Fazey, J. and Hardy, L. (1988). *The inverted-U hypothesis: A catastrophe for sport psychology?* British Association of Sport Sciences Monograph No.1. Leeds: The National Coaching Foundation.

Fillingham, J.K., Sage, K., and Lambon Ralph, M.A. (2006). The treatment of anomia using errorless learning. *Neuropsychological Rehabilitation, 16,* 129-154.

Fillingham, J. K., Hodgson, C., Sage, K., and Lambon Ralph, M. A. (2003). The application of errorless learning to aphasic disorders: A review of theory and practice. *Neuropsychological Rehabilitation, 13,* 337-363.

Frese, M., Albrecht, K., Altman, A., Lang, J., Papstein, P., Peyerl, R., Prumper, J., Schulte-Gocking, H., Wankmuller, I., and Wendel, R. (1988). The effects of an active development of the mental model in the training oprocess: Experimental results in a word processing system. *Behaviour and Information Technology, 7,* 295-304.

Frese, M. and Altmann, A. (1989). The treatment of errors in learning and training. In L. Bainbridge and S.A.R. Quintanilla (Eds.), *Developing skills with new technology* (pp. 65-86). Chichester, UK: Wiley.

Frese, M., Brodbeck, F., Heinbokel, T., Mooser, C., Schleiffenbaum, E., and Thiemann, P. (1991). Errors in training computer skills: On the positive function of errors. *Human Computer Interaction, 6,* 77-93.

Gick, M. L., and McGarry, S. J. (1992). Learning from mistakes: Inducing analogous solution failures to a source problem produces later successes in analogical transfer. *Journal of Experimental Psychology: Learning, Memory, and Cognition, 18,* 623-639.

Guadagnoli, M. A., and Kohl, R. M. (2001). Knowledge of results for motor learning: Relationship between error estimation and knowledge of results frequency. *Journal of Motor Behavior, 33,* 217-224.

Hardy, L., Mullen, R., and Jones, G. (1996). Knowledge and conscious control of motor actions under stress. *British Journal of Psychology, 87,* 621-636.

Hardy, L., and Parfitt, G. (1991). A catastrophe model of anxiety and performance. *British Journal of Psychology, 82,* 163-178.

Hardy, L., Parfitt, G., and Pates, J. (1994). Performance catastrophes in sport: A test of the hysteresis hypothesis. *Journal of Sports Sciences, 12,* 327-334.

Hebb, D. O. (1961). *The organization of behaviour: A neuropsychological theory. Stimulus and response and what occurs in the brain in the interval between them.* New York: Science Editions, Inc.

Heunninckx, S., Wenderoth, N., Debaere, F., Peeters, R., and Swinnen, S. P. (2005). Neural basis of aging: The penetration of cognition into action control. *Journal of Neuroscience, 25,* 6787-6796.

Hodges, N. J., and Franks, I. M. (2002). Modeling coaching practice: The role of instruction and demonstration. *Journal of Sports Sciences, 20,* 793–811.

Hodges, N. J., and Lee, T. D. (1999). The role of augmented information prior to learning a bimanual visual-motor coordination task: Do instructions of the movement pattern facilitate learning relative to discovery learning? *British Journal of Psychology, 90,* 389-403.

Holding, D. H. (1970a). Learning without errors. In L. Smith (Ed.), *Psychology of motor learning.* Chicago: The Athletic Institute.

Holding, D. H. (1970b). Repeated errors in motor learning. *Ergonomics, 13,* 727-734.

Holding, D. H. and Macrae, A. W. (1964). Guidance, restriction, and knowledge of results. *Ergonomics, 7,* 289-295.

Howard, D. V. (1988). Implicit and explicit assessment of cognitive aging. In M. L. Howe and C.J. Brainerd (Eds.), *Cognitive development in adulthood* (pp. 3-37). New York: Springer-Verlag.

Inzelberg, R., Flash, T., and Korczyn, A. D., (1990). Kinematic properties of upper-limb trajectories in Parkinson's disease and idiopathic torsion dystonia. *Advances in Neurology, 53,* 183-189.

Ivancic, K. and Hesketh, B. (2000). Learning from errors in a driving simulation: Effects on driving skill and self-confidence. *Ergonomics, 43,* 1966-1984.

Ivens, C. J. and Marteniuk, R. G. (1997). Increased sensitivity to changes in visual feedback with practice. *Journal of Motor Behavior, 29,* 326-338.

Kaplan, B. J., Wilson, B. N., Dewey, D. M., and Crawford, S. G. (1998). DCD may not be a discrete disorder. *Human Movement Science, 17,* 471-490.

Kay, H. (1951). Learning of serial task by different age groups. *Quarterly Journal of Experimental Psychology, 3,* 166-183.

Kelso, J. A. S., (1995). *Dynamic Patterns: The self-organization of brain and behaviour.* Cambridge, MA: MIT Press.

Lam, W. K., Maxwell, J. P., and Masters, R. S. W. Implicit learning, allocation of attention, and transfer to novel task variations. *Manuscript submitted for publication.*

Larkin, D., and Revie, G. (1994). *Stay in Step: A gross motor screening test for young children K-2,* Printing Headquarters, University of N.S.W.

Li, Y., and Wright, D. L. (2000). An assessment of the attentional demands during random- and blocked-practice schedules. *Quarterly Journal of Experimental Psychology, 53A,* 591-606.

Liao, C., and Masters, R. S. W. (2001). Analogy learning: A means to implicit motor learning. *Journal of Sports Sciences, 19,* 307-319.

Lintern, G., and Gopher, D., (1978). Adaptive training of perceptual motor skills: Issues, results, and future directions. *Journal of Man-Machine Studies, 10,* 521-551.

Lippman, L. G., and Rees, R. (1997). Consequences of error production in a perceptual-motor task. *Journal of General Psychology, 124,* 133-142.

MacMahon, K. M. A., and Masters, R. S. W. (2002). The effects of secondary tasks on implicit motor skill performance. *International Journal of Sports Psychology, 33,* 307-324.

Mané, A. M., Adams, J. A., and Donchin, E. (1989). Adaptive and part-whole training in the acquisition of a complex perceptual-motor skill. *Acta Psychologica, 71,* 179-196.

Marsh, A. P., and Geel, S. E. (2000). The effect of age on the attentional demands of postural control. *Gait and Posture 12,* 105-113.

Masters, R. S. W. (1992). Knowledge, (k)nerves and know-how: The role of explicit versus implicit knowledge in the breakdown of a complex motor skill under pressure. *British Journal of Psychology, 83,* 343-358.

Masters, R. S. W., Eves, F. F., and Maxwell, J. P. (2007). Marginally perceptible (subliminal) outcome feedback promotes motor learning but inhibits accrual of declarative knowledge. *Manuscript submitted for publication.*

Masters, R. S. W., MacMahon, K. M. A., and Pall, H. S. (2004). Implicit motor learning in Parkinson's Disease. *Rehabilitation Psychology, 49,* 79-82.

Masters, R. S. W., and Maxwell, J. P. (2004). Implicit motor learning, reinvestment and movement disruption: What you don't know won't hurt you? In A. M. Williams and N. J. Hodges (Eds.), *Skill acquisition in sport: Research, theory and practice* (pp. 207-228). London: Routledge.

Masters, R. S. W., Poolton, J. M., and Maxwell, J. P. (In press). Stable implicit motor processes despite aerobic locomotor fatigue. *Consciousness and Cognition.*

Mattay, V. S., Fera, F., Tessitore, A., Hariri, A. R., Das, S., Callicott, J. H., and Weinberger, D. R. (2002). Neurophysiological correlates of age-related changes in human motor function. *Neurology, 58,* 630-635.

Maxwell, J. P., and Masters, R. S. W. (2007a). The temporal distribution of errors during learning: Effects on performance and transfer to novel task variations. *Manuscript submitted for publication.*

Maxwell, J. P., and Masters, R. S. W. (2007b). Effects of increased state anxiety on putting performance following errorless or errorful learning. *Manuscript submitted for publication.*

Maxwell, J. P., Masters, R. S. W., and Eves, F. F. (2000). From novice to no know how: A longitudinal study of implicit motor learning. *Journal of Sport Sciences, 18,* 111-120.

Maxwell, J. P., Masters, R. S. W., and Eves, F. F. (2003). The role of working memory in motor learning and performance. *Consciousness and Cognition, 12,* 376-402.

Maxwell, J. P., Masters, R. S. W., and Hammond, J. (2007). The implicit benefits of learning without errors for children: Interactions with movement ability. *Manuscript submitted for publication.*

Maxwell, J. P., Masters, R. S. W., Kerr, E., and Weedon, E. (2001). The implicit benefit of learning without errors. *Quarterly Journal of Experimental Psychology A, 54,* 1049-1068.

Maxwell, J. P., Masters, R. S. W., and Lam, G. (2006a). Errorless learning and transfer to novel task variations: A switch from implicit to explicit control? *Proceedings of the 11th Annual Congress of the European College of Sport Science, Lausanne, Switzerland.*

Maxwell, J. P., Masters, R. S. W., and Lam, G. (2006b). Differential distribution of attentional resources during novel task performance following errorless and errorful learning: Evidence from probe reaction times. *Proceedings of the British Association of Sport and Exercise Sciences Annual Conference, Wolverhampton, UK.*

McClelland, J., Thomas, A. G., McCandliss, B., and Fiez, J. (1999). Understanding failures of learning: Hebbian learning, competition for representational space, and some preliminary data. *Progress in Brain Research, 121,* 75-80.

McGregor, S. J., Nicholas, C. W., Lakomy, H. K. A., and Williams, C. (1999). The influence of intermittent high-intensity shuttle running and fluid ingestion on the performance of a soccer skill. *Journal of Sports Sciences, 17,* 895-903.

Mullen, R., Hardy, L., and Oldham, A., (2007). Implicit and explicit control of motor actions: Revisiting some early evidence. *British Journal of Psychology, 98,* 141-156.

Neisser, U. (1976). *Cognitive and reality: Principles and implications for cognitive psychology.* New York: Appleton-Century-Crofts.

Newell, K. M. (1996). Change in movement and skill: Learning, retention, and transfer. In M. L. Latash and M. T. Turvey (Eds.), *Dexterity and its development* (pp. 393-430). Mahwah, NY: Erlbaum.

Nordstrom, C. R., Wendland, D., and Williams, K. B. (1998). "To err is human": An examination of the effectiveness of error management training. *Journal of Business and Psychology, 12,* 269-282.

Ohlsson, S. (1996). Learning from performance errors. *Psychological Review, 103,* 241-262.

Park, H. L., O'Connell, J. E., and Thomson, R. G. (2003). A systematic review of cognitive decline in the general elderly population. *International Journal of Geriatric Psychiatry, 18,* 1121-1134.

Poolton, J. M., Masters, R. S. W., and Maxwell, J. P. (2005). The relationship between initial errorless learning conditions and subsequent performance. *Human Movement Science 24,* 362-378.

Poolton, J. M., Masters, R. S. W., and Maxwell, J. P. (2007). Passing thoughts on the evolutionary stability of implicit motor behaviour: Performance retention under physiological fatigue. *Consciousness and Cognition, 16,* 456-468.

Poolton, J. P., Maxwell, J. P., Lam, G., and Masters, R. S. W. (2007). Distribution of attentional resources as a function of learning technique: Evidence from probe reaction times. *12th European Congress of Sport Psychology, Halkidiki, Greece.*

Prather, D. C. (1971). Trial-and-error versus errorless learning: Training, transfer, and stress. *American Journal of Psychology, 84,* 377-386.

Prather, D. C., and Berry, G. A. (1970). Comparison of trial-and-error versus highly prompted learning of a perceptual skill. *Proceedings of the 78th Annual Convention of the American Psychological Association, 5,* 677-678.

Raab, M., Masters, R. S. W., Maxwell, J. P., Arnold, A., Tielemann, N., and Poolton, J. M. (In press). Discovery learning in sport - implicit or explicit processes? *International Journal of Sport and Exercise Psychology.*

Reber, A. S. (1993). *Implicit learning and tacit knowledge: An essay on the cognitive unconscious.* New York: Oxford University Press.

Revie, G. and Larkin, D. (1993). Looking at movement: Problems with teacher identification of poorly co-ordinated children. *ACHPER National Journal, 40,* 4-9.

Schank, R. C. (1982). *Dynamic memory: A theory of reminding and learning in computers and people.* New York: Cambridge University Press.

Schmidt, R. A. (1975). A schema theory of discrete motor skill learning. *Psychological Review, 82,* 225-260.

Schmidt, R. A. (1991). Frequent augmented feedback can degrade learning: Evidence and interpretations. In J. Requin and G. E. Stelmach (Eds.), *Tutorials in motor neuroscience* (pp. 59-75). Dordrecht, The Netherlands: Kluwer Academic Publishers.

Schmidt, R. A., and Lee, T. D. (2005). *Motor control and learning: A behavioral emphasis* (4th ed.). Champaign, IL: Human Kinetics.

Schmidt, R. A., Young, D. E., Swinnen, S., and Shapiro, D. E. (1989). Summary knowledge of results for skill acquisition: Support for the guidance hypothesis. *Journal of Experimental Psychology: Learning, Memory, and Cognition, 15,* 352-359.

Seidler, R. D. and Stelmach, G. E. (1995). Reduction in sensorimotor control with age. *Quest, 47,* 386-394.

Shiffrin, R. M. and Schneider, W. (1977). Controlled and automatic human information processing: II. Perceptual learning, automatic attending, and a general theory. *Psychological Review, 84,* 127-190.

Singer, R. N. (1977). To err or not to err: A question for the instruction of psychomotor skills. *Review of Educational Research, 47,* 479-498.

Singer, R. N. and Gaines, L. (1975). Effect of prompted and problem-solving approaches on learning and transfer of motor skills. *American Educational Research Journal, 12,* 395-403.

Singer, R. N. and Pease, D. (1976). A comparison of discovery learning and guided instructional strategies on motor skill learning, retentions, and transfer. *Research Quarterly, 47,* 788-796.

Smeeton, N. J., Williams, A. M., Hodges, N. J., and Ward, P. (2005). The relative effectiveness of various instructional approaches in developing anticipation skill. *Journal of Experimental Psychology: Applied, 11,* 98–110.

Smith, C. D., Umberger, G. H., Manning, E. L., Slevin, J. T., Wekstein, D. R., Schmitt, F. A., Markesbery, W. R., Zhang, Z., Gerhardt, G. A., Kryscio, R. J., and Gash, D. M. (1999). Critical decline in fine motor hand movements in human aging. *Neurology, 53,* 1458-1461.

Smits-Engelsman, B. C. M., Wilson, P. H., Westenberg, Y., and Duysens, J. (2003). Fine motor deficiencies in children with developmental coordination disorder and learning disabilities: An underlying open-loop control deficit. *Human Movement Sciences, 22,* 495-513.

Spielberger, C. D., Gorsuch, R. L., and Lushene, R .F., (1970). *Manual for the State-Trait Anxiety Inventory*. Palo Alto, CA: Consulting Psychologists Press.

Sugden, D. A., and Wann, C. (1987). The assessment of motor impairment in children with moderate learning difficulties. *British Journal of Educational Psychology, 57,* 225-236.

Sullivan, E. A., and Hooper, S. L. (2005). Effects of visual occlusion and fatigue on motor performance in water. *Perceptual and Motor Skills, 100,* 681-688.

Swinnen, S., (1990). Interpolated activities during the knowledge-of-results delay and post-knowledge-of-results interval: Effects of performance and learning. *Journal of Experimental Psychology: Learning, Memory, and Cognition, 16,* 692-702.

Swinnen, S., Schmidt, R. A., Nicholson, D. E., and Shapiro, D. C. (1990). Information feedback for skill acquisition: Instantaneous knowledge of results degrades performance. *Journal of Experimental Psychology: Learning, Memory, and Cognition, 16,* 706-716.

Tailby, R., and Haslam, C. (2003). An investigation of errorless learning in memory-impaired patients: Improving the technique and clarifying theory. *Neuropsychologia, 41,* 1230-1240.

Thach, W. T. (1998). A role for the cerebellum in learning movement coordination. *Neurobiology of Learning and memory, 70,* 177-188.

Thorndike, E. L. (1898/2000). Animal intelligence: An experimental study of associative processes in animals. *Psychological Review Monographs, Supplement 2 (Whole No. 8)*.[Reprinted by Transaction Publishers, New York]

Toates, F. (2006). A model of the hierarchy of behaviour, cognition, and consciousness. *Consciousness and Cognition, 15,* 75-118.

Tunney, N., Taylor, L. F., Gaddy, M., Rosenfeld, A., Pearce, N., Tamanini, J., and Treby, A. (2003). Aging and motor learning of a functional motor task. *Physical and Occupational Therapy in Geriatrics, 21,* 1-16.

Von Wright, J. M. A. (1957). A note on the role of guidance in learning. *British Journal of Psychology, 48,* 133-137.

Waber, D. P., Weiler, M. D., Bellinger, D. C., Marcus, D. J., Forbes, P. W., Wypij, D., and Wolff, P. H. (2000). Diminished motor timing control in children referred for diagnosis of learning problems. *Developmental Neuropsychology, 17,* 181-197.

Ward, N.S., and Frachowiak, R.S. (2003). Age-related changes in the neural correlates of motor performance. *Brain, 126,* 873-888.

West, R.L. (1996). An application of prefrontal cortex function theory to cognitive aging. *Psychological Bulletin, 120,* 272-292.

Willingham, D.B. (1998). A neuropsychological theory of motor skill learning. *Psychological Review, 105*, 558-584.

Winstein, C. J., Pohl, P. S., and Lethwaite, R. (1994). Effects of physical guidance and knowledge of results on motor learning: Support for the guidance hypothesis. *Research Quarterly for Exercise and Sport, 65,* 316-323.

Wulf, G., McNevin, N. and Shea, C. H. (2001). The automaticity of complex motor skill learning as a function of attentional focus. *The Quarterly Journal of Experimental Psychology, 54A,* 1143-1154.

Wulf, G., Shea, C. H. and Whitacre, C. A. (1998). Physical-guidance benefits in a complex motor skill. *Journal of Motor Behavior, 30,* 367-380.

Yerkes, R. M. and Dodson, J. D. (1908). The relationship of strength of stimulus to rapidity of habit formation. *Journal of Comparative Neurology and Psychology, 18,* 459-482.

In: Sport and Exercise Psychology Research Advances   ISBN: 978-1-60456-157-9
Editors: M. P. Simmons, L. A. Foster, pp. 135-155   © 2008 Nova Science Publishers, Inc.

Chapter V

Perceived Challenges in Major Junior Ice-Hockey: The In-Depth Experiences of Athletes in a Remote Region

Tim V. Dubé and Robert J. Schinke[9]
Ben Avery Physical Education Center, School of Human Kinetics,
Laurentian University, Canada

Abstract

The present report overviews the on- and off-ice challenges of elite junior (major junior) hockey players located in one remote region of Canada. The data was gathered with a purposive sample of 10 athletes through semi-structured interviews (Patton, 2002), with the guidance of an advisory panel. There were three stages of data collection and content analysis, with 3-4 respondents elicited during each stage. Based on guidelines espoused by Côté, Salmela, Baria, and Russell (1993) and Schinke and da Costa (2000), the data were segmented into meaning units, coded into a hierarchy of themes, and verified with each respondent. From the data, there is indication that elite junior athletes from ice-hockey can adjust to and benefit from placements within remote locations. Peers, team-mates, coaching staff, billets, and community resources within the remote region offered the aspiring major junior athletes assistance with their adaptation. Implications are provided for applied sport psychology researchers and practitioners interested in placements within remote regions.

Keywords: *Remote Region, Contextual Challenges, Elite Ice-Hockey, Adaptation*

9 Forward all correspondences to: Robert J. Schinke, PhD , B-241B Ben Avery Physical Education Center, School of Human Kinetics, 935 Ramsey Lake Rd., Laurentian University, Sudbury, Ontario, Canada, P3E 2C6, Email: rschinke@laurentian.ca, Telephone: (705) 675-1151 Ext. 1045, Fax: (705) 675-4845.

Many young elite ice-hockey players aspire to the professional ranks, with the pinnacle being performance in the National Hockey League (NHL). A level of performance within Canada's formal hockey system from where NHL players are formally drafted is major junior hockey (Koshan, 2004). Considering the high expectations to impress prospective NHL teams, there is convincing evidence that it takes major junior athletes more than just talent to pursue their ambitions (Bruner, 2002; Koshan, 2004). Major junior athletes are expected to adjust to contextual challenges that include and exceed sport expectations. For instance, there are new team-mates, a new coaching staff, new friends, and a new community with unknown resources. Beyond these obvious adjustment challenges, there are also questions regarding where they are drafted to (e.g., urban, rural, remote location), and perhaps equally compelling, when in age they are asked to do so.

Within the last few years, a few sport scientists have started to examine the multifaceted and high profile context of major junior ice-hockey. Bruner (2002), as one example, considered the hiring of agents, the establishment of contacts with NHL scouts, the pressures of being drafted upward, as well as the balancing of academic demands. Additionally, it is already known that most aspiring hockey players are required to live in locations away from home throughout their teenage years. In his journalistic internship with a major junior team from the same Canadian province as the present report (Ontario), Koshan (2004) noted that of the 24 players on the team's roster, 17 lived with billets (host families that act as surrogate family members). Sport relocation for the aspiring major junior athlete often begins during middle adolescence (15-17 years), a time when most teenagers live with their families, and potentially continues into late adolescence (18-20 years) when the athlete is retained or traded.

Consequently, there is a range of potential contextual challenges that adolescent hockey players are exposed to at the major junior level as they aspire to National Hockey League status. The present report overviews through semi-structured interviews, the contextual challenges and consequent strategies of major junior athletes within one Canadian remote region: Northern Ontario.

Potential Contextual Challenges

More than 10 years ago, Côté and colleagues (1995) teased at the importance of contextual challenges when they considered the knowledge and strategies of expert elite Canadian gymnastic coaches. Precisely, Côté et al.'s coaching model (CM) included three components that reciprocally influenced each other among successful gymnastic coaches: (a) organization, (b) training, and (c) competition. The emerging factors affecting the abovementioned CM's components were the coach's interpersonal characteristics, the athlete's characteristics, and most relevant to this paper, contextual factors. Contextual factors were described as unstable (e.g., variable working conditions). Pertaining to major junior ice- hockey, a few contextual challenges have already been identified by sport scientists as part of the athletes' work conditions. For the purposes of this report, it is at very least important to consider the following contextual challenges: (a) sport demands, (b) academics demands, (c) homesickness, and (d) regional location of placement.

Sport demands. Relevant to OHL players' off-ice demands, Bruner (2002) outlined several sport related challenges. Some of these pertained to off-ice demands, and they include adjusting to new team-mates, developing relationships with coaching staff, coping with the rigours of a busy hockey schedule, and the promotion and retention adjustments associated with making and retaining team membership. On-ice, Bruner indicated that major junior hockey players are also required to attend daily practices, and most times also have mandatory off-ice workouts with their team trainers (Koshan, 2004). Beyond the aforementioned, on a more global level on- and off-ice, Schinke, Draper, and Salmela (1997) learned from a purposive sample of Canadian expert ice-hockey coaches from the professional level, that sport expectations also included fitting within the team, adding to its chemistry, and accepting one's formal and informal roles. Many of these sport related demands have been teased at elsewhere in relation to National Hockey League athletes (Schinke, Gauthier, Dubuc, and Crowder, submitted for publication), though only based on archival data.

Academic demands. As Koshan (2004) learned while traveling with one major junior team, there are pressures that come with trying to balance hockey and school. Without having completed high school or having acquired the necessary pre-requisites for entering university, major junior athletes run the risk of limited education should their futures exclude a professional sport career (Bruner, 2002). Consequently, at least within Canada, 86% of games are played between Thursday and Sunday. The intended purpose of scheduling is meant to limit the number of school days lost by the major junior athlete due to travel (Baker and Schafer, 1988). That said the time demands on major junior athletes are extensive. These challenges are increased when athletes travel far distances (in excess of 400 km each way) regularly over the course of a season (and post-season) to larger urban areas from remote locations. Following, it would appear logical that the major junior athlete's sport demands might impinge on academic development regardless of formal scheduling contingencies.

Homesickness. Adding to the challenges experienced by the aspiring major junior ice-hockey player, are challenges pertaining to loneliness and homesickness. Fisher (1989) defined homesickness as "a complex cognitive-motivational-emotional state concerned with grieving for, yearning for, and being preoccupied with thoughts of home" (p. 426). When Schinke et al. considered the adaptation challenges of Canadian elite Aboriginal athletes (2006) and NHL athletes from various cultures (submitted for publication), it was learned that many struggled after they relocated to a new region and away from family and friends. Homesickness, a form of mal-adaptation, was commonly reflected in the overt behaviour of crying and an internal sense of alienation. It is likely that major junior athletes share many of the same experiences upon leaving their homes to play junior hockey, though at present, one could only presuppose. The question of friendsickness, a sub-component of homesickness, typically happens in the latter teenage years, typically as students leave home to pursue higher education or a professional career, sport or otherwise (see Paul and Brier, 2001). For major junior hockey players relocated to new cities after draft or trade, moving away from established relationships, and developing new friendships can present as a challenge in terms of access to pre-existing social support resources, especially during immediate post-relocation adjustment. It was speculated herein that homesickness can magnify as an adaptation concern when athletes are located to less accessible locations away from their existing social support resources (less immediate access to family and hometown friends).

Regional and remote location placements. Together, the aforementioned challenges build a compelling argument regarding the challenges faced by major junior athletes. Within major junior hockey, the complexities of athletic pursuits are complicated even further when one is traded to a remote location, while also being asked to progress to a new level or retain status. Recently, Gauthier, Schinke, and Pickard (2006) considered the regional challenges associated with sporting life in a remote location, and did so by eliciting the experiences of elite coaches. Gauthier et al. conducted open-ended focus groups and follow-up semi-structured interviews with nationally certified elite Canadian coaches regarding the challenges and strengths of coaching in one northern Canadian region (Northern Ontario). The regional contextual challenges uncovered by Gauthier and colleagues included extensive travel distances, a lack of financial and personnel resources, athlete retention and recruitment, and a lack of competition. Gauthier and colleagues' investigation was initially intended as a project to identify regional challenges. However, the researchers also uncovered that coaches and athletes performing in remote locations acquire unique skill sets. Effective adaptation among the elite coaches (to living in a remote region) entailed developing a positive perspective, a close-knit coaching fraternity, and close ties with members from the community, including fans and media personnel.

The Present Study

As the previous literature would indicate, the aspiring ice-hockey athlete is faced with numerous challenges. Some of these challenges relate solely to sport demands. There are other contextual challenges that address relocation in general and regional placement in specific. Consequently, the present report targets the contextual challenges and consequent strategies experienced by adolescent elite athletes, as these athletes pursue elite sport in a remote region in Northern Ontario, Canada.

Method

Research Assumptions

Prior to the study, the principal investigator (graduate student) conducted an internship placement with an elite junior ice-hockey team within the same region. As part of the experience, I worked with middle adolescent aspiring elite athletes. Throughout the experience, many of my clients were relocated athletes who cycled in and out of the junior team. Inevitably, much of the discussion with the aspiring players and their coaching staff was how to adjust to a new city, new teammates, unfamiliar sport science resources, and new host families. These discussions sparked the author's (my) interest, and consequently a graduate project. Based on observations and consulting experience, the first author (I) anticipated that there would be a variety of contextual challenges associated with being relocated to Northern Ontario (a remote region within Canada). I was uncertain whether (and if so, how) these challenges would be paired with adolescence.

Respondent Group

The respondent group was comprised of major junior hockey players from two OHL teams in Northern Ontario, Canada, both within small cities of less than 150 000 people. The respondent group comprised 10 players (18-23 years). The purpose of interviewing late adolescent players was to capture their retrospective views of the whole OHL experience regarding contextual challenges and social support resources. Participant recruitment was developed employing Patton's (2002) purposive convenience sampling method. According to this sampling strategy, the selection of the participants is first and foremost based on their accessibility to the researcher and, subsequently, for their information rich contributions.

Geographical Context

The study was conducted in Northern Ontario, Canada. Among numerous northern locations, the chosen area covers the northern region of one Canadian province. This area was selected for the current project based on its unique geographical characteristics. Northern Ontario's land covers nearly 89% of the province, but only represents a mere 7.4% of its provincial population (http://www.mndm.gov.on.ca). Northern Ontario's population density is 1.0 person per square kilometre, in comparison to its southern Ontario counterpart at 104.3 persons per square kilometre (http://www.mndm.gov.on.ca). These statistics indicate that much of Northern Ontario is uninhabited wilderness and less populated rural areas and communities.

Question Development

The development of questions included in the interview guide resulted from three group sessions with an advisory panel of four people with an established affiliation to the Ontario Hockey League. Panel members were: one former major junior athlete from the region, one former major junior hockey coach, one league parent, and an OHL player agent. The panel assisted with the preliminary questions in order to ensure the relevance to the OHL players' experiences. For instance, the parent on the panel suggested that one of the probing questions relevant to the contextual challenges should address relationships with girlfriends. In addition, the panel discussion helped clarify and develop contextually relevant wording within the interview guide. Their suggestions, which were maintained in a research logbook, informed the interview protocol. The meetings were audio recorded and the email communications were also documented for note purposes. For instance, revised versions of the interview questions were sent to the panel electronically. The panel subsequently sent their comments and suggestions regarding refined wording of the questions, and changes to the interview guide were made accordingly.

Data Collection

Once informed consent was obtained, the participants were asked to provide demographic information regarding the player's general background information, the player's OHL background, and the player's academic background. Subsequently, each participant was interviewed for approximately 90 minutes adapted from Patton's (2002) semi-structured open-ended interview process. The interviews were conducted in person when possible, however due to respondents' demands, some interviews were also conducted over the telephone (Table 1). During the interviews, participants were probed to ensure adequate understanding and detailed recollections of their lived experiences. Patton's (2002) three types of probes were used to gain thick description. Detail probes (e.g., How did you feel academic pressure?), elaboration probes (e.g., Can you tell me more about dealing with the stress of a busy hockey schedule?), and clarification probes (e.g., You mentioned you did not have time to do things, what do you mean by that?).

The interview was piloted with one former OHL player to refine the interview protocol and gain proficiency in the interview process. The interview was audio taped and transcribed verbatim. It was then reviewed and evaluated by the researcher and his supervisor. The interview transcript was subsequently emailed to the expert panel and to the respondent for verification. In addition, verbal feedback was sought from the respondent. The interview protocol was revised integrating feedback obtained from all sources before further data collection.

Table 1. Interview Guide Questions

Section 1: General sport background	Can you tell me about your general sport background starting from the year or a few months prior to you getting into the OHL leading to the present?
Section 2: Personal and contextual challenges	What sort of challenges do players in the OHL generally face? What sort of challenges do you face? Are there any challenges specific to playing in Northern Ontario? How was that experience relevant during your middle/late adolescent years? Extending from conversations you've had with teammates over the years, can you think of any other challenges that they voiced to you? Are there any challenges that we have not discussed that would benefit the study or better represent your experiences?
Section 3: Debriefing	Are there any other questions or topics that I should have asked about, but didn't regarding your experiences?

Data Analysis

Each interview was transcribed and coded by the interviewer to ensure athlete anonymity, and identifying names and locations were removed. The data was segmented into "meaning units". A meaning unit according to Tesch (1990) is a segment of text that contains a single idea relating to a specific theme. Herein, each meaning unit was labelled using a respondent-based method (e.g., Athlete 1, Athlete 2, etc.). The researcher, with the assistance from the researcher's supervisor, developed a preliminary coding system based on the meaning units from the initial stage of respondents (A1-A4). Each grouping of meaning units was analyzed for similarities and differences using a compare and contrast method with each ensuing stage of respondents (A1-A4, A5-A8, A9-A10), and refinements were made to the larger coding scheme. At the culmination of each stage, the advisory panel vetted the classification tags based on examples of each category and sub-category, and suggested coding refinement in accordance with the context. For example, the category environmental influences became social demands, which subsequently resulted in relationship issues emerging as a sub-category (Table 2).

Trustworthiness Techniques

The researcher ensured the trustworthiness of the study by adhering to validity guidelines set out by Maxwell (2002). To enhance descriptive validity, every interview was recorded using a tape recorder and then cross-verified with the audio recording. For interpretive validity, the present study reflected the lived experiences of OHL players performing in Northern Ontario. To do so, the researcher conducted research meetings with the research project's supervisory committee before and following each stages of data collection. Also for verification purposes, the researcher sent the respondents their transcripts, their coded interviews, as well as an overview of the study's general findings for evaluation. The following respondent provided the researcher with one such refinement, and his changes are italicized:

> I knew it would probably be my best shot *to end up playing with the OHL [team] the quickest. I knew they could watch me play, and if I played well it would pressure them to trade their backup goalie quicker. However if I went back to play Junior B in my hometown of [city], then the [OHL team] would not be able to watch me play and see how I was doing.* So I started with the [Junior A team]. I was there for about a month and a half and they ended up sending the other goalie home and they called me up (A2).

Theoretical validity was enhanced when the researcher coded every interview with emergent categories and sub-categories. Revised versions of the dataset were vetted with the researcher's supervisor and the expert panel until consensus was reached for each stage of data collection and analysis. Afterward, the researcher ensured that all respondents were asked to provide feedback regarding a copy of their coded transcripts, including the separation of categories, and within each, sub-categories. Finally, the goal of the present report was to provide an in-depth understanding of major junior hockey players' contextual challenges while performing in one rural and remote region.

Table 2. Contextual Challenges Categories and Sub-Categories

Categories (Meaning Units)	1st Level Sub-Categories (Meaning Units)	2nd Level Sub-Categories (Meaning Units)
Personal Adjustment (40)	Leaving Home (23)	Missing Family (10) Missing Friends (7) Missing Home (6)
	Living in a New Community (17)	Living with a Host Family (10) Autonomy / Structure (7)
Balancing Educational Demands and Hockey (51)	Sport Demands (28)	Time at the Rink (3) Learning to Balance (25)
	Academic Demands (23)	Settling into a New School (9) School Work / Handing in Assignments (12) Autonomy while Pursuing Post Secondary Education (2)
Social Constraints (10)	General Relationships (4)	General Social Time (4)
	Relationships with Partners (6)	Displacement Concerns (3) Limited Activities (3)
Team and Sport Pressures (102)	Mental Demands (45)	Focus (32) Meeting Expectations (8) Dealing with Injuries (5)
	Physical Demands (40)	Acclimatization to the Speed of Play (33) Physical Training / Schedule (7)
	Interpersonal Demands (17)	Coach-Athlete Dyad (6) Team Dynamics (11)
Regional Challenges (56)	Community Demands (21)	Fan Pressure (7) Social Accountability / Team Representation (14)
	Geographical Demands (35)	Rigors of Travel Schedule (23) Athlete Recruitment / Retention (12)

While the findings of this report are confined to one region, they may be relevant for elite athletes pursuing sport careers in other rural and remote locations.

Results

The present report is intended to present the perspectives of major junior hockey players relevant to the challenges they faced while performing in one remote region: Northern Ontario, Canada. The respondents offered their retrospective and recent experiences across middle and late adolescent stages. For the purpose of this report, similarities across the respondents were classified into five emergent contextual challenges: (a) personal adjustment, (b) balancing educational demands and hockey, (c) social constraints, (d) team and sport pressures, and (e) regional challenges, each with sub-themes (Table 2).

Personal Adjustment

Personal adjustment refers to the changes in interpersonal resources players endure when they have to live away from home to pursue their major junior hockey careers. Within the present report, personal adjustment included leaving home and living in a new community.

Leaving home. The topic of leaving and missing home was frequently discussed in association with being a major junior hockey player, especially during middle adolescence:

> I know a lot of guys have a difficult time when their younger to move away from home…when a 16 year old kid decides that he wants to play in the OHL and you're not sure where you're going to end up playing... probably 90% of the time you're going to end up living away from home and I think at 16 it's a pretty young age to be doing that. (A7)

Interestingly, the same player expressed his disregard of playing on a Northern Ontario team, "I remember saying at 16 that I didn't want to play in [location], [location], or [location] because they were too far from home (A7)". It seemed that relocation concerns were compounded by being situated in a remote location, and that many athletes initially hoped for a more centralized placement. The concerns related to living far away from home and missing family and friends posed a challenge for most, though especially during middle adolescence:

> That's probably the biggest challenge that I faced. If you move away to go to school, the average person moves away at usually 18 or 19. Moving away at 16, you're moving away from all your friends that you've gone to school with and all your friends that you've known your whole life. It's pretty tough because for all those friends that you lost, you got to try and make new ones in a new city. (A4)

Living in a new community. When relocating, the athletes had their first experiences living with a host family, which refers to "guys coming into the OHL from out of town having to live with people they don't know (A1)". Out of the 10 respondents herein, eight lived with billets at one point in their careers. Older players seemed to live more effectively with these families primarily because most were either living with the same families from previous years or had lived with other families prior to joining their present team (and were comfortable with this typical arrangement):

> I think for a young guy coming in, that's one of the big challenges for them, being away from home, having to live in an environment where they don't know people, they don't know what to expect. These people [host families] are really good people. I think once the first couple of weeks are done, they realize that they are there to help them and to take care of them. For the most part the guys feel really comfortable in their homes, and like I said, they have to look at it like their family. They're there for seven or eight months of the year, so they can't turn back really. I think for the first time guy that is a challenge, but it quickly becomes more comforting. (A1)

Another athlete elaborated on his new independence, and suggested that he had to quickly adjust to a more autonomous lifestyle at a young age. He was free of daily parental involvement, and the benefits of structure that previously existed:

> You have to be more responsible on your own. At home, my parents would take me to practice and take me to games. And, now you have to make sure you're up for whatever time you have to be at the rink. There's no one really to look out for you, you're kind of on your own. It's a good thing though, to learn more responsibility and if you're not already grown up, you have to grow up. (A2)

Balancing Educational Demands and Hockey

Many of the athletes experienced challenges as they tried to manage high-school or university, while pursuing their sport careers. The themes that were considered by the athletes when they considered their work-related obligations were sport demands and academic demands.

Sport demands. Many of the players experienced competing obligations during their busy daily schedules. For instance, there was a unanimous reference to the extensive amount of time spent at the rink and on the road, as well as the off-ice training. The following respondent's thoughts on the subject encapsulated the views of all:

> I think for all of us it's a pretty tough thing to do. I mean you're on the ice every single day for at least two hours, and you had the off-ice stuff also. You're at the rink probably three hours a day and a lot of the weekends you're on the road, so a lot of the guys find it hard to balance out the school work and hockey, but it's something that you have to manage while playing. (A1)

Even though the respondents improved their time management skills, it was noted that all of the athletes struggled with competing time demands throughout their careers. Learning to organize their priorities while playing at the elite level was reflected by the highest number of meaning units:

It's very hard to do your homework on these road trips because you have pre-game skates, you have team meals, and team bonding events. It's very hard to keep both the academic and athlete; you have to either pick one or the other or you know you're going to be left with nothing in both aspects. So my main focus is hockey and then I try to focus also on school whenever I have time. So it's basically a full time job going to hockey. (A5)

Academic demands. The pressures of performing at the elite level in hockey undermined adjusting to a new school, the completion of school assignments in accordance with timelines, and catching up after a lengthy road trip, especially during playoffs in middle adolescence:

I was 17, in high school in grade twelve, especially when we got to the end of the year in the playoffs. We were playing every other day, it was pretty well impossible to get to school every day. I found that really tough, especially when we have to go home and transfer schools. When you come home and go into the same class, they might have already covered some stuff that you missed from being in [city]. That was probably the toughest thing in school, was when I came back home. (A2)

The pressure of performing academically for many of the respondents, when discussing their middle adolescence, was compounded when their coaches emphasized the importance of (and followed-up regarding) schooling:

As a 17 year old, you're trying to get through high school. It's harder because you're now in a higher league and you want to get better in hockey first, then in the schooling. But, you don't know how to do both because the coaches always put more pressure on the younger guys to get through school. So, you want to get good marks but at the same time you want to become a better hockey player. (A3)

Once reaching late adolescence, the athletes were expected to be self-directed. It seemed that coaches encouraged this transition to autonomy:

I think the challenge as an older player in the OHL is to continue your education. A lot, probably around 90% of the guys finish their high school in the OHL. I think the challenge for the older guys is to have the self motivation to go out there and want to do university classes or want to college classes. I've been taking probably one or two a semester for the last 3 years and that's just because I chose to. There's really no, well in the OHL they don't really tell you to do university credits, it's kind of on your own accord that you do that. I would say the biggest challenge for an older guy is deciding that he wants to do it and find the time in his day to do it. (A7)

Social Constraints

Relationships were constrained because of the players' daily sporting involvement, including sport demands and relationships with partners.

General social time. The respondents all expressed the limited time they had for social activities outside of hockey. The following athlete's experience reflected the perspective of the others with regards to making the necessary sacrifices in terms of social life:

> We had curfew every single night, and that cuts into your social time for sure. It's a sacrifice you have to make. For a lot of the guys this is their life and the place they want to go is the NHL. They're willing to make those sacrifices to be there someday. (A1)

Having a girlfriend. Taking one example closer to home that spanned developmental stages, many of the players discussed the topic of maintaining an intimate relationship. The following experience denoted the feelings of many:

> Having a girlfriend, it's tough. You don't really have a lot time. So, if they're not the type of girlfriend that's really there to support you all the time, you get frustrated. I had to give up a girlfriend when I was 16, just about 17; just because there was no time. (A3)

Another respondent provided his retrospective view of having girlfriends from middle to late adolescence in relation to ongoing relocation:

> I know a lot of guys have girlfriends and moving away is tough, especially when you're younger. You're moving away from them and you don't really get to see them. The past couple of years I just didn't have a girlfriend because I knew I would be bouncing around quite a bit. I think it's something I just kind of avoided the past couple years because I didn't know where I'd be the next 3 months and it wasn't fair to start up a relationship. (A7)

Team Pressures and Sport Adjustment

The respondents spoke of team related pressures as a result of their participation on major junior teams. The emergent sub-themes were mental demands, physical demands, and sport adjustment.

Mental demands. Many of the respondents identified personal pressure and mental focus as part of their athletic experience, and some even mentioned mental exhaustion. Mental exhaustion was considered often, though especially in relation to middle adolescence:

> I think it's tough mentally; just trying to go to the rink everyday and you've got to work hard. They demand a lot out of you. Personally, some aren't ready mentally to do that, but some are. For me, some days I'm tired because they push you to the extreme. That's the one challenge that I face everyday is trying to stay focused and trying to stay on the top line. (A4)

Another respondent pointed out that mental demands make or break a player's career based on level of commitment because, "a lot of guys realize that they don't have a career in this sport and then they tend not to focus (A7)". Upon following-up, the respondent described his struggles while aspiring to a career in the professional ranks during his tenure:

When you're young you have high school, you have girls, you have friends, and then you throw hockey on top at a very high level. So I think there's a high stress level there. To me, as I get older, I'm trying to make a career. When you don't plan well or if you're cut or traded or whatever it is then you kind of take it to heart. Am I really going to be a hockey player, is this really going to be my direction? ...so there are those stresses as to what you're going to do later in life. (A7)

The pressures of dealing with setbacks were spoken of during middle adolescence where players were making an effort to thrive at the OHL level while aspiring making the jump to the NHL:

When you go into the OHL, I think everybody thinks that they can go to the NHL. When you're 16 years old and you just started playing in the OHL, you still have that feeling in your mind that I'm on my way here and then next progression is to get drafted to the NHL. I think a lot of guys realize in the first couple of years whether or not they're going to be hockey players. Then they're going to determine, based on that, what their level of commitment is. (A7)

The same respondent expanded his view in relation to late adolescence regarding the notion of overcoming setbacks and staying on track with personal goals:

I think it kind of goes one way or another as you become an older player. A lot of guys realize that they don't have a career in this sport and then they tend to not focus on it as much in the off season or during the season. And then you'll find other guys who want a career out of it and their training to become professional hockey players, training twice a day in the summer and then every single day after workouts. (A7)

Another sub-theme within mental demands involved the difficulties and expectations the athletes experienced across developmental stages related to succeeding. There were the expectations the players had for themselves, and also, the expectations from others:

People are asking all the time "What happened?" or "What's going on?" or "How come things didn't work out?" Everybody's just expecting you, since you've already dominated your whole life and you get into trouble, people just can't seem to understand what's going on and some people just expect too much. (A10)

The last sub-theme within the mental demands category refers to dealing with injuries. There was consensus across the respondents that overcoming the mental strains of getting injured was integral to their rehabilitation and their return to the line-up:

Especially if your coping with injuries, if you have had a pull or something. It's hard for sure, just to recover. I hurt my shoulder this year. You can't let it be a mind game. If you let it get to your head you just start thinking bad things, especially for kids that are going into the draft. You can't let it put you down mentally. You're obviously going to be down physically but all you can do is rehab and think positive, "It's going to get better, I'm going to get healthy enough to play". (A8)

Physical demands. There were also physical demands spoken of in relation to daily practices, off-ice workouts, and adjusting to the speed of the game. The pressures of on- and off-ice training were most often experienced during middle adolescence where players were making an effort to fit in to the OHL environment:

> To be 16 years old and to be playing 20 year olds...obviously you're not going to be as strong as them...you might be at a little disadvantage at a pushing match or a shouting match or a fight. Also, it's definitely a grind at 16 being scheduled 34 games on the road and 34 at home. (A9)

The players also had to adapt to the speed of play during games at this level, especially considering that they were playing against higher quality players:

> When I first came in the league, there were definitely some very good players. It's pretty tough because a lot of those guys are ready for the next level, but you're just kind of starting into the level that they've already exceeded. So, it's really a challenge to try and keep up with those guys and to try and do the things that they do. Last year, the team had won and I think they had about five guys that have gone on to play in the NHL this season. (A4).

Interpersonal demands. There were also interpersonal challenges spoken of in relation to coach-athlete relationships and team dynamics. Many referred to the challenges of adjusting to different coaching styles and as part of the adjustment, the challenges associated with developing a relationship with the coach:

> I definitely think guys respond differently to different styles of coaching. I think you know a player's coach, which is a little easier going, a little free flowing. Or you have an older style coach that it's kind of his way and that's it. So it's definitely, you have to adjust how you react because everybody has a boiling point and everybody's eventually just going to snap. (A9)

It at least seemed that the coach-athlete relationship evolved during late adolescence:

> I think the older you get the less that you want to be friends with the coach. Well not friends but, I think when you're younger you kind of look at them as a very, very key person in your life almost. Whereas when you're older you realize he's just my hockey coach, to take what you can from him, learn as much as you can but really, he's just my hockey coach. I think when you're 16, 17 you look at them as more important people in your life. As you get older there's a much more professional kind of feel between a player and a coach. (A7)

Team dynamics as a sub-theme refers to the interactions the respondents discussed in relation to making friends on the team and team bonding events. For instance, in terms of making friends on the team, the following respondent's view was shared by many others when recalling their experiences as middle adolescent athletes:

On the teams I played on, the rookies were a group and all the other players were another group. I just thought that team wise and chemistry wise, it didn't work out. I was aware when I was a rookie that there were two groups and I just hated it. It felt like I couldn't talk to the older guys. (A10)

Another respondent echoed the previous respondent's view and extended this point explaining the role many of the respondents shared as they got older:

In terms of making friendships, it was mostly that rookies were friends with rookies then as you get older you become friends with everybody, especially when you just sort of step in. You're on the same kind of boat as another guy, you automatically have that friendship, bonded no matter what. As you get older, I just try to be friends with everybody because it's tough in a lot of instances. I think for a team to be successful you have to get along. I think that was probably one of my jobs as I got older. (A7)

Remote Regional Challenges

Social concerns and pressures were experienced by all of the respondents as they lived in small rural locations. As a consequence of playing with a team from a remote location, there were community demands and a rigorous travel schedule.

Community demands. The players felt as if they were always in the spotlight as a result of their recognition as a result of their participation on a major junior hockey team in a remote community:

I think another challenge that some players would face is within the community they're playing in. There are some people that absolutely love the players representing their city. But at the same time they're some that don't agree with what we do and think that we shouldn't be doing it because we get too much given to us. It all depends how good the team is doing I guess in the cities. For example, when I first got to the [location], the team wasn't doing very well. So, when you go out in public people that you don't even know off the street would know who you are because you play for the [team name]. And they would look at you like you're a bad person. (A4)

The middle adolescent experiences the players denoted suggested that they had a harder time coping with community expectations. For instance, this player offered his view of this social accountability as a younger athlete:

Hockey's a big part of being in Northern Ontario, everyone knows about the [team name] or the [team name]. Then certain names come up with the team and if something happens where it's a bad thing, it's hard to change peoples minds about it. (A6)

Rigours of the travel schedule. There were also rigours associated with travel schedules as the athletes were transported to and from road games. The respondents, without exception, discussed the difficulties of traveling when from a remote location:

I think it's more difficult for sure. There were a quite a few times we had to play at 2:00 in [city] and we'd leave at 6:30 in the morning. It's pretty hard to play a hockey game on six hours of rest, you try to sleep on the bus but you have four hours to the game. We had a couple times where we had that and then we'd have a game the next day. I think it's much more demanding playing up North than say [location] where there is relatively no travel and you have most games within a two hours radius. (A7)

When the athletes were asked to discuss the traveling challenge and its significance while situated in their geographical location, many stated something along these lines: "it's a matter of how you cope with it and how you react to it because some people will react positively and it won't really bother them (A9)". He went on to explain that, "you can use the travel time to your advantage whether it's just preparation time on the bus or maybe get that extra little sleep on the bus (A9)". This skill seemed to have been learned as the athletes matured and became more accustomed to road trips.

Discussion

The results from the present study delineated the challenges experienced by elite ice-hockey players performing in one remote geographical region - Northern Ontario, Canada. Contextual factors are documented within the elite sport literature. Côté et al. (1995) first indicated the relevance of contextual factors when he developed a coaching model (CM) from the views of expert Canadian gymnastic coaches. Elaborating on "contextual factors" Côté and colleagues indicated that elite sport environments are variable due to the presence of "influx" circumstances. For instance, he noted that training and competition environments and their associated demands may vary within each sport discipline and furthermore within each location. Data from the immediate report reflected five overarching categories of challenges encountered by the athletes within one remote region in relation to sport demands. These were (a) personal adjustment, (b) competing work demands, (c) social demands, (d) within team pressures, and (e) remote region challenges.

Personal Adjustment

Personal adjustment challenges include the stresses associated with having to move to a new community and having to leave close friends behind (Fisher, 1989; Paul and Brier, 2001). Homesickness, one facet of the more general challenge, was studied previously with different elite sport samples including Canadian Aboriginals (Schinke et al., 2006) and National Hockey League athletes (Schinke et al., submitted for publication). In both instances, there was indication of effective adaptation strategies that combined positive ties within the immediate sporting context and the larger community. The present report is the first to uncover the topic of homesickness overtly with elite adolescent athletes (major junior athletes achieve elite status before adulthood). Herein, the adjustment to leaving close friends behind proved to be difficult for the major junior athletes, specifically during middle adolescence. As a consequent strategy, peer group affiliation within and outside of sport facilitated adaptation. Most among the respondents suggested that they were compelled to forge ties with their peers (as were their peers with them) because they resided in a close-knit community. Focusing specifically on peers within their team, the respondents indicated that loneliness caused by relocation was a shared reality for most, and that the adversity forged meaningful long-term friendships, friendships that continued after team status ended.

Competing Work Demands

A second challenge related to the struggles balancing educational demands while pursuing elite sport endeavours. As mentioned earlier in this report, work demands were previously found to be contextually relevant to major junior hockey by Bruner (2002) and Koshan (2004). Bruner's report delineated the academic goals and the education packages related to the experiences of middle adolescents. Koshan briefly outlined this challenge in his journalistic internship with one OHL team located in a larger urban location. Within the present report, the in-depth perspectives and elaborate descriptions by our purposive sample provided more detail regarding how sport and academic demands were experienced across major junior careers. Precisely, the balancing of school and hockey remained a significant challenge across developmental stages. Competing work challenges were complicated further for those within the present report, in part because of the long hours spent traveling (e.g., distractions on the bus, early morning and late night bus trips, lack of quality homework time). It also appears that educational demands increased for the late adolescent athletes. These demands were often at a time when post-secondary pursuits conflicted with sport advancement and a potential sport career. Consequently, the ability to develop effective time management skills during each week, and also during lengthy trips was necessary adaptation strategies, especially in the latter part of careers.

Social Demands

Adolescence is regarded as a time when one's social development requires extensive interactions with peer groups (Brown, 1993; Fisher, 1989), and where peer pressures are prominent (Feldman and Elliott, 1990). Bruner (2002) and Koshan (2004) have already documented that major junior athletes encounter constrained social time away from sport, and so, a slightly different developmental experience from the adolescent norm. At the onset of major junior careers, the athletes within this report recognized (and considered) the many sacrifices they had to make such as following a curfew and curtailing their social time with peers outside of ice-hockey. However, as the athletes progressed to late adolescence, they were keenly aware that in order to make it to retain their status, or progress to the next level of professional sport, ongoing social sacrifices would be necessary. Such recognitions were also reflected in personal relationships. For those able to manage personal relationships, there were challenges associated with limited time allotment, and the possibility of relocation due to trade, promotion, or demotion. Consequently, it would seem that what was gained in athletic development and status was countered by atypical and limited (possibly limiting) social opportunities.

Within Team Pressures

Contextual challenges included the mental and physical pressures emanating from on- and off-ice expectations. Within the literature, authors have eluded to the team related adjustment challenges as athletes experience promotion (Bruner, 2002) or maintenance (Koshan, 2004) within major junior ice-hockey. These demands included the adjustment to high quality players, a faster game, and the internal pressures associated with status retention (see also Baker and Schafer, 1988). When Schinke et al. (submitted for publication) considered these same team pressures among rookie and veteran NHL athletes, a place many of our respondents aspired to, similar themes emerged. Precisely, the athletes (rookie and veteran alike) were selected for and accepted within their new professional teams contingent on performance. Within the present report, team pressures again consisted of the difficulties and expectations related to achieving a continuously high level of performance. Among the pressures, the athletes were also concerned about meeting the coach's expectations as athletes and as team representatives. In later years on the team (perhaps a new team), the athletes were also expected to set an example and standard of conduct for younger team-mates, and in most instances to don formal and informal roles within the group. The importance of such roles has already been documented from the views of expert ice-hockey coaches (Schinke, Draper, and Salmela, 1997). The present work again, has supported that there are stated and un-stated team pressures within elite ice-hockey, and further, that athletes are very aware of what those expectations are.

Being in a Remote Region

There has been recent indication that where one is geographically located, also, can be regarded as a sport-related challenge. Previously, Gauthier and colleagues (2006) reported that pursuing elite sport within a remote region of Canada posed as a challenge and a benefit. Gauthier et al. learned from the views of nationally certified elite coaches from Northern Ontario, Canada, that there were challenges recruiting and retaining talented athletes across sport disciplines. Further, it was noted that there was extensive travel associated with pursuing competition, when located (and relocated) away from larger urban centres. Similar to the coaches' views discussed in Gauthier and colleagues, and most likely reflective of the fact that both respondent groups were from the same region, the major junior hockey players in this report echoed many of the same regional challenges. Precisely, the athletes herein identified travel distances and its impingement on academic and social development as challenging. In addition, there was indication that athlete recruitment and retention is also on the minds of transitional athletes when they consider relocating, not just coaches.

Countering the limitations of being located within a remote region, in keeping with previous work by Gauthier and colleagues, the present report also identified placement benefits. For instance, the athletes within this report all indicated that there were a wide number of social support resources that contributed to their adaptation to a new level, a new location, or both. Team-mates were supportive resource, and it was said that shared loneliness facilitated a tight knit experience among team members. In addition, coaching staff and community members were also regarded as supportive of the athletes, especially because there was an understanding of the challenges associated with being from (and now a part of) a remote community.

Limitations

The limitations with the present study pertain to participant recruitment and access, generalizability of the findings, and retrospective interviewing.

Participant recruitment. Participant recruitment and access refers to the difficulties this researcher faced when approaching team management and league executives while attempting to seek endorsement of the study. It seems as though this limitation, which was previously reported by Bruner (2002), regarding the unwillingness "to participate in research for fear of exposing a weakness in their organization or the OIIL" (p. 60), continues to hold true within elite ice-hockey. As such, the first author was constrained to a limited pool of athletes, recruited by word of mouth as opposed to more formal means (e.g., coaching staff).

Transferable results. The current study provides several unique contributions to the literature. For instance, the results from this report target major junior hockey players from one league (Ontario Hockey League), and within, from one remote region (Northern Ontario, Canada). Studies about elite sport experiences from such regions uncover fascinating adaptation challenges, and consequently, creative problem solving. However the strength of the study can also be regarded as its weakness. For instance, a region specific case study can be regarded as unrepresentative of more general adaptation challenges experienced by major junior athletes across regions of Canada, the United States, and Europe. That said it is hoped that this report will provide insight into the experiences and perceptions that are relevant to aspiring elite junior ice-hockey players from remote locations during their adolescence.

Interviewing in retrospect. Retrospective interviewing does not always allow for critical insight into respondent's psychological processes. This is mainly attributed to the higher level of critical thinking required as well as the level of detail in the recall of past experiences. Retrospection, however still can bring forth relevant information related to respondents' views. For the purpose of this study, all of the respondents are still within their late adolescence, and the three types of probing previously discussed enhanced the reliability of the data.

Recommendations for Applied Practice

The goal of the research was to learn from the players' lived experiences and their perspectives of adapting at the major junior level within one remote regional location. It is assumed by these authors that many countries are exemplified by elite athletes (and teams of elite athletes) located well outside of urban centers. As such, the present report can provide helpful suggestions for athletes and their personal support resources, coaches, and sport psychologists. For athletes located in remote locations, there is indication that community resources can offset the physical demands associated with extensive travel. The present report exemplifies the importance of the athletes' perspectives, which can certainly help current and aspiring elite ice-hockey players alike recognize and cope with developmental challenges while they perform (and develop) in smaller remote communities. Some of the effective pathways to athlete adaptation within a remote region included the development of strong sport and community peer affiliation. In addition, it has become clear that the aspiring major junior athlete can also garner emotional support from a wide array of sport and community based resources while they acclimate to relocation challenges.

Parents, coaches, and community resources involved with major junior athletes could also benefit from the present report. For parents, there is indication that the challenges of physical relocation, especially before adulthood, could be offset by an encouragement of meaningful relationships with host families, coaching staff, and community resources. Coaches within remote locations can enhance the athlete's experience first, by using their remoteness as a selling point to recruit aspiring athletes. Once athletes have relocated, the major junior coaches and other resources can also become more effective in helping the athletes access effective support mechanisms within the team and within the larger community. The applied sport psychology consultant working with athletes located in remote communities ought to encourage a delicate balance between community assimilation, sport, and educational development, especially during middle adolescence. Lastly, it is possible for the information gathered from this study to be used as research and teaching material within national coaching certification programs.

References

Baker, T., and Schafer, R. (1988). Major junior or U.S. college? *Hockey Coaching Journal, 1*(5), 20-21.

Brown, B. B. (1993). Peer groups and peer cultures. In S. S. Feldman and G. R. Elliott (Eds.), *At the threshold: The developing adolescent* (171-196). Cambridge: Harvard University.

Bruner, M. (2002). An investigation of the cognitive, social, and emotional development of major junior OHL hockey players. Unpublished master's thesis document, University of Windsor, Windsor, Ontario, Canada.

Côté, J., Salmela, J. H., Baria, A., and Russell, S. J. (1993). Organizing and interpreting unstructured qualitative data. *The Sport Psychologist, 7,* 127-137.

Côté, J., Salmela, J. H., Trudel, P., Baria, A., and Russell, S. J. (1995). The coaching model: A grounded assessment of expert gymnastic coaches' knowledge. *Journal of Sport and Exercise Psychology,* 17, 1-17.

Feldman, S., and Elliott, G. (1990). Capturing the adolescent experience. In S. S. Feldman and G. R. Elliott (Eds.), *At the threshold: The developing adolescent* (pp. 1-13). Cambridge: Harvard University.

Fisher, S. (1989). *Homesickness, cognition, and health.* Brighton: Erlbaum.

Gauthier, A., Schinke, R. J., and Pickard, P. (2006). Coaching adaptation: Techniques learned and taught in one northern Canadian region. *The Sport Psychologist, 20,* 449-464.

Koshan, T. (2004, November 10 and 11). A room with a view: A week with the Brampton Battalion. *The Toronto Sun,* S12-S15, S8-S11.

Maxwell, J. (2002). Understanding and validity in qualitative research. In M. A. Huberman, and M. B. Miles (Eds.). *The qualitative researcher's companion* (pp.37-63). Thousand Oaks: Sage.

Ministry of Northern Development and Mines Website. (2005, April 15). Retrieved June 3, 2005, from http://www.mndm.gov.on.ca/mndm/nordev/redb/sector_profiles/ Northern_ontario_e.pdf.

Patton M. Q. (2002). *Qualitative research and evaluation methods* (3rd ed.). Thousand Oakes, CA: Sage.

Paul, E. L., and Brier, S. (2001). Friendsickness in the transition to college: Precollege predictors and college adjustment correlates. *Journal of Counseling and Development, 79,* 77-88.

Schinke, R. J., and da Costa, J. (2000). Qualitative research in the sport psychology. *Avante, 6,* 38-45.

Schinke, R. J., Draper, S. P., and Salmela, J. H. (1997). A conceptual model of team building in high-performance sport as a season-long process. *Avante, 3,* 47-62.

Schinke, R. J., Gauthier, A., Dubuc, N. G., and Crowder, T. Understanding adaptation in professional hockey through an archival source. Submitted for publication.

Schinke, R. J., Michel, G., Gauthier, A., Danielson, R., Peltier, D., Enosse, L., et al. (2006). The adaptation to elite sport: A Canadian Aboriginal perspective. *The Sport Psychologist, 21,* 435-448.

Tesch, R. (1990). *Qualitative analysis types and software.* New York: Falmer.

In: Sport and Exercise Psychology Research Advances   ISBN: 978-1-60456-157-9
Editors: M. P. Simmons, L. A. Foster, pp. 157-174   © 2008 Nova Science Publishers, Inc.

Chapter VI

Examining Third Order Effects on Adolescents' Sport Participation and Motivation

Enrique García Bengoechea[10] and William B. Strean[2]
1. McGill University, Montreal, Quebec, Canada
2. Faculty of Physical Education and Recreation, University of Alberta, Edmonton, Alberta, Canada

Abstract

In this study we examined the perceptions of a group of adolescents representing a variety of sport experiences regarding the motivational impact of what Bronfenbrenner (1979) called "second party" or "third order" effects, in allusion to the influence of other members of the social group on the interactions between two people. Qualitative analyses of semi-structured interview data highlighted several circumstances where participants took an active role in negotiating multiple interpersonal influences in the context of their sport participation. Specifically, exercising personal judgment and choice when faced with conflicting information and seeking to compensate the motivational deficits associated with particular relational contexts were two ways through which participants negotiated multiple influences and became active agents of their socialization and development in sport. We situate the findings and suggest avenues for future research in the context of a systems-style approach (Bugental and Goodnow, 1998) for the study of socialization processes in youth sport.

Keywords: *Adolescence, motivation, socialization, interpersonal dynamics, youth sport.*

10 Corresponding author: Enrique García Bengoechea, PhD, Assistant Professor, Department of Kinesiology and Physical Education, McGill University, 475 Pine Avenue West Montreal, Quebec, Canada, H2W 1S4, Phone: (514) 398-4184 ext. 0541 Fax: (514) 398-4186, E-mail: enrique.garcia@mcgill.ca.

Introduction

Organized sport is a valued context of participation and development for many adolescents across North America. For example, statistics indicate that over 7.1 million U.S. students participate in high school sports (National Federation of State High School Associations, 2007) and many North American adolescents participate regularly in organized sports in their leisure time. A key factor in determining the nature of the youth sport experience as well as its outcomes is the motivation of participants to remain involved in and to achieve in sport (e.g., Fry, 2001; Weiss and Williams, 2004). Reeve (1995) explained that the study of motivation addresses more than just the problems of students'--or athletes' for that matter--lack of interest, low effort, and disengagement. Rather, Reeve argued, it is also about fostering psychological growth and healthy development. Indeed, several motivation theorists have posited the existence in the human being of an innate energy or tendency to grow and develop as competent and well adjusted individuals (e.g., Deci and Ryan, 1985; Harter, 1978; Maslow, 1987; White, 1959). Such an innate tendency, however, can be either nurtured or thwarted in the course of an individual's daily interactions with his/her environment. Therefore, as Vallerand (2001) has suggested, motivation should be seen in terms of an ongoing transaction between individuals and their environments.

Researchers studying the influence of the social environment on adolescents' sport motivation have mainly focused on the independent influence of significant others such as parents, coaches, and peers (e.g., Allen and Howe, 1998; Babkes and Weiss, 1999; Smith, 1999). In recent years, researchers have taken an interest in how significant others interact or combine to produce an impact on children's and adolescents' sport motivation. For example, Averill and Power (1995) examined the relation between parental childrearing attitudes and children's experiences in sport. Their results showed that an adequate understanding of the outcomes of the interaction between the coach and the athlete cannot be obtained without taking into consideration the nature of the parent-athlete interaction. Specifically, their findings revealed that mothers and fathers who reported the highest level of involvement in their child's soccer experience had children reporting the lowest level of cooperation with the coach. Van Yperen (1995) underscored the buffering effect of parental support against the impact of low individual performance levels on perceptions of team interpersonal stress in elite male youth soccer players. More recently, Vazou, Ntoumanis, and Duda (2006) found additive effects on several indices of young athletes' motivation as a result of their perceptions of the coach-and peer-created motivational climate. However, they did not find significant interaction effects. As a possible explanation, Vazou and colleagues advanced that since within each team both coach and peer climates were rated as being more task-involving than ego-involving, there was no within team incompatibility between coach and peer motivational climates. In another study dealing with the motivational implications of youth soccer players' perceptions of their relationships with parents and peers, Ullrich-French and Smith (2006), on the other hand, reported both additive and interactive effects. In terms of the latter, for example, the results revealed that self-determined motivation is positively related with the quality of the athlete-mother relationship when the quality of the athletes' friendships with peers is relatively lower, but is not related with mother relationship quality when friendship quality is relatively higher. In light of these results, Ullrich-French and

Smith concluded that considering the combination of parent, peer group and friendships relationships is critical when it comes to understand the link between motivation and social relationships in youth sport.

Adopting a qualitative approach, García Bengoechea and Strean (2007), sought to understand how a group of adolescents representing a variety of sport experiences made sense of the interpersonal environment and its motivational influence in sport. García Bengoechea and Strean found that participants perceived other individuals around them as playing five major motivational roles, namely providers of support, sources of pressure and control, sources of competence-relevant information, agents of socialization of achievement orientations, and models to emulate. Further, the participants saw a fairly large number of individuals besides parents and coaches (e.g., siblings, relatives, team mates, opponents, elite athletes, school peers, school teachers, spectators) as involved in playing these roles.

As the previous studies show, a focus on multiple interpersonal influences and their dynamic interplay helps us to better understand the nature and outcomes of sport participation in children and adolescents. One way of conceptualizing and making sense of this interplay that has proven useful is what Bronfenbrenner (1979) called "second party" or "third order" effects. These effects concern the indirect influence of other parties (e.g., parents) on the interactions between members of a dyad (e.g., coach-athlete). Thus, and since each member of a microsystem (i.e., a pattern of interpersonal relations experienced on a face to face basis) influences every other member, Bronfenbrenner (1989) argued that it is important to take into account the influence of each relationship on other relationships. The appropriate design for this purpose, according to Bronfenbrenner, is one in which each relationship is considered as a context for processes taking place in the other. Bronfenbrenner's view is consistent with Bugental and Goodnow (1998), who argued that the specific research strategies for exploring the impact of the social group may vary, but the common aim is "to create some merger between a focus on interactions between two people and the recognition that other members of the social group are also a part of that interaction" (p. 440).

Two qualitative studies illustrate the merits of using such an approach when studying adolescents in sport. As part of a larger study examining coaches' perceptions of contextual factors in youth sport, Strean (1995) recounted the experience of two coaches who coached in the same soccer club and held similar objectives. The first coach, who had poor relations with parents and little support, struggled to coach his team. For example, this coach had to direct much of his energy and attention during games to screaming parents. Having developed rapport with parents and created a structure of parental support, on the other hand, the second coach found his situation very favourable and experienced few tensions as he coached his young players throughout the season. More recently, Jowett and Timson-Katchis (2005) investigated the impact of parents on the relationship between female adolescent competitive swimmers and their coaches. Based on interviews with 5 sets of coach-athlete-parent-triads from Greece and Cyprus, Jowett and Timson-Katchis concluded that over-involved parents elicited negative feelings from the coach and the athlete. Similar to the Averill and Power's study (1995), these findings stress the importance of parents keeping their involvement in their children's sport experience in perspective.

Despite the valuable insights provided by the studies previously reviewed, the dynamic interplay of significant others in the interpersonal environment of adolescent sport participants is still poorly understood. This is particularly true if we consider the adolescents' perspective or the meaning they attach to the interpersonal environment and its motivational influence in sport. Consequently, and building upon the initial findings of García Bengoechea and Strean (2007), the purpose of this study was to examine the perceptions of a group of adolescents representing a variety of sport experiences regarding the impact of third parties on their relationships with other individuals and its motivational consequences in sport.

Method

Participants

Consistent with a maximum variation sampling strategy (Patton, 1990; Seidman, 1998), the participants were twelve athletes, aged 13-17, who represented a variety of experiences in terms of sport and competitive level. Specifically, the athletes included one 13-year-old female ("Sheryl" [11]), who took part in basketball, fastball, and volleyball; two 14-year-old females: "Kirsten" (swimming), and "Miriam" (badminton); three 14-year-old males: "Samuel" (swimming), "Nelson" (swimming, basketball), and "Ralph" (soccer, volleyball); two 15-year-old females: "Sarah" (badminton), and "Jill" (track and field, soccer); one 15-year-old male: "Daniel" (soccer, snowboarding); one 16-year-old male: "Brian" (football, basketball); one 17-year-old male: "Neil" (soccer, football); and one17-year-old female: "Anna" (tennis). Of these, Sheryl, Ralph, Jill, Daniel, Brian, and Neil participated mostly in leagues and contests at the city level. Kirsten, Miriam, Samuel, Nelson, Sarah, and Anna had reached the more demanding provincial level. Miriam, Sarah, and Anna also had experience competing at the elite national level in their respective age groups.

We recruited all participants from a variety of youth sport settings in a large Western Canadian City. In compliance with standard ethical procedures, participants and one of their parents filled out an informed consent form.

Data Collection and Analysis

Drawing on insights from an interpretative phenomenological approach (e.g., Smith, 1995) we collected data through semi-structured interviews. Trying to understand the content and complexity of the meanings that people attach to their experiences is a central concern within a phenomenological framework. This involves the investigator engaging in an interpretative relationship with the transcript.

Specifically, each participant took part in two semi-structured interviews, which were conducted by the first author. All interviews were audio-recorded and transcribed verbatim. After a series of questions to facilitate rapport and get to know better the participants from a motivational standpoint (e.g., "Tell me about your goals as an athlete"), the first interview dealt broadly with the individuals that the participants perceived as being influential on their

---

[11] All participants' names are pseudonyms.

sport motivation and how they were influential. This part of the interview consisted of an initial open-ended question, which was the same for all the participants: "Think of people who have an influence on your motivation as an athlete... How do these people have an influence?" Following this initial question, subsequent questions and the order in which they were asked varied for each participant. This was done so as to not to constrain the participants' evocation of individuals perceived as being influential and the order in which they came to their minds. When appropriate, following-upon the participants' responses, the interviewer asked questions intended to understand how the participants perceived third parties as being influential on their relationships with other individuals in sport (e.g., "...what did your father say when your coach did that?"). The second interview with each participant provided an excellent opportunity to ask clarification and elaboration questions to shed light on issues that remained unclear in the first interview and to address new topics of interest.

Consistent with Polkinghorne's (1995) concept of analysis of narratives, data analysis proceeded through different phases aimed to identify major patterns in the data. The relatively low number of participants allowed us to do so while still being able to maintain a sense of the individuality of each participant. After several readings of the transcripts, the first major analytic phase of the research consisted of coding the data (Charmaz, 1995). Initial codes were used to start breaking the data into meaningful units and to begin to see processes and phenomena of interest in general at work. Focused codes that made the most analytic sense and that encompassed the data most accurately and completely were then used to sort through larger amounts of data.

Categories were developed from meaningful fragments or units of data that were identified in the data set (see Merriam, 1998). The process of filling out emergent categories was assisted by constant comparison procedures in which one respondent's experiences and perceptions where compared with another respondent's in an iterative process, using the look/feel alike criteria proposed by Lincoln and Guba (1985). In such a process, subsequent units were compared to units already coded and integrated into emerging categories and were either added to them or used eventually to develop new categories. In sum, the search for emerging categories entailed a recursive movement between noted similar instances in the data and the emerging categories during the process of organizing the data according to their commonalties (Polkinghorne, 1995). This recursive movement was carried out until a particular category was saturated, that is until no new information about this category seemed to emerge during the coding process (Strauss and Corbin, 1998).

In addition, we adopted several strategies outlined by Rossman and Rallis (2003) to ensure that our analysis was rigorous and credible. These included a peer debriefing strategy in which the second author helped the first author clarify the basis for his emerging interpretations and conclusions; member checking of emerging interpretations during the second interview with each participant; provision of rich description of the circumstances in which the data were found to hold; and prolonged immersion in the data as the first author endeavoured to make sense of the large amounts of available information through the procedures previously described.

Results

The analyses highlighted several instances in which the participants perceived third parties as being influential on their interactions with other people in sport. At the outset of the analytic strategy, we grouped these instances in two overarching categories, which we labelled, respectively, "competing messages" and "compensatory effects." Further, compensatory effects occurred within the context of the role of others as providers of informational, emotional, and companionship support, and as sources of competence-relevant information.

Competing Messages

Participants reported how, occasionally, parents and coaches gave technical information that clearly contradicted or conflicted with what each other were suggesting to athletes. This happened, for example, when parents and coaches held different points of view as to how specific skills should be performed or about what aspects of the game the athletes should be paying more attention to. Nelson, for example, recalled a time when his basketball coach gave him instructions that clashed with what his father had taught him and he himself believed was the best to do in that particular situation:

> That was an awkward situation because he [coach] did expect me to do that [stand in front of a taller player in the post and try to deny the pass] and I knew for a fact that he was wrong on that. And I went to my dad to get help on what should I do there. And I think he had a talk with the coach eventually. But I showed the coach that it could be done another way.

Conversely, Neil reminisced about a situation in which he favoured his coach's technical advice when it conflicted with his mother's:

> A lot of goalies have to jump to make the save because they have poor footwork and they are not at the right place at the right time to make the easy saves. This is what I have to say to counter her [mother]. My coach tells me "don't jump unless you have to, don't dive unless you have to." So I am always trying to be at the right place at the right time to make the easy save. My mom always says "you are not jumping around as the other goalies."

Parents and coaches sent also contradictory or conflicting information when they disagreed about the evaluation of an athlete's performance and in the subsequent feedback that they gave to him/her. This was the case of Daniel, who mentioned that his parents sometimes tell him that he has played an "awesome" game while his coach thinks he has just played a "bad" one.

Although finding themselves in awkward situations occasionally, receiving contradictory information from parents and coaches about, for example, what to do in specific game scenarios did not necessarily place participants in a position in which they experienced conflict or pressure to abide by the expectations of either of them. When put in a similar situation, participants in this study typically reported considering both points of view and using their own judgment to decide what to do. Some participants also explained that they brought up and discussed with their coaches the technical advice that their parents had given to them in order to avoid potential controversies. Nelson and Sarah offered their perspective on these particular issues: "It's pretty much my own judgment that I have to go. Only my team mates, occasionally, but usually my own judgment, or I take a combination of the two [coach and father's advice]" (Nelson); "… and if there is [conflicting information], then I'll discuss it with either of them [father and coach] and ask why and then do whatever I feel comfortable with doing." (Sarah). Similarly, Sheryl stated:

And even if my mom mentions something extra, I usually put a little extra focus on that too. Just because if she thinks that it's a little inadequate maybe I should be working on it even if my coach doesn't bring it up. Or I'll ask my coach if I should be working on that as well.

More often than not, however, participants reported that they took the coaches' technical advice rather than the parents' when both were in opposition. Samuel, for example, said, "I just do what I think I should do, but I usually take the coaches' [advice]." In the same vein, Miriam admitted:

I react differently to what my coach says rather than, like compared to what my dad says sometimes. Maybe when my coach says something, my dad has said it before, but I will pay more attention to it if my coach says it.

Competing messages were also evident in situations in which participants faced mixed messages from others regarding their sport abilities. Interestingly, these participants seemed able to maintain an overall sense of athletic worth by deliberately choosing to pay more attention to messages indicating competence rather than incompetence. This leads us directly into the next section.

Compensatory Effects

Focusing on the motivational influence of third parties on dyadic relationships revealed the existence of compensatory effects. Specifically, athletes actively attempted to compensate for the motivational deficits of a particular relationship by relying more on other relationships.

The development of compensatory effects occurred both over relatively short (up to the duration of a sport season) and long (spanning an athlete's sport career) periods of time. As an example of the former, Sheryl recalled how relying on her team mates and friends compensated to some degree the negative motivational influence that one of her coaches exerted on her one particular season:

I am really a social person… and having a group of 12 girls around [on the team] is like heaven . . . And, especially with sports, because I somehow ended up with a group of friends who are almost completely non-athletic. I have got three friends that play sport with me. So being around so many people who have the same interests as me is really fun… And your coach, you kind of get over. It balances out. They balance each other out.

As an example of the latter, Neil elaborated on the circumstance that his mother is not "as big motivation as she was before" in the following terms:

When I started off, when I was young, my parents weren't concerned about us winning or anything, go there and have fun, that's all that was about for me. And right now a lot of times it's still about fun, going out and having fun, but at this competitive level it comes more about winning, and so your coaches and sometimes your team mates have to motivate you to win. My mom, she is not an expert, but she says what she can to help me out.

The development of compensatory effects was most evident within the context of the role of other individuals as providers of informational, emotional, and companionship support, and as sources of competence-relevant information.

Compensatory Effects within the Role of others as Providers of Informational Support

Compensatory effects in relation to the role of coaches and parents as providers of task specific informational support were manifest in two specific circumstances. First, athletes compensated for the lack of attention from coaches by actively seeking technical feedback from other sources such as team mates and knowledgeable family members (e.g., parents, siblings, and cousins). This mainly happened when the number of athletes that coaches were in charge of and/or the complexity of certain game situations in team sports made it difficult for them to keep an eye on all the players all or most of the time. For example, Kirsten, noted that since her coach cannot watch everybody in the water, "[sometimes] I would ask her [team mate] to help me and see if I can do anything better than [name of coach] may not have seen." Similarly, Sarah remarked that "players coach each other too, especially when the coach can't be watching everyone. Just watching a game and giving each other feedback."

Second, when coaches or parents were not perceived by athletes as being knowledgeable enough about the sport or about particular aspects of it, other individuals in the athletes' network perceived as more knowledgeable were likely to take on their role as primary sources of technical information for athletes. Jill, for instance, recalled in regard to this:

We go to soccer together, and then hockey I go there, and basketball sometimes she [younger sister] comes to watch me. So we are always there for each other, and we can pick up more things that happened than our parents, because we know what is going on (laughs). So we can help each other out, how to improve, and what went wrong or what's good, and lots of good stuff, I guess, for improvement and to keep us into the game.

The case of another athlete, Nelson, provides an excellent example of a father becoming the main technical point of reference for an athlete over and beyond the coach. Nelson explained the reasons why he usually takes his father's side rather than his coach's when the advice of both clashes:

> So I really have to rely on my own judgment to decide what's best to do, but a lot of the times this year I have gone with my dad's advice because I know he knows what he's doing, especially in the area I play. That's where he always used to play. He knows it very well, and I know for a fact that my coach never played there. He is more of an outside player.

Compensatory effects within the context of the role of others as providers of informational support also occurred in relation to the role of fathers and mothers. The story of Neil constitutes a case in point in that it shows that, even when they are not perceived as being particularly knowledgeable about sports, mothers can eventually take on some of the roles that fathers typically played in this study when, for different reasons, the latter are not often around. This circumstance can be seen in the following comment, in response to the question of whether he talks after the games about his performance with his father, in the rare occasions when the latter attended Neil's games:

> Yes, I do, but my dad hasn't been involved in soccer really or in any of my sports in a long time. So I kind of feel like when I talk to him he just kind of, he doesn't exactly know where I am at, in terms of skill and competition and all that. I would rather talk to my mom about soccer and sports.

Compensatory Effects within the Role of others as Providers of Emotional and Companionship Support

An analysis of the influence of others on the participants' motivation revealed the importance of the availability of people who understand as an "outlet" for athletes to talk about what they are going through in their sport practice. This was particularly true for female athletes in this study (see García Bengoechea and Strean, 2007). Likewise, such an analysis highlighted the importance for athletes of having others in their networks with whom to share social and recreational activities within the context of casual relationships or friendships. Compensatory effects within the role of others as providers of emotional support were necessary to offset the negative motivational influence coming from school peers who did not show an interest for or an understanding of athletes' sport participation. Likewise, compensatory effects developed in order to counteract the negative impact of peers who criticized what athletes were doing (e.g., putting so much time into training and competing) or the sport they were taking part in. As an example of this, Sarah shared her negative experiences with some school peers: "A negative influence[on my sport motivation] is badminton being sort of a new not very popular sport lots of people sort of criticize it . . . people in school. Like basketball, volleyball, and hockey those are the real sports." In a similar vein, Anna recalled:

It is harder to be friends with some people at school just because they don't understand where you are coming from and they don't understand why you are doing what you are doing, they don't really have a care or an interest for it.

Specifically, athletes made up for the lack of interest in and/or understanding about their sport practice from peers by talking about what they were going through with family members involved in their sport participation (e.g., parents, siblings). Likewise, they did so by talking about their sport practice to people, such as team mates and coaches, with whom they shared the same interests and experiences:

Not many of my school friends play badminton, so they don't really know what it is like. They play sports and they know about tournaments and competitive sports, but they don't really know how to play badminton, so I don't talk to them much about it. I will just say "it was good" or . . . I don't really go into depth with them, as I do with my friends from [name of city], who actually play badminton. (Miriam)

Kirsten referred specifically to the buffering effect that interacting with her coaches has against the negative influence of some of her school peers, who do not understand what she does and sometimes criticize her sport (e.g., by saying "swimming is stupid"):

You know you don't want to be around them, but you are because you are in class with them. You have to. And then, sometimes, they have an effect on you, and that doesn't help you very much. But then, when you are around the coaches and staff they always have a positive influence on us, so we get the back up. But sometimes, just being around our friends at school [is a negative motivational influence] because they don't understand that they don't help you at all.

Compensatory effects within the role of others as providers of companionship support emerged also as a response to the progressive loss of social life that was eventually associated with increasing time demands in terms of training and competition. Spending more and more hours training and competing made it difficult at times for athletes to keep up with friends and acquaintances that were not involved in sport. In compensation, friends made through sport took increasingly the role of school or other friends as companions to "hang out" with and share spare time activities together. The case of Anna, however, was particularly interesting because it raises the possibility that the development of compensatory effects may not always be fully successful in making up for a given affective or motivational lack:

You are surrounded by the people that you have been going to school with for like the last eight years, and it is sort of hard to see it slip away . . . You meet a few new players at practice and you can become pretty good friends over the year. But after the year ends, you don't really keep in touch. But the people that really mean a lot are the people that you see every day at school. So it is a little bit, it is like a give and take on both sides, but it is more of a loss than it is a gain, I would say.

Compensatory Connections within the Role of others as Sources of Competence-Relevant Information

Lastly, the development of compensatory effects was also apparent in situations in which athletes faced conflicting messages from others regarding their sport abilities. Indeed, the process of data analysis brought to light several instances in which athletes seemed able to maintain an overall sense of athletic competence by paying more attention to or giving more weight to messages from others that were indicative of one's ability rather than of one's lack of skill. This was the case of Samuel, who despite receiving negative messages about his sport competence and worth from some school peers and, occasionally, from his sister (e.g., "they discourage me saying that I can't do it or that it would be too hard," "they say I'm stupid and I can't do anything right") was able to maintain a belief in his possibilities to achieve his goals also by relying strongly on positive competence messages from his parents and his coach (e.g., saying to him "there is no limits to what you can do," " you have the ability to do it and you might just do if you work really hard"). In a related vein, despite recognizing that most of his coaches had, in a way or another, sent him the message that he is not a good player, Daniel, made, nevertheless, the following assertion when elaborating about his perceived soccer competence: "So, I don't know, I enjoy it [soccer] lots because I'm really good at it, some people say, and, well, my mom does, and my brother does too."

Discussion

A characteristic of contexts often emphasized in analyses of socialization within socio-cultural perspectives is the degree to which there is homogeneity or heterogeneity, consensus or diversity in the information about the world that is available to individuals in a given group (Bugental and Goodnow, 1998). Once thought of as an automatic source of difficulty, the presence of a variety of messages and positions is increasingly seen as an open window for benefit and mutual facilitation and as offering the individual an opportunity for exploring alternatives and making choices (e.g., Bugental and Goodnow, 1998; Corsaro and Eder, 1990). As per their accounts, athletes in the present study were in most cases able to deal with competing technical messages from coaches and athletes in a constructive manner through the exercise of personal judgment and choice. This finding can be interpreted as an indication that adolescent athletes are active contributors to their own socialization in sport rather than passive recipients of external influences (see Bugental and Goodnow, 1998). Nevertheless, it is also possible that the circumstance that parents of athletes in this study were not typically perceived as being over-involved or negatively involved in their children's participation may have contributed to ease potential tensions. Thus, a challenge for future studies in this area is to shed light on the possible consequences of facing messages that are overly competitive with or antagonistic to one another and are accompanied by pressure to abide by the expectations of the sender.

The finding that athletes attempted to compensate for the motivational shortfalls of a particular relationship by investing more energy into or relying more on other relationships is particularly significant on several grounds. For example, Parke and Buriel (1998) contended that the challenge for future work within comprehensive system-style approaches to socialization is to determine the circumstances under which "strong, weak, or compensatory connections might be expected between relationship systems" (p. 485). In this study, one of such circumstances deserving particular attention concerns the dynamics within the role of others as providers of task specific informational support. For example, although athletes typically reported taking the coach's advice when the technical information they receive from parents and coaches collides, there was some evidence that this trend may be reversed when the coach is not perceived as being as knowledgeable as one of the parents. Likewise, there was some indication that traditional gender roles in regards to patterns of parental involvement in youth sport in North America may be inverted to some extent when fathers are away from home for different circumstances. As Coakley (2001) acknowledged, these traditional gender roles imply that fathers are typically more involved on technical and administrative issues than mothers are. In addition, the results highlight the important role that peers (e.g., team mates) may be called to play when, because of not being able--or willing--to pay enough attention to his/her athletes, the coach does not adequately meet the athletes' needs for skill-relevant information at a given time.

The significance of examining the phenomenon of motivational compensation is further emphasized when one considers the development of compensatory effects that occurred between relationships operating in two or more settings. Within the framework of his hierarchical model of motivation, Vallerand (2001) proposed that "the dynamic interplay between motivational processes in different life contexts may also lead to what may be called the compensation effect" (p. 313). Specifically, Vallerand (2001) suggested that it is possible that losses of motivation in one life context may be made up for by motivational gains in a second life context. For instance, some evidence exists that losses of motivation in the education context can be compensated for to a certain degree by gains in motivation in the sport context (see Vallerand, 2001). We also found evidence that the progressive loss of social life that was in some cases associated with increasing training and competition demands can be compensated for to a certain extent by an increasing reliance on team mates as companions and friends. As Brandstätter (1998) stated, human development over the life course appears as a story of gain and loss, of success and failure. Therefore, Brandstätter (1998) explained, efforts to keep this balance favorable are an essential aspect of human activity whose outcomes have a profound impact on individuals' self-perceptions and future expectations.

The results also revealed that negative sport-specific motivational influences from peers at school were, to some extent, "balanced out" by positive motivational influences from peers and coaches on the sport team and family members at home. In this manner, the present findings also provide evidence that motivation in youth sport is not only the result of influential relationships within this particular setting, but also of influential relationships in other settings such as school and home and of their respective linkages. Thus, these results provide support for the relevance of considering relations or linkages between two or more settings in which the developing person participates in order not only to understand processes of human development in general but also motivational issues in particular (e.g., Bronfenbrenner, 1989; García Bengoechea, 2002).

Several authors (e.g., O'Connor and Rosenblood, 1996; Vallerand, 2001) have proposed that a homeostasis mechanism within the self seems to exist in order to restore a general equilibrium of the self in the case of losses in one particular life context. The results indicate that a similar mechanism may be at play to restore a general equilibrium of the self in the case of motivational losses in one particular relationship directly or indirectly related to participation in organized youth sport. Work by Harter, Waters, and Whiteshell (1998) on relational self-worth provides indirect support for this argument. Specifically, Harter et al. found that adolescents' perceived worth as a person varied depending upon which interpersonal contexts one considers (e.g., relationships with parents, teachers, or friends). For example, the perceived worth of some adolescents was high around their friends but low around their parents. Importantly, the adolescents' perceived worth in a particular interpersonal context (e.g., with teachers) was strongly associated with their perceptions of support from others in that interpersonal context (i.e., from teachers). It seems then, as the results illustrate, that adolescent sport participants may actively seek to compensate the psychological deficits associated with a lack of support from others (e.g., school peers) in one particular relational context by investing more "relationship energy" (see Parke and Buriel, 1998) into other interpersonal contexts (e.g., with team mates).

The previous considerations raise a critical issue when looking at the socialization of sport motivation during adolescence. The conception of individuals as active contributors to their own development is prominent in contemporary theories and models of motivation, socialization, and human development in general (e.g., Brandstätter, 1998; Bronfenbrenner, 1989; Bugental and Goodnow, 1998; Deci and Ryan, 1985; Ford and Lerner, 1992; Lerner, 1998). For example, Deci and Ryan (1985) postulated that organismic motivation theories such as self-determination theory (Deci and Ryan, 1985; 1991) tend to view the individual as active, that is, as being volitional or intentional and initiating behaviours rather than being pushed around by the interaction of physiological drives and environmental constraints. Likewise, Bugental and Goodnow explained that there is a common concern in contemporary accounts of socialization about how to make sure that individuals are portrayed as actively influencing the settings that they encounter. Within the framework of an action-theoretical perspective on human development, Brandstätter contended that activities of intentional self-development must be viewed within the larger context of processes that serve to actualize and stabilize one's identity.

Also important in this respect, as Brandstätter (1998) noted, are intentional processes that protect and defend the self against events and changes that the individual perceives as dissonant with his/her existing self-schema. In this study, we found some evidence that participants were able to maintain an overall sense of athletic competence by relying more on information from others that signified high rather than low ability when faced with mixed messages from different people. This, according to Brandstätter, can be seen as an instance of activities of self-verification (Swann, 1983) through which the individual intentionally and preferentially selects social or informational contexts that are likely to provide self-congruent feedback on those dimensions of the self-concept that define one's personal identity.

Finally, the finding that the development of compensatory connections may be examined both over the short-and the long-terms is also important. Indeed, it appears to provide a basis for explaining and interpreting changes in the motivational roles and the relative importance of others in adolescents' sport motivation as the latter develop over time. What is more, it also reinforces the view of motivation as an ongoing transaction between the individual and his/her environment (Vallerand, 2001).

Conclusion

The present study constitutes an effort to move beyond current accounts of the socialization of motivation in adolescent sport participants by adopting a comprehensive perspective that takes multiple sources of perceived influence into consideration and presents the developing individual as an active contributor to his/her own socialization. Taken as a whole, the findings illustrate the significance, and even the necessity, of adopting frameworks for the study of socialization processes in youth sport that move us beyond the analysis of one-way, single source effects to take into account the dynamics within multiple sources of mutual influence. In other words, this study illustrate the benefits, both from a theoretical and a practical perspective, of adopting a systems-style approach (e.g., Bugental and Goodnow, 1998) for the study of socialization processes in youth sport in general and for the study of the socialization of motivation in adolescent sport participants in particular. System-style models of socialization are mainly concerned with the dynamics within a social context and have been prominent in analyses that attempt to describe the interconnections among members of a family and the various parts of a social context (Bugental and Goodnow; see also Parke and Buriel, 1998). Briefly, system-style models of socialization propose that any social context can be seen as forming a whole such that change in any one part flows on to change in others, either dampening or heightening the conditions already existing, until a new but temporal stabilization is achieved (Bugental and Goodnow, 1998).

Several important issues, however, still remain regarding the socialization of motivation in adolescents involved in sport within a systems-style framework. Notably, since the present study constitutes an initial, but by no means definitive, attempt to examine some of the dynamics--in the form of third order effects--within the perceived role of others on adolescents' sport motivation, future studies using both qualitative and quantitative methodologies are needed to further explore some of these dynamics. In relation with the interpersonal dynamics identified in the present study, more research is needed to ascertain the degree to which consensus/homogeneity or diversity/heterogeneity in the messages that significant others send to athletes prevail in youth sport contexts, the ways in which these features are manifested, and the consequences in either case. Likewise, more work is needed to determine the conditions under which compensatory connections among relationships might be expected to develop in order to offset existing motivational deficits. In particular, future efforts should attempt to shed more light on the critical question of whether young sport participants can fully compensate for the motivational shortfalls of a given relationship by investing more energy (Parke and Buriel, 1998) into other relationships. Furthermore, studies are needed that clarify the conditions under which compensatory connections are more or less likely to be successful and the motivational consequences in the case the compensatory attempts do not totally achieve their purposes.

With regard to the development of compensatory connections over extended periods of time, research that looks at how the relative motivational roles of influential others around young sport participants shift across development would be most welcomed. Having an adequate picture of how these roles shift as participants develop would allow us to focus on the important question of whether it is possible to characterize youth sport settings in terms of the relative importance of various relationships at different points in time (see Parke and Buriel, 1998; see also Horn, 2004).

Our understanding of the socialization of motivation in adolescent sport participants would also benefit considerably from expanding the range of our analyses from the level of face-to-face interactions in order to include elements from the broader social and cultural context. Recognition that relationships are embedded in a variety of social settings is critical to understand variation in the functioning of these relationships and the meanings that the social actors attach to them (e.g., Bronfenbrenner, 1989; Parke and Buriel, 1998). In this regard, it is important to note that the participants in this study came mainly from white, intact, middle-to-upper class urban North American families, and therefore the meanings they attached to their experiences and relationships may not adequately represent those of adolescents from different backgrounds. Ultimately, as Vallerand (2001) has suggested, acknowledging the complexity involved in social life should lead us to move from simply studying sport participants as "athletes" to studying whole individuals who in addition to being athletes are students and members of a social--and cultural--matrix.

Finally, future studies on the socialization of motivation in adolescent sport participants should continue to pay attention to documenting the different ways in which individuals contribute to their own socialization and play an active role in their own developmental trajectories in sport. In the present study, exercising personal judgment and choice in the presence of conflicting information and seeking to compensate the motivational deficits associated with particular relational contexts were two specific ways through which adolescents became active agents of their own socialization and development in sport. The ideal result of such continued efforts would be a more complete picture and an enhanced understanding of the processes through which young athletes are able to take advantage of their inner motivational resources (Reeve, 1996) in order to generate their own sport motivation.

References

Allen, J. B., and Howe, B. L. (1998). Player ability, coach feedback, and female adolescent athletes' perceived competence and satisfaction. *Journal of Sport and Exercise Psychology, 20,* 280-299.

Averill, P. M., and Power, T. G. (1995). Parental attitudes and children's experiences in soccer: Correlates of effort and enjoyment. *International Journal of Behavior* Development, 18, 263-276.

Babkes, M. L., and Weiss, M. R. (1999). Parental influence on children's cognitive and affective responses to competitive soccer participation. *Pediatric Exercise Science*, 11, 44-62.

Brandstäter, J. (1998). Action perspectives on human development. In W. Damon (Series Ed.) and R. M. Lerner (Vol. Ed.), *Handbook of child psychology:* Vol. 1. *Theoretical models of human development* (5th ed., pp. 807-863). New York: John Wiley and Sons.

Bronfenbrenner, U. (1979). *The ecology of human development: Experiments by nature and design.* Cambridge, MA: Harvard University Press.

Bronfenbrenner, U. (1989). Ecological systems theory. In R. Vasta (Ed.), *Six theories of child development: Revised formulations and current issues* (pp. 185-246). Greenwich, CT: JAI.

Bugental, D. B., and Goodnow, J. J. (1998). Socialization processes. In W. Damon (Series Ed.) and N. Eisenberg (Vol. Ed.), *Handbook of child psychology:* Vol. 3. *Social, emotional, and personality development* (pp. 389-462). New York: John Wiley and Sons.

Charmaz, K. (1995). Grounded theory. In J. A. Smith, R. Harré, and L. Van Langenhove (Eds.), *Rethinking methods in psychology* (pp. 27-49). London: Sage.

Coakley, J. (2001). *Sport in society: Issues and controversies* (7th ed.) Boston: McGraw-Hill.

Corsaro, W. A., and Miller, P. J. (Eds.). (1992). *Interpretive approaches to socialization.* San Francisco: Jossey-Bass.

Deci, E. L., and Ryan, R. M. (1985). *Intrinsic motivation and self-determination in human behavior.* New York: Plenum.

Deci, E. L., and Ryan, R. M. (1991). A motivational approach to self: Integration in personality. In R. A. Dienstbier (Ed.), *Nebraska symposium on motivation:* Vol 38. *Perspectives on Motivation* (pp. 237-288). Lincoln, NE: University of Nebraska Press.

Ford, D. H., and Lerner, R. M. (1992). *Developmental systems theory: An integrative approach.* Newbury Park, CA: Sage.

Fry. M. D. (2001). The development of motivation in children. In G. C. Roberts (Ed.), *Advances in motivation in sport and exercise* (pp. 51-78). Champaign, IL: Human Kinetics.

García Bengoechea, E. (2002). Integrating knowledge and expanding horizons in developmental sport psychology: A bioecological perspective. *Quest,* 1-20.

García Bengoechea, E., and Strean, W. B. (2007). On the interpersonal context of adolescents' sport motivation. *Psychology of Sport and Exercise,* 8, 195-217.

Harter, S. (1978). Effectance motivation reconsidered. *Human Development, 21,* 34-64.

Harter, S., Waters, P., and Whiteshell, N. R. (1998). Relational self-worth: Differences in perceived worth as a person across interpersonal contexts among adolescents. *Child Development, 69,* 756-766.

Horn, T. S. (2004). Developmental Perspectives on self-perceptions in children and adolescents. In M. R. Weiss (Ed.), *Developmental sport and exercise psychology: A lifespan perspective* (pp. 101-143). Morgantown, WV: Fitness Information Technology.

Jowett, S., and Timson-Katchis, M. (2005). Social networks in sport: The influence of parents on the coach-athlete relationship. *The Sport Psychologist, 19,* 267-287.

Lerner, R. M. (1998). Theories of human development: Contemporary perspectives. In W. Damon (Series Ed.) and R. M. Lerner (Vol. Ed.), *Handbook of child psychology*: Vol. 1. *Theoretical models of human development* (5th ed., pp.1-24). New York: John Wiley and Sons.

Lincoln, Y. S., and Guba, E. G. (1985). *Naturalistic inquiry.* Newbury Park: Sage.

National Federation of State High School Associations. (n.d.). *NFHS high school athletics participation history*. Retrieved April 11, 2007 from http:// www.nfhs.org/web /2006/08 /publications_index.aspx

Maslow, A. H. (1987). *Motivation and personality* (3rd ed.). New York: Harper and Row.

Merriam, S. B. (1998). *Qualitative research and case study applications in education*. San Francisco: Jossey-Bass.

O'Connor, S. C., and Rosenblood, L. K. (1996). Affiliation motivation in everyday experience: A theoretical comparison. *Journal of Personality and Social Psychology, 70,* 513-522.

Patton, M. Q. (1990). *Qualitative evaluation and research methods* (2nd ed.). Newbury Park: Sage.

Parke., R. D., and Buriel, R. B. (1998). Socialization in the family: Ethnic and ecological perspectives. In W. Damon (Series Ed.) and N. Eisenberg (Vol. Ed.), *Handbook of child psychology:* Vol. 3. *Social, emotional, and personality development* (5th ed. pp. 463-552). New York: John Wiley and Sons.

Polkinghorne, D. E. (1995). Narrative configuration in qualitative analysis. International Journal of Qualitative Studies in Education, 8(1), 5-23.

Reeve, J. (1996). *Motivating others. Nurturing inner motivational resources*. Boston: Allyn and Bacon.

Rossman, G. B. and Rallis, S. F. (2003). *Leaning in the field: An introduction to qualitative research* (2nd ed.). Thousand Oaks, CA: Sage.

Seidman, I. E. (1998). *Interviewing as qualitative research: A guide for researchers in education and the social sciences* (2nd ed.). New York: Teachers College Press.

Smith, A. L. (1999). Perceptions of peer relationships and physical activity participation in early adolescence. *Journal of Sport and Exercise Psychology, 21,* 329-350.

Smith, J. A. (1995). Semi-structured interviewing and qualitative analysis. In J. A. Smith, R. Harré, and L. Van Langenhove (Eds.), *Rethinking methods in psychology* (pp. 9-26). London: Sage.

Strauss, A., and Corbin, J. (1998). *Basics of qualitative research: Techniques and procedures for developing grounded theory*. Thousand Oaks, CAL: Sage.

Strean, W. B. (1995).Youth sport contexts: Coaches' perceptions and implications for intervention. *Journal of Applied Sport Psychology, 7,* 23-27.

Swan, W. B. (1983). Self-verification: Bringing the social reality in harmony with the self. In J. Suls and A. G., Greenwald (Eds.), *Psychological perspectives on the self* (vol, 2, pp. 33-66). Hillsdale, NJ: Erlbaum.

Ullrich-French, S., and Smith, A. L. (2006). Perceptions of relationships with parents and peers in youth sport: Independent and combined prediction of motivational outcomes. *Psychology of Sport and Exercise, 7,* 193-214.

Vallerand, R. J. (2001). A hierarchical model of intrinsic and extrinsic motivation in sport and exercise. In G. C. Roberts (Ed.), *Advances in Motivation in Sport and Exercise* (pp. 263-320). Champaign, IL: Human Kinetics.

Van Yperen, N. W. (1995). Interpersonal stress, performance level, and parental support: A longitudinal study among highly skilled young soccer players. *The Sport Psychologist, 9,* 225-241.

Vazou, Z., Ntoumanis, N., and Duda, J. L. (2006). Predicting young athletes' motivational indices as a function of their perceptions of the coach-and peer-created climate. *Psychology of Sport and Exercise, 7,* 215-233.

Weiss, M. R., and Williams, L. (2004). The *why* of youth sport involvement: A developmental perspective on motivational processes. In M. R. Weiss (Ed.) *Developmental sport and exercise psychology: A lifespan perspective* (pp. 223-268). Morgantown, WV: Fitness Information Technology.

White, R. W. (1959). Motivation Reconsidered: The concept of competence. *Psychological Review, 66,* 297-333.

In: Sport and Exercise Psychology Research Advances   ISBN: 978-1-60456-157-9
Editors: M. P. Simmons, L. A. Foster, pp. 175-190   © 2008 Nova Science Publishers, Inc.

Chapter VII

Transition out of Elite Sport: A Dynamic, Multidimensional, and Complex Phenomenon

Yannick Stephan[12] and Virginie Demulier
JE 2494, Paris XI University, Orsay, France

Abstract

Interest in the area of sport career termination has grown considerably in recent years among sport psychology researchers. Over 270 references could be identified on the topic of career transitions in sport during the last three decades. The present chapter aims to review and update existing research and to present some future theoretical and methodological issues emerging from recent advances in this field. Existing research have been guided by three main interests. The first is related to the identification of the nature of retirement from elite sport. Second, a descriptive view has been adopted by researchers to identify athletes' reactions to sport career termination. A third main question in the area of sport career termination concerns the mechanisms and variables playing a role in athletes' reactions and adaptation. The number of explanatory variables identified has grown during the last years, and hypothesized risk or facilitating factors span an enormous range, from individual characteristics to cultural determinants, taking also into account several transition-related variables. The present chapter proposes a reorganisation of the many explanatory variables in two interrelated categories, pre-conditions and transitional factors, which determine the quality of adaptation to retirement. Its appears that transition out of elite sport is a dynamic, complex, and multidimensional phenomenon, given the crucial importance of time in its definition, and the number of variables playing a role in the adaptation process of former athletes.

Keywords: *transition, sport, dynamic, multidimensionality, adaptation*

12 Address for correspondence: Yannick Stephan, PhD, Université Paris XI, JE 2494, Bat. 335 91405 Orsay cedex, France , E-mail: yannick.stephan@u-psud.fr.

Introduction

The standards of high-level performance in sport and its associated demands has increased considerably throughout the years. During the sport career, elite athletes invest a great part of their lives in training, with additional time devoted to traveling and competition. They narrow external activities to achieve optimal athletic performance, which becomes their major life focus (Crook and Robertson, 1991) and, as a result, "it is impossible for him [or her] to be much else" (Werthner and Orlick, 1986, p. 337). However, this athletic involvement, despite its potential benefits for sport achievement, could also have some potential psychological consequences when athletes are faced with sport career termination. Thus, this area of research has received a great interest from sport psychologists desired to better understand the consequences of this phenomenon.

Over the last decades, retirement from elite sport has received considerable attention from scholars (see Lavallee, Wylleman, and Sinclair, 2000; Wylleman, Alfermann, and Lavallee, 2004, for reviews). As emphasized by Lavallee et al. (2000), over 270 references could be identified on the topic of career transitions in sport. Existing research have been guided by three main interests, such as the identification of the nature of retirement from elite sport, identification of athletes' reactions to sport career termination and the mechanisms and variables playing a role in athletes' reactions and adaptation. The present chapter aims to review and update existing research and to present some future theoretical and methodological issues emerging from recent advances in this field.

The nature of retirement from elite sport: From a discrete event to a transitional process

A first axis of research in the area of retirement from elite sport has been interested in the nature of this event. The two first framework used in the area of retirement from elite sport are related to socio-gerontological and thanatological theories (Hill and Lowe, 1974; Lerch, 1981; Rosenberg, 1981). According to these frameworks, the athletic career was seen as a singular, discrete event, portrayed as traumatic, negative, and dysfunctional. However, Coakley (1983) argued that retirement is not an isolated event, but one that occurs for a given person, at a given time, for certain reasons. This author further described that retirement often involves new opportunities and the potential for growth and development. McPherson (1980) states that this perspective must be replaced by a process-oriented approach. Thus, researches re-appraised the termination of the athletic career as a transitional process that initiates a process of adaptation. Retirement is a normative transition that involves elite athletes coping strategies to adapt to their live after leaving top level competition (Stambulova, 2000). It introduces a discontinuity in one's life (Crook and Robertson, 1991) and begins a transition during which athletes are faced with dramatic changes in their personal, social, and occupational lives (Taylor and Ogilvie, 1994).

It is now widely established that transition out of elite sport is often marked by an initial sense of loss leading to a period of personal growth and adaptation (Crook and Robertson, 1991; Kerr and Dacyshyn, 2000; Werthner and Orlick, 1986). A transition is an event or non event which results in a change in assumptions about oneself and the world and thus requires a corresponding change in one's behaviour and relationships (Schlossberg, 1981, p.5). Exiting a career is a major life change that transforms one's social and physical worlds, with changes in roles, relationships, and daily routines (Kim and Moen, 2001). The transformations induced by any transition may well affect how individuals perceive themselves, their abilities and the quality of their lives (Kim and Moen, 2001).

Transitions naturally occur over time. Inherent in the word transition is the notion of change, both internal psychological change, as well as external, behavioural change. Life transitions such as role shifts, or other major life changes often bring about adjustments in existing trajectories. Thus, while athletes may vary in their response, they face several stages that force them to make psychosocial adjustments. This period of transition is a "turning point" (Ebaugh, 1988) in which athletes review their identities, roles, and motivations (Danish, Owens, Green, and Brunelle, 1997). The adjustment process involves a shift in identity, from the identity and orientation of athlete, to a state of disorientation and loss of identity, and finally to a re-orientation and new definition of self (Kerr and Dacyshyn, 2000). Former athletes did not just simply add a new piece to their identity; instead they are found to reorganize existing aspects of self and to establish a more coherent self in different roles.

Transition out of elite sport could be considered as a dynamic phenomenon, that is an evolutive process, where time is a central criteria (Stephan., Bilard, Ninot, and Delignières, 2003a; 2003b). Athletes' adaptation to their retirement is not immediate, but is temporally organized, commencing prior to and continuing well after the event. As emphasized by Danish et al. (1997), retirement from elite sport begin from the time it is anticipated, through its occurrence, until its aftermath has been determined and assessed. This assumption is supported by several studies. Lally (2007) revealed that athletes progressively change their self-identity from pre- to post-retirement. During an initial period, most athletes seem to dangle in a time of uncertainty and disorientation (Kerr and Dacyshyn, 2000; Stephan et al., 2003b). Retirement triggers a series of internal reorganization in the individual's life, with adjustment of references to retirement-induced changes (Stephan et al., 2003a; 2003b). Kerr and Dacyshyn (2000) labelled new beginnings this period following uncertainty and disorientation. In summary, retirement from elite sport is a transitional process, which begins before the actual retirement event, and pursue up to a complete adaptation. Thus, it could be considered as a dynamic process that evolves over time, and where time and changes are of crucial importance.

The Outcomes of Transition out of Elite Sport: A Descriptive View of Reaction and Adaptation Patterns

The descriptive perspective is designed to quantify and illustrate athletes' experience with retirement and the number of athletes concerned with such reactions. The main finding emerging from these studies is that the relationship between retirement and athletes reactions is complex. Reports on the effects of retirement have been inconclusive, and heterogeneity in reactions seems to be the rule.

As Lavallee, Nesti, Borkoles, Cockerill, and Edge (2000) emphasized, an estimated amount of 20% of retired athletes report major problems with their life after the sport career, opposed to 80% who report a healthy career transition. But, three main kind of reactions have been observed and described. A first axis suggests that retirement from elite sport is related to positive reactions or no reactions at all, which could be label the relief hypothesis (Blinde and

Greendorfer, 1985; Coakley, 1983; Greendorfer and Blinde, 1985). Werthner and Orlick (1986) found that 21% of athletes express no difficulties, and Ungerleider (1997) confirms that 18% of athlete in their sample also did not express difficulties. Sinclair and Orlick (1993) found that 74% of athletes were satisfied with their life since retirement, and 63% found that retirement have changed their lives in a quite positive fashion. A second pattern of reactions is illustrated by other studies, which have emphasized that athletes express only moderate difficulties (Alfermann, Stambulova, and Zemaytite, 2004; Stephan et al., 2003a; 2003b). Werthner and Orlick (1986) revealed that this kind of reactions concerns 46% of athletes, and Ungerleider (1997) report the same for 42% of their sample. And a final report suggests that retirement from elite sport results in major difficulties for some athletes, such as identity crisis or strong negative affects (Alfermann et al., 2004; Lally, 2007; Grove, Lavallee, Gordon, and Harvey, 1998; Ogilvie and Howe, 1986). In addition to this heterogeneity in athletes' psychological reactions, interindividual differences have been found for time needed to adapt (Sinclair and Orlick, 1993). For example, Sinclair and Orlick (1993) found that 23% were adapted in the first two or three months after retirement, 32% took were adapted between 6 months and one year, and 22% needed more than two years.

However, these descriptive studies did not take into account the dynamic nature of transition out of elite sport. In fact, and based on the nature of the retirement, it seems likely that athletes' reactions change over time. This conceptualization as a temporal process imply that reactions are likely to change across time, as it is revealed for global self-esteem and subjective well-being (Stephan et al., 2003a; 2003b). As emphasized by Stephan et al. (2003a; 2003b), these dimensions showed initial disequilibrium, followed by a return to their initial levels. These studies illustrated and quantify the different stages of transition out of elite sport, and described the shift in psychological reactions which occurs over time. However, how to explain that some athletes experience major negative reactions, whereas other show moderate ones, or no or positive reactions?

Explanatory Models

A third main question in the area of sport career termination concerns the mechanisms and variables playing a role in athletes reactions and adaptation. More precisely, what are the explanatory factors which could complete the description of athletes reactions? The last decade have resulted in an increase in the number of theoretical models developed for the career transition processes. These models have explanatory potential of the reactions and adaptation pattern observed among athletes.

Sport psychologists first looked outside of the athletic domain for conceptual frameworks by focusing on transition models such as the Schlossberg's Model of Human Adaptation to Transition (Schlossberg, 1981). This model explain the process and outcomes of a transition by an interaction of four sets of factors, including the situation (event or non event transition), the self (individual characteristics of the athlete), the support (the kind of support received), and the strategies used to cope with the transition. The strategies to cope with the transition are key elements of the model and the other three factors can be seen as factors influencing coping. This model have been applied by some sport-related specific studies

(Swain, 1991). However, it was found to lack operational detail of the specific components related to adjustment process among athletes (Taylor and Ogilvie, 1994). The athletic career transition model (Stambulova, 1997; 2003) have been developed to understand career transitions as a whole and have also been used to explain retirement from elite sport (Alferman et al., 2004; Stambulova, Stephan, and Japharg, 2007). It emphasized that effectiveness of coping with transitions is dependent on the dynamic balance between transition resources and barriers. Transition resources imply internal and external factors which facilitate coping process, whereas transition barriers cover internal and external factors, which interfere with effective coping. However, this model lacks specificity for the study of sport career termination.

The Taylor and Ogilvie'(1994) athletic career termination model built upon Schlossberg's model by applying it to sport and operationalizing the personal and situational factors that affect retirement and athlete's ability to adapt to retirement. It deals specifically with retirement from elite sport and proposes that quality of the transition is dependent upon the reasons for termination, factors related to adaptation (developmental experiences, self-identity, perceptions of control, social identity, and tertiary contributors) and available resources (coping skills, social support and pre-retirement planning). These three models have been applied to a wide range of studies on sport career termination, and have highlight the interindividual differences in reaction and adaptation pattern. They place coping as key outcome, depending on several factors.

A Dynamic, Multidimensional, and Complex View of Transition out of Elite Sport

However, since Taylor and Ogilvie (1994) model, a great number of variables have been related to transition outcomes, and this model needs to be updated according to recent advances. In fact, the number of variables identified has grown during the last years, and hypothesized risk or facilitating factors span an enormous range, from individual characteristics to cultural determinants, taking also into account several transition-related variables. In the present chapter, the organization of these variables is based on the ideas of complexity and multidimensionality of the transition process, emphasized by several authors (Crook and Robertson, 1991; Fernandez, Stephan, and Fouquereau, 2006). Previous research have emphasized that the process of adjustment to sport career termination is multifaceted and complex (Baillie and Danish, 1992) and have suggested that the course of athletic retirement and adaptation call for a complex and multifaceted perspective between athletic and non athletic factors (Cecic Erpic, Wylleman, and Zupancic, 2004). This idea of complexity is also supported by Stambulova et al. (2007) which revealed that the transition process imply a number of factors interplayed. Multidimensionality means that the quality of adaptation depends not only of a single variable, but that many different variables could be involved. Complexity means that these several variables could interact with each other to determine athletes' reaction and adaptation patterns. Thus, in the present chapter, retirement is considered as a complex process where a network of individual as well as contextual factors interacts with each other, and determines the athletes' reactions and adaptation.

The present chapter proposes an organization of these variables in two main interrelated categories, named pre-conditions and transitional factors, and suggested that athletes reactions and adaptation could result from complex interactions between variables within these categories. According to this organization, pre-conditions could influence athletes' adaptation, through the transitional factors. The general assumption is that retirement from elite sport causes changes in psychological well-being and that these activate adaptive mechanisms that seek to reduce the impact of this event.

Pre-Conditions

The first set of explanatory variables is related to pre-conditions for the transition (Stambulova et al., 2007). They correspond to antecedents of transition out of elite sport, individual, and cultural factors, and could be considered as the main influence of athletes' reactions and adaptation.

Reasons for retirement are one of the most emphasized influences on the effectiveness of coping with transition out of elite sport. Initially, four main causes of ending a career, namely age, deselection, injury, and free choice were identified (Taylor and Ogilvie, 1994). These causes were further dichotomized between freely chosen and externally forced retirement. The freedom of choice contributes to differences in emotional adaptation to the transition process, and adaptation is optimized after freely ending the career than after involuntary retirement (Alfermann, 2000). Athletes who terminated their career voluntarily more often reported positive emotions, whereas involuntary decision leads to more negative emotions (Alfermann, 2000).

However, studies have emphasized the multi-causal nature of transition out of elite sport, which results from a long process of reasoning and decision-making. For instance, in Koukouris' study (1991) investigating the disengagement process among elite Greek male athletes, 38 causes were identified, including inadequate financial support from the club or the federation, lack of success, excessive time commitment required for top performance, lack of adequate athletic facilities, injury. As suggested by Fernandez et al. (2006), the reasons for deciding to end a sporting career resemble the chaos theory model: numerous, varied and cumulative. Researchers have dichotomized the reasons according to their voluntary versus involuntary nature (Alfermann, 2000; Crook and Robertson, 1991; Webb, Nasco, Riley, and Headrick, 1998; Werthner and Orlick, 1986). However, these classifications have recently been called into question. For example, Kerr and Dacyshyn (2000) demonstrated that the distinction between freely chosen (voluntary) and forced (involuntary) retirement is not always clear because of the diversity and the nature of the potential factors, which determine why athletes retire. Recently, Fernandez et al. (2006) have suggested a new organization of the retirement decision-making. These authors have emphasized that the decisional process leading to sport career termination is based on a complex interaction and balance between push factors (e.g., injury), pull factors (e.g., to spend more time with their family), anti-push factors (e.g. the desire to pursue the sports career because of still feeling able to perform, or the elite athlete's attachment to social status), and anti-pull factors (e.g. uncertainty of the post-sports life or to the anxiety induced by feeling unable to succeed in a new socioprofessional setting).

Pre-retirement planning has been also emphasized as a crucial influential factor for both reactions and adaptation to the transition process. Athletes, who plan retirement in advance, do not waste their energy in wrong directions and, hence, are able to mobilise and use their resources more effectively than athletes who do not plan their retirement. Pre-retirement planning gives athletes a feeling of subjective control over the situation and increases his/her self-efficacy with regard to successful post-career adaptation (Alfermann et al., 2004; Taylor and Ogilvie, 1994). Athletes who planned their retirement in advance feel higher perceived control over the retirement process and have higher self-efficacy in regard of post athletic career adaptation (Alfermann, 2000; Alfermann et al., 2004; Blinde and Stratta, 1992; McPherson, 1980; Taylor and Ogilvie, 1994; Webb et al., 1998). Alfermann et al. (2004) showed that planned retirement is associated with more positive and less negative emotional reactions to sport career termination, shorter duration of the transitional period, lesser use of distraction strategies, and higher current life satisfaction.

Cecic Erpic et al. (2004) found that the degree of athletic identity and its prevalence over other social roles has also a significant effect on the quality of the retirement process from sports, more particularly on the degree of psychological difficulties experienced and the degree of difficulties related to the organization of post-sports life. Brewer, Van Raalte, and Petitpas (2000) and others (Pearson and Petitpas, 1990; Werthner and Orlick, 1986) support the view that athletes with a strong athletic identity experience more intense and more frequent difficulties during the process of retirement from sport, such as social and emotional adjustment difficulties (Baillie and Danish, 1992; Brewer., Van Raalte, and Linder, 1993). These post-retirement difficulties could be explain because those who strongly commit themselves to the athlete role may be less likely to plan for post-athletic career opportunities prior to their retirement from sport (Gordon, 1995; Pearson and Petitpas, 1990), with anxiety about career exploration and decision making (Grove, Lavallee, and Gordon, 1997). Athletic identity have also been related to athlete's resources used during the transition. A strong athletic identity was related to venting of emotions, mental disengagement, behavioral disengagement, and reliance on denial, seeking instrumental support, suppression of competing activities, and seeking of emotional support (Grove et al., 1997). It exhibit also correlations with time taken to adjust, both emotionally and socially (Grove et al., 1997).

Athletes' nationality is also a strong pre-condition for a successful transition and adaptation process. Recent research have found cross-cultural differences in pre-conditions, coping resources, and quality of adaptation to the transition process. More precisely, Alfermann et al. (2004) and Stambulova et al. (2007) found that athletes from different countries differ in their reasons for career termination, planning for retirement, emotional reactions to sport career termination, coping strategies and time for adaptation. Thus the cultural context of the transition out of elite sports, e.g. elite sports climate, mass media attention, job possibilities for athletes, availability of athletic retirement services, living standard and cultural traditions, are pre-conditions which need to be taken into account when studying repercussions of transition out of elite sport.

The complexity of the retirement process emerged also from interactions between pre-conditions variables. For example, research have found that a substantial negative relationship between athletic identity and pre-retirement planning (Grove et al., 1997). It seems also that nationality is related to reasons for retirement and pre-retirement planning (Alfermann et al., 2004; Stambulova et al., 2007) Thus, there is not a single pre-condition, or predisposing factor which determine the quality of adaptation, but it seems more to be the result of a complex interaction between several risks factors.

Transitional Factors

Pre-conditions are related to athletes' reactions and adaptation, though a second set of factors which emerged during the transitional process, after the actual retirement event. They could be considered as transitional factors, which are factors which take place during the transition process, such as life changes and athletes' use of coping resources to face with these changes.

Transitional Changes

The new situation following retirement from elite sport could also be considered as a complex interaction of stressors (Ogilvie and Taylor, 1993). It is recognized that the transition process is multidimensional, with changes in several spheres of live (Stambulova et al., 2007; Stephan and Bilard, 2003; Stephan et al., 2003a; 2007). Thus, more than being attributable to the transition and the retirement event per se, athletes reactions and adaptation could result from the changes in different area of their lives resulting from the transition. For example, bodily changes, socioprofessional changes, as well as life style and life rhythm changes are factors that could explain how and why retirement from elite sport could be particularly distressful for some athletes (Stephan et al., 2003a, 2003b). The socioprofessional transition marks the passage from "something they knew very well to something new" (Werthner and Orlick, 1986, p. 358), with the individual descending from the heights of the extraordinary into the mundane world of ordinariness (Sparkes, 1998). Feelings of competence and self-efficacy are called into question by confrontation with the demands of normal working life (Gearing, 1999). The physical skills that athletes have perfected for so long may now seem useless (Thomas and Ermler, 1988), and they have to learn all over again to be competent at something new (Werthner and Orlick, 1986). Doubts about their competence in the new situation may also affect subjective well-being. The bodily transition, with related changes in physical condition, weight gain, or somatic manifestations have an influence on global self-esteem (Stephan et al., 2003a). Changes in life style, and associated feelings of void of sensations and stimulations, with changes in important competencies, could be related to decrease in subjective well-being (Stephan et al., 2003b).

In addition, as emphasized by Cecic Erpic et al. (2004), aspects of athletes' lives are closely connected and mutually interdependent with regard to the career transition. These authors showed that the quality of the sports career termination is affected by non-athletic factors, more particularly by non-athletic transitions, such as family transitions or educational transitions. Moreover, transition-related changes are likely to interact with each other, and the changes in one area could influence changes in other area. For example, the involvement in a new professional situation could induce changes in life style, with new daily routines, timetables and habits (Stephan et al., 2003b) resulting in bodily changes with weight gain, loss of physical condition. Conversely, positive bodily changes and experiences during the transition are likely to influence positively job involvement (Stephan et al., 2003b).

Coping Resources

The extent to which transition out of elite sport could potentially be a source of distressful reactions depends on athletes' resources to cope with these changes. Thus, athletes resources combine to match the environmental challenges. The resources imply all internal and external factors, which facilitate the coping process (e.g., the athlete's self-knowledge, skills, personality traits, motivation, availability of social and/or financial support). Studies have emphasized that social resources, including the social support system are influential for athletes' smooth or problematic adaptation (Alfermann et al., 2004; Sinclair and Orlick, 1993; Stephan et al., 2003b; Stambulova et al., 2007; Swain, 1991). The coping process is central in a transition and includes all strategies the athlete use in order to adjust to particular transition demands and changes. Successful transition is associated with effective coping when the athlete is able to recruit/use or rapidly develop necessary resources. The complexity of retirement from elite sport is illustrated by the fact that these resources are determined mainly by pre-conditions, such as retirement planning, reasons for retirement, or athletic identity. For example, planned retirement was associated with less use of refusing to believe in retirement, less use of drugs, less giving up, and more use of accepting retirement (Stambulova et al., 2007). Athletes who terminated their career voluntarily and who had made a conscious decision more often reported a more active coping process (Alfermann, 2000). Involuntary retired athletes reported more passive coping strategies and a higher need for social support than did voluntarily retired athletes (Alfermann, 2000). Thus, pre-conditions play a role in the degree to which transitional changes could be distressful for athletes, because they determine the effective or non-effective development and use of these resources. In other words, they could provide athletes with some skills to face with transitional changes. In this case, if athletes possess adequate resources, transitional changes could induce only moderate reactions, with a temporary decrease in self-esteem. Conversely, a lack of adequate resources to face with changes, could result in an escalation of negative reactions, and could hinder the adaptation, resulting in a longer time of adjustment, and less satisfaction with the new setting.

The dynamic, multidimensionality and complexity of transition out of elite sport exists also at the level of athletes' resources to face with the transition demand. Transitional athletes did not use only one strategy to face with the transition demands. In line with a view that coping is a complex, dynamic process (Carver, Scheier, and Weintraub, 1989; Lazarus and Folkman, 1984) it has been found that retired athletes use a combination of strategies, from emotion-focused one, to problem-focused and social support seeking ones (Grove et al., 1997; Stambulova et al., 2007; Stephan et al., 2003b). Coping strategies shift also during the transitional process. For example, it has been demonstrated that the transitional athletes changed from avoidance strategies to the strategy of training and/or exercising during the transition process, which moderate bodily changes (Stephan et al., 2003b). Thus, there is a point during the transition where individuals begin to perceive more control and change their coping strategies (Stephan et al., 2003b). It seems that this is not the kind of strategy which is beneficial for the adjustment process, but the coping effectiveness depends on when it is used. This ability to flexibly adjust the coping strategies to changing conditions is likely to depend on pre-conditions, such as individual differences variables.

Athletes' Adaptation

According to existing research, the adaptation of former athletes is related to several pre-conditions. Thus, it has been demonstrated that pre-retirement planning and low athletic identity are related to lower time needed for adaptation (Grove et al., 1997; Stambulova et al., 2007) and planned retirement is associated with higher life satisfaction nowadays (Alfermann et al., 2004). However, pre-conditions influence athletes' adaptation because they provide them resources to face with transitional changes, and to quickly adapt. Thus, more than a direct relationship between pre-conditions and adaptation indicators, it seems that the resources provided by pre-conditions play a mediational role between retirement from sport and adaptation outcomes.

Directions for Future Research

Elite Athletes' Views of Retirement

One area of research which have received little attention from researchers is related to active elite athletes view of retirement. It is established in other field such as workplace retirement, that retirement anxiety, which refers to a general feeling of apprehension or worry regarding the potentially disruptive consequences of retirement, is related to a low level of pre-retirement planning and is likely to interfere with coping and adaptive behaviour (Taylor and Shore, 1995). Positive attitudes toward retirement are expected to be related to an adequate anticipation and planification of retirement, and as a result to later adjustment to retirement and satisfaction with a new life. Thus, the identification of active athletes' view of retirement is likely to provide some insights about the determinants of some crucial pre-conditions, such as pre-retirement planning. In addition, it could be hypothesized that positive attitudes toward retirement could explain why some athletes proactively diminished their athletic identity prior to retirement, which preclude a major identity crisis upon and during the retirement process (Lally, 2007).

Level of Participation and Gender Differences

Another theoretical question is related to the level of participation of the samples studied. It seems possible that adaptation to transition out of elite sport differ as a function of level of participation. However, no research has yet tested for potential comparison between student-athletes and Olympic or professional athletes. The main problem is that a negative correlation between sample size and sport level seems to exist. That is, that as the number of athletes increases, the athletic level of the sample decreases. Research must also take into account potential gender differences in the quality of adaptation. Previous research have reported inconsistent findings, with some studies having found gender differences in pre-conditions and coping strategies (Stambulova et al., 2007) whereas other have failed to find any differences (Alfermann, 2000). Thus, this question needs further clarification.

Individual Pre-Conditions

Individuals' psychological factors, could be important pre-conditions variables to take into account for quality of the adaptation to transition out of elite sport. Studies have suggested that the nature of athletes' motives for sport participation, such as passion for the activity, could influence athletes' reactions during the transition (Amiot, Vallerand, and Blanchard, 2006). Studies conducted in other field has emphasized the influence of personality traits on positive and negative aspects of adjustment and coping strategies (Kling, Ryff, Love, and Essex, 2003). However, no research has yet tested the influence of either individuals' motives or personality traits on adjustment to the transition process. Additional individual psychological factors could provide a more complete picture of the pre-conditions for a successful or difficult adaptation to transition out of elite sport. For example, personality traits such as openness to experience or neuroticism could determine the adaptation process, through their influence on individual resources and coping. These individuals' psychological factors could influence how the transition is anticipated, how its associated changes are perceived and faced with, and as a result could determine the time needed for adaptation and future life satisfaction.

Transitional Factors

Evidence exists now on the multidimensionality of transition out of elite sport (Stambulova et al., 2007; Stephan et al., 2003b). However, no studies have yet tested for the unique influence of different changes on athletes' psychological well-being, and how specific coping resources could be used to meet the unique demand of each change. Moreover, further researches are needed to better capture the complexity of these transitional factors. Only one qualitative study have shown that the professional transition induces life rhythm changes, and as a result bodily changes (Stephan et al., 2003b). There is a need to further explore the interaction between these changes across time and how they facilitate or hinder athletes' adaptation, and how resources use could dampen them. Finally, the mediational role of these transitional factors between pre-conditions and the quality of adaptation should be verified and confirmed.

Methodological Perspectives

Several methodological limitations emerge from the existing literature. Although adaptation to transition out of elite sport is a dynamic process, few studies have examined the dynamic nature of the phenomenon. Studies have investigated the psychological repercussions of this transition using a retrospective design, despite the inherent problems associated with memory decay and recall bias and the clear risk of significant information being neglected (Kerr and Dacyshyn, 2000; Squire, 1989). Moreover, the few studies which have used a longitudinal design have found that athletes' reactions change and evolve over time (Stephan et al., 2003a, 2003b). Thus, retrospective accounts of athletes' transitional reactions are limited by their inability to adequately capture this dynamic. The dynamic nature of transition out of elite sport imply a in vivo process-oriented approach, with longitudinal design which begin prior to retirement and extend up to the adaptation point. This kind of method could allow the complete investigation of the influence of pre-conditions on athletes' adaptation, and how this influence is mediated by transitional factors. No research to our knowledge, have investigated transition out of elite sport using such a method. Adequate measurement must be developed to adequately capture the multidimensionality and complexity of variables involved in this process.

As Baillie and Danish (1992) emphasized, the process of adjustment to sport career termination is an individual phenomenon. Thus, intra-individual longitudinal studies could be appropriate to identify several specific patterns of reactions and adaptation, related to individual-specific set of pre-conditions and resources. Diary study design may be helpful to track and examine athletes' intraindividual changes immediately before and after their retirement. Methodological approaches in past research on transitions in general, and on retirement from competitive sport in particular, have included quantitative and qualitative methodologies. As emphasized by previous researches, there is a need for a multimethod approach to the study of transition out of elite sport, using qualitative procedures to complement the more quantitative approach, in order to achieve a better understanding of this process (Grove et al., 1997; Stephan et al., 2003b).

Conclusion

The present chapter aims to review existing research, and to update existing models according to recent advances. It appears that transition out of elite sport is a dynamic process, where time and changes are crucial, a multidimensional phenomenon, given the number of potential variables playing a role in the adaptation process, which supposes complex interaction between these variables. Despite the substantial number of publications during the last decades, many perspectives for future research exist and are worth to consider. The main is to adjust the methods used to the nature of this phenomenon, to better capture athletes reaction and adaptation patterns, and to provide an in-depth understanding of the determinants of a successful vs difficult transition out of elite sport.

References

Alfermann, D. (2000). Causes and consequences of sport career termination. In D. Lavallee, and P. Wylleman (Eds.), *Career transitions in sport: International perspectives* (pp. 45-58). Morgantown, WV: Fitness Information Technology.

Alfermann, D., Stambulova, N., and Zemaityte, A., (2004). Reactions to sport career termination: A cross-national comparison of German, Lithuanian and Russian athletes. *Psychology of Sport and Exercise, 5*, 61-75.

Allison, M. T., and Meyer, C. (1988). Career problems and retirement among elite athletes: The female tennis professional. *Sociology of Sport Journal, 5*, 212-222.

Amiot, C., Vallerand, R.J., and Blanchard, C. (2006). Passion and psychological adjustment: A test of the Person-Environment fit hypothesis. *Personality and Social Psychology Bulletin, 32*, 220-229.

Baillie, P., and Danish, S. (1992). Understanding career transition of athletes. *The Sport Psychologist, 6*, 77-98.

Blinde, E. M., and Greendorfer, S. L. (1985). A reconceptualization of the process of leaving the role of competitive athlete. *International Review For Sociology of Sport, 20*, 87-93.

Blinde, E. M., and Stratta, T. M. (1992). The "sport career death" of college athletes: Involuntary and unanticipated sport exits. *Journal of Sport Behavior, 15*, 3-20.

Brewer, B. W., Van Raalte, J. L., and Linder, D. E. (1993). Athletic identity: Hercules' muscles or Achilles' heel? *International Journal of Sport Psychology, 24*, 237-254.

Brewer, B. W., Van Raalte, J. L., and Petitpas, A. J. (2000). Self-identity issues in sport career transitions. In D. Lavallee, and P. Wylleman (Eds.), *Career transitions in sport: International perspectives* (pp. 29-43). Morgantown, WV: Fitness Information Technology.

Carver, C. S., Scheier, M. F., Weintraub, J. K. (1989). Assessing coping strategies: a theoretically based approach. *Journal of Personality and Social Psychology, 56*, 267-283.

Cecic Erpic, S., Wylleman, P., and Zupancic, M. (2004). The effect of athletic and non-athletic factors on the sports career termination process. *Psychology of Sport and Exercise, 5*, 45-60.

Coakley, J.J. (1983). Leaving competitive sport: Retirement or rebirth? *Quest, 35*, 1-11.

Crook, J. M., and Robertson, S. E. (1991). Transition out of elite sport. *International Journal of Sport Psychology, 22*, 115 - 127.

Curtis, J., and Ennis, R. (1988). Negative consequences of leaving competitive sport? Comparison findings for former elite-level hockey players. *Sociology of Sport Journal, 5*, 87-106.

Danish, S. J., Owens, S. S., Green, S. L., and Brunelle, J. P. (1997). Building bridges for disengagement: The transition process for individuals and teams. *Journal of Applied Sport Psychology, 9*, 154-167.

Ebaugh, H. R. F. (1988). *Becoming an ex: The process of role exit*. Chicago: University of Chicago Press.

Fernandez, A., Stephan, Y., and Fouquereau, E. (2006). Assessing reasons for sport career termination : Development of the Athletes' Retirement Decision Inventory (ARDI). *Psychology of Sport and Exercise, 4*, 407-421.

Gearing, B. (1999). Narratives of identity among former professional footballers in the United Kingdom. *Journal of Aging Studies, 13*, 43-58.

Gordon, S. (1995). Career transitions in competitive sport. In T. Morris and J. Summers (Eds.), *Sport psychology: theory, applications, and issues* (pp. 474-501). Brisbane, Australia: Jacaranda Wiley.

Greendofer, S.L., and Bline, E.M. (1985). "Retirement" from intercollegiate sport: Theoretical and empirical considerations. *Sociology of Sport Journal, 2*, 101-110.

Grove, J. R., Lavallee, D., and Gordon, S. (1997). Coping with retirement from sport: The influence of athletic identity. *Journal of Applied Sport Psychology, 9*, 191-203.

Grove, J. R., Lavallee, D., Gordon, S., and Harvey, J. H. (1998). Account-making: A model for understanding and resolving distressful reactions to retirement from sport. *The Sport Psychologist, 12*, 52-67.

Hill, P., and Lowe, B. (1974). The inevitable metathesis of the retiring athlete. *International Review of Sport Sociology, 4*, 5-29.

Hopson, B., and Adams, J. D. (1977). Toward an understanding of transition: Defining some boundaries for transition. In J. Adams, J. Hayes, and B. Hopson (Eds.), *Transition: Understanding and managing personal change*. London: Martin Robertson.

Kerr, G., and Dacyshyn, A. (2000). The retirement experiences of female elite gymnasts. *Journal of Applied Sport Psychology, 12*, 115-133.

Kim, J. E., and Moen, P. (2001). Is retirement good or bad for subjective well-being? *Current Directions in Psychological Science, 10*, 83-86.

Kleiber, D. A., and Brock, S. C. (1992). The effect of career-ending injuries on the subsequent well-being of elite college athletes. *Sociology of Sport Journal, 9*, 70-75.

Kling, K. C., Ryff, C. D., Love, G., and Essex, M. (2003). Exploring the influence of personality on depressive symptoms and self-esteem across a significant life transition. *Journal of Personality and Social Psychology, 85,* 922-932.

Koukouris, K. (1991). Quantitative aspects of the disengagement process of advanced and elite Greek male athletes from organised competitive sport. *Journal of Sport Behavior, 14*, 227-246.

Lally, P. (2007). Identity and athletic retirement: a prospective study. *Psychology of Sport and Exercise, 8*, 85-89.

Lavallee, D., Nesti, M., Borkoles, E., Cockerill, I., and Edge, A. (2000). Intervention strategies for athletes in transition. In D. Lavallee and P. Wylleman (Eds.). *Career transitions in sport. International perspectives* (pp.111-130). Morgantown: Fitness Information Technology.

Lavallee, D., Wylleman, P., and Sinclair, D. (2000). Career transitions in sport: An annotated bibliography. In D. Lavallee and P. Wylleman (Eds.). *Career transitions in sport. International perspectives* (pp. 207-258). Morgantwon, WV: Fitness Information Technology.

Lazarus, R.S., and Folkman, S. (1984). Stress, appraisal, and coping. *American Psychologist*, *46*, 819-834.

Lerch, S. H. (1981). The adjustment to retirement of professional baseball players. In S. L. Greendorfer and A. Yiannakis (Eds.), *Sociology of Sport: Diverse perspectives* (pp. 138-148). West Point, NY: Leisure Press.

McPherson, B. D. (1980). Retirement from professional sport: The process and problems of occupational and psychological adjustment. *Sociology Symposium*, *30*, 126-143.

Ogilvie, B. C., and Howe, M. (1986). The trauma of termination from athletics. In J. M. Williams (Ed.), *Applied sport psychology: personal growth to peak performance* (pp. 365-382). Palo Alto, CA: Mayfield.

Pearson, R. E., and Petitpas, A. J. (1990). Transitions of athletes: Developmental and preventive perspectives. *Journal of Counselling and Development*, *69*, 7-10.

Rosenberg, E. (1981). Gerontological theory and athletic retirement. In S. L. Greendorfer and A. Yiannakis (Eds.), *Sociology of sport: Diverse perspectives* (pp. 118-126). West Point, NY: Leisure Press.

Schlossberg, N. (1981). A model for analysing human adaptation to transition. *The Counselling Psychologist*, *9*, 2-18.

Sinclair, D. A., and Orlick, T. (1993). Positive transitions from high-performance sport. *The Sport Psychologist*, *7*, 138-150.

Sparkes, A. C. (1998). Athletic identity: An Achilles' heel to the survival of self. *Qualitative Health Research*, *8*, 644-664.

Squire, L. R. (1989). On the course of forgetting in very long-term memory. *Journal of Experimental Psychology: Learning, Memory, and Cognition*, *15*, 241-245.

Stambulova, N. B. (1997). Transitional period of Russian athletes following sports career termination. In R. Lidor and M. Bar-Eli (Eds.), *Proceedings of the 9th World Congress Of Sport Psychology* (pp. 658-660). Netanya: International Society of Sport Psychology.

Stambulova, N. (2000). Athlete's crises: A developmental perspective. *International Journal of Sport Psychology*, *31*, 584-601.

Stambulova, N. (2003). Symptoms of a crisis-transition: A grounded theory study. In N. Hassmen (Ed.), *SIPF Yearbook 2003* (pp. 97-109). Örebro: Örebro University Press.

Stambulova, N., Stephan, Y, and Japharg, U. (2007). Athletic retirement: A cross-national comparison of elite French and Swedish athletes. *Psychology of Sport and Exercise*, *8*, 101-118.

Stephan, Y., and Bilard, J. (2003). Repercussions of transition out of elite sport on body image. *Perceptual and Motor Skills*, *96*, 95-104.

Stephan, Y., Bilard, J., Ninot, G., and Delignieres, D. (2003a). Bodily transition out of elite sport: A one-year study of physical self and global self-esteem among transitional athletes. *International Journal of Sport and Exercise Psychology*, *2*, 192-207.

Stephan, Y., Bilard, J., Ninot, G., and Delignieres, D. (2003b). Repercussions of transition out of elite sport on subjective well-being: A one-year study. *Journal of Applied Sport Psychology*, *4*, 354-371.

Stephan, Y., Torregrosa, M., and Sanchez, X. (2007). The body matters: Psychophysical impact of retiring for elite sport. *Psychology of Sport and Exercise*, *8*, 73-83..

Swain, D. (1991). Withdrawal from sport and Scholssberg's Model of transitions. *Sociology of Sport Journal*, 8, 152-160.

Taylor, J., and Ogilvie, B. C. (1994). A conceptual model of adaptation to retirement among athletes. *Journal of Applied Sport Psychology*, 6, 1-20.

Taylor, M. A., and Shore, L. M. (1995). Predictors of planned retirement age: An application of Beehr's model. *Psychology and Aging*, 10, 76–83.

Thomas, C. E., and Ermler, K. L. (1988). Institutional obligations in the athletic retirement process. *Quest*, 40, 137-150.

Ungerleider, S. (1997). Olympic athletes' transition from sport to workplace. *Perceptual and Motor Skills*, 84, 1287-1295.

Webb, W. M., Nasco, S. A., Riley, S., and Headrick, B. (1998). Athlete identity and reactions to retirement from sports. *Journal of Sport Behavior*, 21, 338-362.

Werthner, P., and Orlick, T. (1986). Retirement experiences of successful Olympic athletes. *International Journal of Sport Psychology*, 17, 337-363.

Wylleman, P., Alfermann, D., and Lavallee, D. (2004). Career transitions in sport: European perspectives. *Psychology of Sport and Exercise*, 5, 7-20.

In: Sport and Exercise Psychology Research Advances   ISBN: 978-1-60456-157-9
Editors: M. P. Simmons, L. A. Foster, pp. 191-205   © 2008 Nova Science Publishers, Inc.

Chapter VIII

Social Contacts and Cohesion in a Group Exercise Context

Mark A. Eys[131] and Shauna M. Burke[2]
[1] School of Human Kinetics, Laurentian University, Canada
[2]University of Western Ontario, Canada

Abstract

Despite the highly recognized benefits of exercise, 51% of Canadian adults do not achieve a level of physical activity equivalent to walking 30 minutes per day (Cameron et al., 2005). These low activity rates have prompted the development of strategies to increase physical activity (Burke, Carron, Eys, Ntoumanis, and Estabrooks, 2006). One strategy has been to enhance perceptions of cohesion among group exercisers. Cohesion has been shown to be positively related to adherence (Carron et al., 1996) and negatively related to dropout behavior (Spink and Carron, 1993). Carron and Spink (1993) suggested that one method to increase perceptions of cohesion is to provide greater opportunities for social interaction. The *quantity* of social contacts represents a construct termed structural social support (Sarason, Sarason, and Pierce, 1994) and has been theorized to be linked to relational outcomes such as cohesion (Holt and Hoar, 2006). Consequently, the primary purpose of the present study was to examine the relationship between perceptions of cohesion and the percentage of social contacts that exercisers (a) knew, and (b) interacted with in a group exercise context. Importantly, the percentage of social contacts does not necessarily provide an indication of the *quality* of those relationships. Therefore, a secondary purpose of the study was to examine perceived social support as a potential mediator of the social contacts-cohesion relationship. Adult exercisers ($N = 87$; $M_{age} = 34.47 \pm 13.23$) completed measures of cohesion (GEQ; Carron et al., 1985), perceived social support (adapted SPS; Cutrona and Russell, 1987), and a sociogram of their exercise class used to indicate the percentage of other group members

13 Address correspondence to: Mark Eys, School of Human Kinetics, Laurentian University, Sudbury, Ontario, Canada, P3E 2C6, Telephone: (705) 675-1151 ext. 1203, Fax: (705) 675-4845, Email: meys@laurentian.ca, Date of first submission: September 24, 2007.

whom they knew and interacted with. Results demonstrated that the percentage of group members *known* to the participants was positively related to the cohesion dimensions of Attractions to the Group-Social and Group Integration-Social. The percentage of other group members with whom the participants *interacted with* was negatively related to the cohesion dimension Attractions to the Group-Task. Furthermore, the social support function Opportunity for Nurturance was found to be a mediator of the social contacts-cohesion relationship. Specifically, the percentage of group members known to participants was positively related to perceptions of being relied upon by others which, in turn, was positively related to the Attractions to the Group-Social dimension of cohesion. Results are discussed in relation to group dynamics theory and applied relevance.

Keywords: *Social Interaction, Cohesion, Social Support, Exercise, Physical Activity*

The benefits of regular physical activity are well established. The United States Department of Health and Human Services (USDHHS; 2004) and the Canadian Fitness and Lifestyle Research Institute (CFLRI; 2007) concur that regular physical activity increases strength, facilitates weight control, and enhances well-being/quality of life. In addition, individual studies have demonstrated support for numerous physiological (e.g., Haskell, 1994), cognitive (e.g., Etnier, Salazar, Landers, Petruzzello, Han, and Nowell, 1997), and psychological (e.g., Landers and Petruzzello, 1994) benefits for individuals of all ages (Carron, Hausenblas, and Estabrooks, 2003).

Despite these well-known benefits, participation in physical activity in North America remains low. Cameron, Craig, and Paolin (2005) found that 51% of Canadians are not moderately active, which is the equivalent of walking 30 minutes on a daily basis. Coincidentally, recent research by the CFLRI (2007) found that 51% of Canadians could be classified as overweight or obese. In the United States it is estimated that 85% of adults do not meet the recommendations for a minimal amount of daily exercise and 40% do not engage in any leisure time physical activity (USDHHS, 2004).

These low rates of participation have prompted the development of many strategies and protocols to enhance involvement in and commitment to physical activity (Burke, Carron, Eys, Ntoumanis, and Estabrooks, 2006). These strategies have been implemented and assessed in a number of contexts including worksites, medical settings, community groups, schools, and within families and include group and individual-based programs (e.g., Atienza, 2001; Dishman and Buckworth, 1996; Kahn et al., 2002; Lox, Martin Ginis, and Petruzzello, 2006). It should be noted that there has been some debate as to the comparative utility of group versus individual-based physical activity programs in terms of adherence and compliance. While it is not the purpose of the present study to discuss this debate at length, recent literature has provided evidence about the effectiveness of utilizing the group context to promote physical activity adherence, whether the strategy incorporates strictly a group approach (Burke, Carron, Eys, Ntoumanis, and Estabrooks, 2006; Carron, Hausenblas, and Mack, 1996) or utilizes the group as a first step toward developing greater self-regulation. An example of this latter approach would be the group-mediated cognitive-behavioral intervention developed and described by Brawley, Rejeski, and Lutes (2000).

More interesting, in their meta-analysis examining the optimal contexts with which to offer exercise programs, Burke, Carron, Eys, Ntoumanis, and Estabrooks (2006) found that it wasn't necessarily just the group setting that was effective but rather tight-knit, *cohesive* groups were more successful at retaining their members for the duration of the programs. In addition, another meta-analysis conducted by Carron et al. (1996) found that task and social cohesion were significantly related to adherence behavior. Cohesion has been considered the most important small group variable (Lott and Lott, 1965) and is defined as "a dynamic process that is reflected in the tendency for a group to stick together and remain united in the pursuit of its instrumental objectives and/or for the satisfaction of member affective needs" (Carron et al., 1998, p. 213). Evolving from this definition, Carron, Widmeyer, and Brawley (1985) suggested that there are four dimensions of cohesion: (a) Individual Attractions to the Group-Task (i.e., the individual's perceptions of his/her personal involvement in task aspects of the group), (b) Individual Attractions to the Group-Social (i.e., the individual's perceptions of his/her involvement in social aspects of the group), (c) Group Integration-Task (i.e., the individual's perceptions of the degree of unity the group possesses surrounding task aspects), and (d) Group Integration-Social (i.e., the individual's perceptions of the degree of unity the group possesses regarding social aspects).

Clearly, based on the abovementioned literature, it is safe to conclude that cohesion plays an important role within exercise groups. The next question is how does one develop cohesion in an exercise context in the most effective manner? A number of physical activity intervention programs (e.g., Carron and Spink, 1993; Estabrooks and Carron, 1999; Estabrooks, Fox, Doerksen, Bradshaw, and King, 2005; Spink and Carron, 1994) have utilized all or part of a framework developed by Carron and Spink (1993). This framework was developed from previous group dynamics theory and assumes that the foundation of cohesion lies in (a) the type of environment the group operates in, (b) the group's structure, and (c) the processes it engages in. Consequently, practical intervention suggestions are geared toward these three areas. First, Carron and Spink suggested that developing the group's sense of distinctiveness (i.e., through developing a group name, common clothing, etc.) is a major aspect to incorporate within the group's *environment*. Second, focusing on the geographical location of the group members (e.g., where and how individuals will be placed) and the development of group norms (e.g., shared expectations for all group members such as being on time or having similar goals for weight loss) are examples of group *structure*. Finally, interaction among and sacrifices made by group members represent two examples of group *processes* that could be developed in an exercise setting.

While the utility of the above framework in promoting exercise adherence has been demonstrated (e.g., Carron and Spink, 1993), it is not clear which specific aspects of the cohesion intervention program are contributing most to its success. This is not uncommon in research of this kind. In fact, Lox et al. (2006) stated that "Most tests of the effectiveness of social approaches to increasing physical activity have consisted of examining the effects of simultaneously delivered, multiple...interventions delivered along with other behavioral or informational interventions" (p. 171). Furthermore, while the suggestions and framework are based on sound theory, a number of theoretical links (i.e., the relationship between specific group processes to cohesion in an exercise setting) have yet to be demonstrated. As just one exception, a study by Eys, Hardy, and Patterson (2006) found that the presence of normative expectations within exercise groups was positively related to perceptions of the task dimensions of cohesion (i.e., Attractions to the Group–Task and Group Integration–Task).

Another prescription that is invariably associated with any cohesion intervention program is to enhance interaction and communication among group members. Burke, Carron, Eys, Ntoumanis, and Estabrooks (2006) highlighted the potential importance of social contacts in an exercise setting and concluded that "participants benefit most from physical activity when they are given the opportunity to interact with others" (p. 32). However, a review of literature demonstrates that this specific strategy has yet to be examined. Consequently, the primary purpose of the present study was to examine the relationships between the percentage of social contacts individuals perceived to have in an exercise class (i.e., the percentage of other exercisers *known to the individual*), the percentage of other exercisers the individuals *interacted with* during the class, and their perceptions of task and social cohesion.

The number or percentage of social contacts an individual has is a concept that falls under the structural dimension of social support (Holt and Hoar, 2006). More specifically, structural social support refers to the presence of and connections between social contacts. Structural social support is one of three social support dimensions presented by Holt and Hoar in their conceptualization of the social support process. The two remaining dimensions include functional social support (i.e., that which is actually/objectively provided to a recipient) and perceptual social support (i.e., that which the recipient *perceives* as being given to him or her). These three dimensions of support are conceptually linked, through two proposed social support mechanisms (i.e., buffering effect or main effect), to both instrumental and relational outcomes. One such relational outcome presented in their model is cohesion. However, one caveat should be presented. Holt and Hoar are clear that past literature has advised that examining isolated dimensions of social support (i.e., only structural social support) presents a limited picture of its influence (e.g., Pierce, Sarason, Sarason, Joseph, and Henderson, 1996). Consequently, a secondary purpose of the present study was to examine individual perceptions of the social support received (i.e., perceptual social support) in relation to the percentage of participant social contacts, interaction, and cohesion. This was carried out using a multidimensional measure of social support that assesses six social functions proposed by Weiss (1974): Reliable Alliance (i.e., tangible aid), Reassurance of Worth (i.e., esteem support), the Opportunity for Nurturance (i.e., increased sense of self-worth as a result of assisting others), Social Integration (i.e., network support), Attachment (i.e., emotional support), and Guidance (i.e., informational support; Duncan and McAuley, 1993). In the context of the present study (and in relation to Holt and Hoar's conceptualization of social support), these provisions provide insight into the nature and quality of support that each individual perceives as being given to him or her (i.e., perceptual social support).

Three general hypotheses were advanced based on the previous literature presented. First, it was predicted that both task and social dimensions of cohesion would be positively related to the percentage of fellow classmates known to the exercisers and the percentage of fellow classmates with whom they interacted. Second, the percentage of classmates known and interacted with was expected to be positively related to perceptions of social support received. Third, based on the above two hypotheses, it was considered reasonable to generally expect that perceived social support would mediate the social contacts–cohesion relationship. Specifically, it was expected that a greater percentage of social contacts known and interacted with would result in a higher perception of social support received which, in turn, would result in enhanced perceptions of cohesion.

Method

Participants

Eighty-seven adult exercisers (males = 33, females = 52, gender not indicated = 2) from a northeastern Ontario (Canada) community with a mean age of 34.47 ± 13.23 years participated in the present study. The exercisers were members of group spin (i.e., stationary exercise bicycle activity; $n = 40$), aerobic ($n = 35$), and aquafit (i.e., water-based aerobic activity; $n = 10$) classes.

Measures

    Cohesion. Exercisers' perceptions of group cohesion were measured via the Group Environment Questionnaire (GEQ; Carron, Widmeyer, and Brawley, 1985) that was modified for the exercise environment. This measure assesses the four dimensions of cohesion previously discussed on a 9-point Likert-type scale anchored at 1 (strongly disagree) and 9 (strongly agree). Specifically, these dimensions include (a) Individual Attractions to the Group–Social (ATG-S; 4 items; example item "Some of my best friends are in this group"; α = .65), (b) Individual Attractions to the Group–Task (ATG-T; 4 items; example item "This group does not give me enough opportunities to improve my personal fitness"; α = .79), (c) Group Integration–Social (GI-S; 4 items; example item "Our group would like to spend time together outside of class"; α = .87), and (d) Group Integration–Task (GI-T; 4 items; example item "Our group is united in trying to reach its fitness goals"; α = .40). While previous research has supported the reliability and validity of the GEQ in a variety of contexts (see Carron et al., 1998 for a review), the Cronbach alpha value for the GI-T dimension was considered inadequate to consider it for further analyses based on recommended suggestions by Nunnally (1978).

    Social support. Perceived social support was assessed using the Social Provisions Scale developed by Cutrona and Russell (1987). This scale has been adapted to the exercise domain by Duncan and colleagues (e.g., Duncan and McAuley, 1993) and has been shown to be both valid and reliable (Courneya and McAuley, 1995). As indicated in the introduction, this measure has six subscales assessing perceptions of (a) Reliable Alliance (4 items; example item "While I was exercising with others during the last month, there was someone I could depend on for aid if I really needed it"; α = .74), (b) Reassurance of Worth (4 items; example item "While I was exercising with others during the last month, other people viewed me as competent"; α = .76), (c) Opportunity for Nurturance (4 items; example item "While I was exercising with others during the last month, there were people who depended on me for help"; $\alpha = .81$), (d) Social Integration (4 items; example item "While I was exercising with others during the last month, there were people who enjoyed the same social activities I do"; $\alpha = .74$), (e) Attachment (3 items; example item "While I was exercising with others during the last month, I felt a strong emotional bond with at least one other person"; $\alpha = .70$), and (f) Guidance (5 items; example item "While I was exercising with others during the last month, there was someone I felt comfortable talking about problems with"; $\alpha = .88$). Each item was responded to on a 4-point Likert-type scale anchored at 1 (strongly disagree) and 4 (strongly agree).

Exercise class social contacts and interaction. A brief sociogram designed specifically for the present study was presented to all participants. This diagram (see Figure 1 for an example questionnaire) highlighted the various positions occupied by exercisers within their class. All participants were then asked to indicate (a) their position in the group with an 'X', (b) the degree to which they knew each member of the group on a 1 (complete stranger) to 9 (close friend) Likert-type scale, and (c) the degree to which they interacted with each member of the group on a 1 (never) to 9 (all the time) Likert-type scale. From this information, two scores were calculated for each participant. First, the percentage of individuals known to each participant in the class was calculated by dividing the number of people of whom each participant had some knowledge of (i.e., not 'complete strangers') into the total number of individuals in the class. Second, the percentage of individuals each participant interacted with was calculated by dividing the number of people with whom each participant interacted with to some degree (i.e., not those with a '1' on the interaction scale) into the total number of individuals in the class. For the sake of brevity, these two measures shall herein be referred to as *'Percent Known'* and *'Percent Interaction'*.

Procedure

After ethical approval for the present study was obtained, participants were recruited from exercise facilities within the northeastern part of the province of Ontario (Canada). Initially, approval from the exercise facilities was obtained to approach members to volunteer for the study. The investigators explained the general purpose of the study and the participants read the letter of information and, if interested, signed a consent form. Upon return of the consent form, each participant was given a questionnaire to complete. Data collection occurred approximately 3-5 weeks into the exercise programs to allow for some group development to occur. In addition, data collection occurred after an exercise session. Finally, each participant was given five dollars as incentive and as a token of appreciation for their involvement in the study. Access to the general results of the study upon its completion was guaranteed to all participants.

Data Analysis Strategy

To test the three hypotheses outlined in the introduction, two separate types of analyses were required. First, to test the relationships between (a) cohesion and social contact variables (i.e., Percent Known and Percent Interaction) and (b) perceived social support and social contact variables, standard multiple regression analyses were utilized. Specifically, Percent Known and Percent Interaction represented the independent variables while the (a) three dimensions of cohesion and (b) six dimensions of social support represented the two separate groups of dependent variables.

The following diagram highlights the various positions within your exercise class. Please indicate the following:

1) Your position in the group. Please mark the appropriate circle with an **"X"**.
2) How well do you know the other members of your group? On the line within each circle marked "How well?" please indicate a number from 1-9 based on the following scale.

| 1 | 2 | 3 | 4 | 5 | 6 | 7 | 8 | 9 |

Complete Stranger   **Close Friend**

3) How well do you know the other members of your group? On the line within each circle marked "How well?" please indicate a number from 1-9 based on the following scale.

| 1 | 2 | 3 | 4 | 5 | 6 | 7 | 8 | 9 |

Never   **All the time**

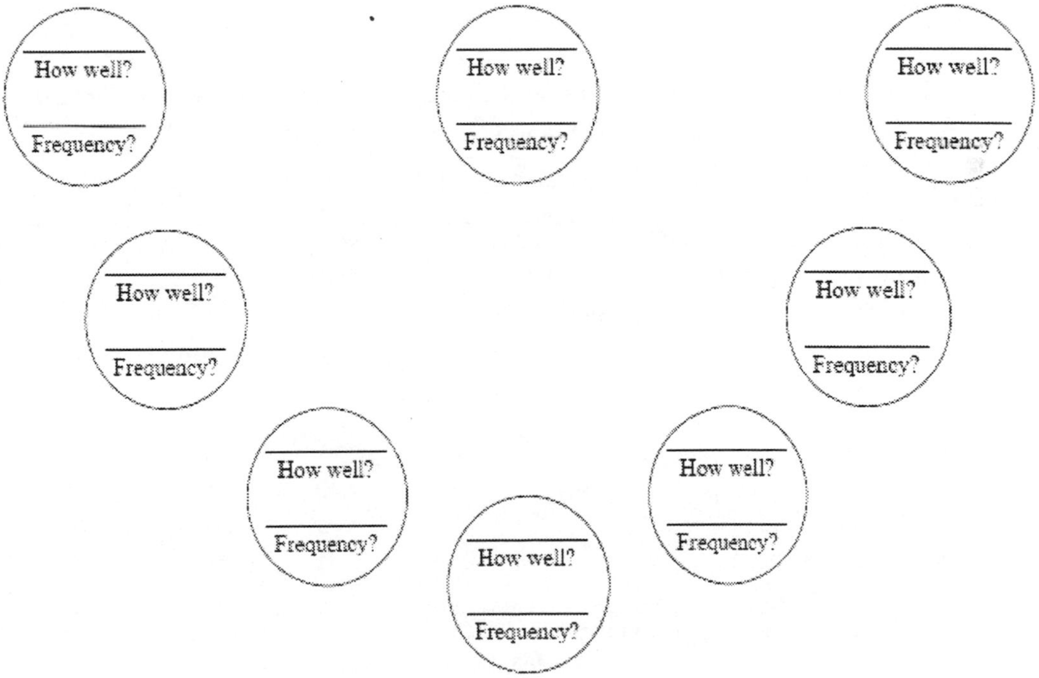

Figure 1. Example sociogram questionnaire for a spin (stationary bicycle activity) class.

In order to address the third general hypothesis, Baron and Kenny's (1986) regression approach to mediation was employed. According to this approach, a mediating pathway exists if the following four criteria are met: (a) the predictor variable (social contact variables) must be significantly related to the dependent variable (cohesion dimensions); (b) the predictor variable must be significantly related to the proposed mediator (perceived social support dimensions); (c) the proposed mediator must be significantly related to the dependent variable when the predictor variable is controlled for; and (d) once the relationship between the mediator and the dependent variable is controlled for, the association between the predictor variable and the dependent variable is non-significant (complete mediation) or lower (partial mediation) in comparison to its original relationship to the dependent variable.

Results

Descriptive Statistics

Descriptive statistics (means, standard deviations, and alpha coefficients if necessary) for all variables are presented in Table 1. On average, participants knew approximately 47% of their exercise classmates and interacted with approximately 59% of them. In addition, mean perceptions of cohesion ranged from 4.48 (Group Integration–Social) to 7.39 (Attractions to the Group–Task) on the 9-point scale. Finally, mean values for perceived social support dimensions ranged from 2.40 (Opportunity for Nurturance) to 3.03 (Social Integration) on the 4-point scale.

Table 1. Means, Standard Deviations, and Cronbach α Values for Social Contact, Perceived Social Support, and Cohesion Variables (N = 87)

Variable	Mean	SD	α
Individuals known to participant (%)	46.81	36.24	n/a
Individuals interacted with (%)	58.55	39.33	n/a
Attractions to the Group – Social (cohesion)	5.06	2.09	.62
Attractions to the Group – Task (cohesion)	7.39	1.46	.79
Group Integration – Social (cohesion)	4.48	2.34	.87
Reliable Alliance (social support)	3.02	.54	.74
Reassurance of Worth (social support)	2.93	.55	.76
Opportunity for Nurturance (social support)	2.40	.64	.81
Social Integration (social support)	3.03	.51	.74
Attachment (social support)	2.51	.67	.70
Guidance (social support)	2.76	.69	.88

Note. Scores for cohesion dimensions can range from 1 (low cohesion) to 9 (high cohesion). Scores for social support variables range from 1 (low social support) to 4 (high social support).

Bivariate correlations are presented in Table 2. It should be noted that there was a moderately high ($r = .77$, $p < .01$) correlation between Percent Known and Percent Interaction. Further, small to moderate intercorrelations ($-.17 \leq r \leq .46$) were demonstrated among cohesion variables while moderately high intercorrelations were found among perceived social support dimensions $(.39 \leq r \leq .76)$.

Table 2. Bivariate Correlations Between Social Contact, Perceived Social Support, and Cohesion Variables (n = 87)

Variable	1.	2.	3.	4.	5.	6.	7.	8.	9.	10.	11.
1. Individuals known to participant	---	.77**	.23*	-.14	.39**	.11	.16	.27*	.20	.08	.20
2. Individuals interacted with		---	.15	-.31**	.18	.10	.20	.34**	.13	.04	.19
3. ATG-S			---	.17	.46**	.53**	.33**	.38**	.47**	.50**	.53**
4. ATG-T				---	-.17	.16	.05	-.03	.24*	.11	.09
5. GI-S					---	.31**	.19	.18	.28**	.19	.22*
6. Reliable Alliance						---	.51**	.39**	.69**	.59**	.76**
7. Reassurance of Worth							---	.57**	.64**	.40**	.58**
8. Opportunity for Nurturance								---	.48**	.45**	.55**
9. Social Integration									---	.65**	.75**
10. Attachment										---	.75**
11. Guidance											---

Note. ATG-T = Individual Attractions to the Group-Task, ATG-S = Individual Attractions to the Group-Social, GI-T = Group Integration-Task, GI-S = Group Integration-Social. Original = original version of questionnaire, Positive = revised questionnaire. Correlations/alpha values for the undergraduate sample (n = 195) are presented in the upper right portion of the table whereas correlations/alpha values for intramural sample (n = 81) can be found in the lower left portion. * p < .05, ** p < .01.

Social Contact and Cohesion Relationships

An examination of the social contact variables and cohesion dimensions demonstrated only three relationships. Specifically, Percent Known was positively related to the cohesion dimensions Attractions to the Group–Social, R^2_{adj} = .04, F(1,74) = 4.23, p < .05, and Group Integration–Social, R^2_{adj} = .14, F(1,74) = 13.33, p < .01. In addition, Percent Interaction was negatively related to Attractions to the Group–Task, R^2_{adj} = .08, F(1,74) = 7.89, p < .01.

Social Contacts and Perceived Social Support

An examination of the social contact variables and perceived social support dimensions demonstrated only two relationships. Specifically, both Percent Known, R^2_{adj} = .06, $F(1,75)$ = 6.01, $p < .05$, and Percent Interaction, R^2_{adj} = .10, $F(1,75)$ = 9.50, $p < .001$, were positively related to the social support dimension Opportunity for Nurturance.

Mediational Relationship

The first two criteria set forth by Baron and Kenny (1986) for testing mediational effects requires relationships to be present between the predictor, mediator, and dependent variables. Based on these criteria and the results presented in the previous sections, only one mediational pathway was tested further. This pathway consisted of the relationship between Percent Known and Attractions to the Group-Social (ATG-S) being mediated by the perceived social support variable Opportunity for Nurturance. As was noted, the first two criteria in the mediational analysis were satisfied in that (a) the predictor (Percent Known) was significantly related to the dependent variable (ATG-S) and (b) the predictor variable was significantly related to the mediating variable (Opportunity for Nurturance). A further regression analysis was performed to test the final two criteria. With regard to criterion 'c', it was found that ATG-S was significantly predicted by Opportunity for Nurturance when Percent Known was controlled for, $\beta = .30$, $t(2, 73) = 2.66$, $p < .01$. Finally, with regard to criterion 'd', the relationship between Percent Known and ATG-S when the mediator-dependent variable relationship was controlled for was non-significant, $\beta = .16$, $t(2, 73) = 1.38$, $p > .05$. Consequently, it can be suggested from these results that Opportunity for Nurturance mediates the Percent Known-ATG-S relationship.

Conclusion

The purpose of the present study was to examine the relationships between the percentage of social contacts individuals perceived to have in an exercise class (i.e., the percentage of other exercisers *known to the individual*), the percentage of other exercisers the individuals *interacted with* during the class, and their perceptions of task and social cohesion. In addition, a secondary purpose was to examine individual perceptions of the social support received (i.e., perceptual social support) in relation to the above variables. Overall, it was demonstrated that the percentage of other exercisers known to individuals was positively related to social aspects of group cohesion while the percentage of other exercisers individuals interacted with was negatively related to the cohesion dimension Attractions to the Group-Task. Finally, it was shown that the social support variable Opportunity for Nurturance mediated the relationship between the percentage of other exercisers known to the individual and Attractions to the Group–Social. A number of issues warrant further discussion in relation to the results of the present study.

First, the results indicating a general positive association between the percentage of other exercisers known and perceptions of social cohesion falls in line with our a priori hypothesis and suggestions from previous research highlighting the benefits of group exercise interventions. Specifically, getting to know others plays a significant role in group intervention strategies developed by Carron and Spink (1993) and Brawley, Rejeski, and Lutes (2000). Carron and Spink (1993) provide examples within their model such as: encourage group members to become fitness friends, ask regular members to help incoming members, use partner work, and provide opportunities for individuals to introduce themselves to other members. Within the group-mediated cognitive-behavioral intervention developed by

Brawley and colleagues, the development of a buddy system plays a vital role through many weeks of their program. From the results of the present study, appropriate use of these strategies should be effective in optimizing group social cohesion and creating a positive atmosphere in general.

Interestingly, and contrary to our a priori hypothesis, the percentage of other exercisers participants interacted with was negatively related to perceptions of task cohesion (i.e., ATG-T) and constitutes a second issue worthy of some discussion. While not aligned with our initial predictions, this result reflects concerns outlined in the introduction of the present study; specifically, that there is a need to understand the foundation and contributions of individual intervention strategies designed to develop group cohesiveness and, consequently, individual adherence to exercise. In other words, the complexity of the exercise context may be such that some general intervention strategies (e.g., increase interaction) may not be as effective as first thought.

In the present case, it seems reasonable to suggest that the general strategy to increase interactions among group exercisers may work at odds with its intended goal (i.e., increasing cohesion). Possible explanations for this finding are advanced. First, the present study investigated interactions among exercisers at a very general level (i.e., the degree to which they interacted with each member of the group) and did not delve into what specific *types* of interactions were taking place. For example, an aspect that might moderate the interaction-cohesion relationship is the degree to which members engage in *task related* vs. *non-task related* communications. It might be the case that task-oriented individuals (i.e., those who were very focused on the exercise program) may become distracted by non-task related discussion they are forced to engage in within the group environment. While this situation is purely speculative at this stage, the issue of proper balance in terms of task and social pursuits has arisen in previous group research in a physical activity environment. For example, Hardy, Eys, and Carron (2005) found sport participants perceived that "an ideal team-building intervention is one that creates a balanced task versus social atmosphere" (p. 184). Consequently, an overemphasis on social interaction (i.e., non-task related) may detract from the goals of many exercisers and, in the end, lower their attraction to the group.

A second possible explanation is based on the discrepancy between the mean percentage values of individuals known to the participants (i.e., approximately 47%) and those interacted with (i.e., approximately 59%). This difference gives the impression that individuals may be interacting with others in the exercise environment who they would list as "complete strangers". It is unknown through the methods of the present study whether or not this is a situation that is desired by the participants (i.e., do they *want* to interact with people they don't know?). Recent literature (e.g., Beauchamp, Carron, McCutcheon, and Harper, 2007; Burke, Carron, and Eys, 2006, 2007) has highlighted the importance of considering the contextual preferences of individuals within the exercise environment (i.e., how they like to engage in physical activity) and it may be worthwhile to consider not only the general delivery of an exercise program (i.e., in a group vs. individual setting) but also (a) the task vs. social orientations of the participants and (b) the degree to which they desire to interact with their co-exercisers.

A third issue that arose through our results was the salience of one aspect of social support; namely, Opportunity for Nurturance. Defined as an increased sense of self-worth as a result of assisting others (Weiss, 1974), it could be implied that getting to know others in the exercise environment (or exercising with people we are already familiar with) provides the opportunity to be relied upon which, in turn, increases our own enjoyment on a social level. The mediational pathway demonstrated in the present study seems to support this (i.e., knowing others---greater opportunity for nurturance---greater attraction to social aspects of the group). In essence, this result suggests that giving support is, at the very least, as important as receiving support in an exercise setting. This makes sense in light of previous group research. For example, Baumeister and Leary (1995) discussed the potential importance of mutuality (i.e., reciprocity in affect, concern, etc.) in relationships with regard to the fundamental need to belong. Their summary of this concept included studies (e.g., Hays, 1985) demonstrating that people tend to prefer relationships in which they can give and receive support (i.e., care and concern).

The importance of helping others in terms of positive perceptions and adherence in the exercise environment has also been noted in recent physical activity literature. For example, Burke, Shapcott, Carron, and Eys (2007) conducted a qualitative examination of reasons why a group setting (i.e., either a structure environment such as an exercise class or a non-structured environment such as an informal running group) was preferable to a sub-set of adult exercisers. A predominant reason noted by the participants was that knowing others depended on them to be physically active (e.g., for motivation or travel to an exercise setting) actually motivated them to maintain their activity regimen.

The previous discussion gives rise to possible future research directions. First, it is suggested that specific aspects of simultaneously delivered multiple interventions be explored. While examples of these types of broad interventions have been shown to be successful, it is always possible to refine approaches to create an environment that will be more appealing to more people, in addition to increasing the efficiency of intervention program delivery. Previous research has been conducted on specific aspects of interventions including the use of buddy systems (e.g., Tucker and Irwin, 2006) and normative expectations (Eys et al., 2006). However, further research could continue to examine in more depth the independent influence of other strategies aimed at developing the group's distinctiveness, structure (i.e., individual positioning), and processes (i.e., member sacrifices and group communication/interaction).

Ultimately, the outcome that exercise scientists are interested in improving is the adherence of participants to an exercise or physical activity regimen. The present study provides evidence that there seems to be a link between the percentage of individuals known and interacted with in the exercise context and perceptions of cohesion. Given previous research indicating a link between perceptions of cohesion and adherence (Carron et al., 1996), it is not unreasonable to suggest that the issue of social contacts within the exercise class may play an important role in the adherence patterns of its participants. Consequently, a second suggested research direction is to further examine the link between social contacts and adherence in an exercise setting.

Finally, the present study only examined perceptions of members of formal, structured exercise groups. This represents only one of many forms of physical activity (both group and individual) that individuals have opportunities to engage in. In fact, depending on the age of participant (Burke, Carron, and Eys, 2006, 2007) and the cohort with which they are exercising (Beauchamp et al., 2007), the structured group exercise environment may represent a scenario that is not preferable for a majority of people. Consequently, it would be worthwhile to consider the ideal (a) number and types of social contacts and (b) amount and modes of interaction within other contexts such as unstructured groups (e.g., a group of friends going for a run) and 'individual conditions' whereby people exercise alone but do so with easy access to others (e.g., running on a treadmill at an exercise facility).

Author Note

The authors would like to thank Laurentian University and the Laurentian University Research Fund (LURF) for its support of this project.

References

Atienza, A. A. (2001). Home-based physical activity programs for middle-aged and older adults: Summary of empirical research. *Journal of Aging and Physical Activity, 9*, S38-S58.

Baron, R. M., and Kenny, D. A. (1986). The moderator-mediator variable distinction in social psychology research: Conceptual, strategic, and statistical considerations. *Journal of Personality and Social Psychology, 51*, 1173-1182.

Baumeister, R. F., and Leary, M. R. (1995). The need to belong: Desire for interpersonal attachments as a fundamental human motivation. *Psychological Bulletin, 117,* 497-529.

Beauchamp, M. R., Carron, A. V., McCutcheon, S., and Harper, O. (2007). Older adults' preferences for exercising alone versus in groups: Considering contextual congruence. *Annals of Behavioral Medicine, 33*, 200-206.

Brawley, L. R., Rejeski, W. J., and Lutes, L. (2000). A group-mediated cognitive-behavioral intervention for increasing adherence to physical activity in older adults. *Journal of Applied Biobehavioral Research, 5,* 47-65.

Burke, S. M., Carron, A. V., and Eys, M. A. (2006). Physical activity context: Preferences of university students. *Psychology of Sport and Exercise, 7*, 1-13.

Burke, S. M., Carron, A. V., and Eys, M. A. (2007). *Adults' preferences for physical activity contexts.* Manuscript in preparation.

Burke, S. M., Carron, A. V., Eys, M. A., Ntoumanis, N., and Estabrooks, P. A. (2006). Group versus individual approach? A meta-analysis of the effectiveness of interventions to promote physical activity. *Sport and Exercise Psychology Review, 1,* 19-35.

Burke, S. M., Shapcott, K., Carron, A. V., and Eys, M.A. (2007). *A qualitative examination of individual preferences for aerobic physical activity contexts.* Manuscript in preparation.

Canadian Fitness and Lifestyle Research Institute (2007). *2006 Physical Activity Monitor.* Ottawa, ON: Canadian Fitness and Lifestyle Research Institute.

Cameron, C., Craig, C.L., and Paolin, S. (2005). *Local opportunities for physical activity and sport: Trends from 1999 – 2004.* Ottawa, ON: Canadian Fitness and Lifestyle Research Institute.

Carron, A. V., Brawley, L. R., and Widmeyer, W. N. (1998). The measurement of cohesiveness in sport groups. In J. L. Duda (Ed.), *Advances in sport and exercise psychology measurement* (pp. 213-226). Morgantown, WV: Fitness Information Technology.

Carron, A. V., Hausenblas, H. A, and Estabrooks, P. A. (2003). *The psychology of physical activity.* New York: McGraw-Hill.

Carron, A. V., Hausenblas, H. A., and Mack, D. E. (1996). Social influence and exercise: A meta-analysis. *Journal of Sport and Exercise Psychology, 18,* 1-16.

Carron, A. V., and Spink, K. S. (1993). Team building in an exercise setting. *The Sport Psychologist, 7,* 8-18.

Carron, A. V., Widmeyer, W. N., and Brawley, L. R. (1985). The development of an instrument to assess cohesion in sport teams: The group environment questionnaire. *Journal of Sport Psychology, 7,* 244-266.

Courneya, K. S., and McCauley, E. (1995). Reliability and discriminant validity of subjective norm, social support, and cohesion in an exercise setting. *Journal of Sport and Exercise Psychology, 17,* 325-337.

Cutrona, C. E., and Russell, D. W. (1987). The provisions of social relationships and adaptation to stress. In W. H. Jones, and D. Perlman (Eds.), *Advances in personal relationships* (pp. 37-67). Greenwich, CT: JAI Press.

Dishman, R. K., and Buckworth, J. (1996). Increasing physical activity: A quantitative synthesis. *Medicine and Science in Sports and Exercise, 28,* 706-719.

Duncan, T. E., and McAuley, E. (1993). Social support and efficacy cognitions in exercise adherence: A latent growth curve analysis. *Journal of Behavioral Medicine, 16,* 199-218.

Estabrooks, P. A., and Carron, A. V. (1999). Group cohesion in older adult exercisers: Prediction and intervention effects. *Journal of Behavioral Medicine, 22,* 575-588.

Estabrooks, P. A., Fox, E. H., Doerksen, S. E., Bradshaw, M. H., and King, A. C. (2005). Participatory research to promote physical activity at congregate-meal sites. *Journal of Aging and Physical Activity, 13,* 121-144.

Etnier, J. L., Salazar, W., Landers, D. M., Petruzzello, S. J., Han, M., and Nowell, P. (1997). The influence of physical fitness and exercise upon cognitive functioning: A meta-analysis. *Journal of Sport and Exercise Psychology, 19,* 249-277.

Eys, M. A., Hardy, J., and Patterson, M. M. (2006). Group norms and their relationship to cohesion in an exercise environment. *International Journal of Sport and Exercise Psychology, 4,* 43-56.

Hardy, J., Eys, M. A., and Carron, A. V. (2005). Exploring the potential disadvantages of high cohesion in sports teams. *Small Group Research, 36,* 166-187.

Haskell, W. L. (1994). Physical/physiological/biological outcomes of physical activity. In H. A. Quinney, L. Gauvin, and A. E. T. Wall (Eds.), *Toward active living* (pp. 17-23). Champaign, IL: Human Kinetics.

Hays, R. B. (1985). A longitudinal study of friendship development. *Journal of Personality and Social Psychology, 48,* 909-924.

Holt, N. L., and Hoar, S. D. (2006). The multidimensional construct of social support. In S. Hanton and S. D. Mellalieu (Eds.), *Literature reviews in sport psychology* (pp. 199-225). Hauppauge, NY: Nova Science Publishers, Inc.

Iverson, D. C., Fielding, J. E., Crow, R. S., and Christenson, G. M. (1985). The promotion of physical activity in the United States population: The status of programs in medical, worksite, community, and school settings. *Public Health Reports, 100*, 212-224.

Kahn, E. B., Ramsey, L. T., Brownson, R. C., Heath, G. W., Howze, E. H., Powell, K. E., et al. (2002). The effectiveness of interventions to increase physical activity: A systematic review. *American Journal of Preventive Medicine, 22*, 73-107.

Landers, D. M., and Petruzzello, S. J. (1994). The effectiveness of exercise and physical activity in reducing anxiety and reactivity to psychosocial stressors. In H. A. Quinney, L. Gauvin, and A. E. T. Wall (Eds.), *Toward active living* (pp. 77-82). Champaign, IL: Human Kinetics.

Lott, A J., and Lott, B. E. (1965). Group cohesiveness as interpersonal attraction: A review of relationships with antecedent and consequent variables. *Psychological Bulletin, 64,* 259-309.

Lox, C. L., Martin Ginis, K. A., and Petruzzello, S. J. (2006). *The psychology of exercise: Integrating theory and practice* (2nd ed.). Scottsdale, AZ: Holcomb Hathaway Publishers.

Nunnally, J. C. (1978). *Psychometric theory.* New York: McGraw-Hill.

Pierce, G. R., Sarason, B. R., Sarason, I. G., Joseph, H. J., and Henderson, C. A. (1996). Conceptualizing and assessing social support in the context of family. In G. R. Pierce, B. R. Sarason, and I. G. Sarason (Eds.), *Handbook of social support and the family* (pp. 3-23). New York: Plenum Press.

Sarason, I. G., Sarason, B. R., and Pierce, G. R. (1994). Social support: Global and relationship-based levels of analysis. *Journal of Social and Personal Relationships, 11,* 295-312.

Spink, K. S., and Carron, A. V. (1993). The effects of team building on the adherence patterns of female exercise participants. *Journal of Sport and Exercise Psychology, 15,* 39-49.

Spink, K. S., and Carron, A. V. (1994). Group cohesion effects in exercise classes. *Small Group Research, 25,* 26-42.

Tucker, P., and Irwin, J. D. (2006). Feasibility of a campus-based "buddy system" to promote physical activity: Canadian students' perspectives. *Journal of Physical Activity and Health, 3,* 323-334.

U.S. Department of Health and Human Services. (2004). *Health People 2010.* Washington, DC: U.S. Government Printing Office.

Weiss, R. S. (1974). The provisions of social relationships. In Z. Rubin, (Ed.), *Doing unto others* (pp.17-26). Englewood Cliffs, NJ: Prentice Hall.

In: Sport and Exercise Psychology Research Advances　　ISBN: 978-1-60456-157-9
Editors: M. P. Simmons, L. A. Foster, pp. 207-219　　© 2008 Nova Science Publishers, Inc.

Chapter IX

The Athletes' Retirement Decision Inventory (ARDI): Preliminary Findings

Anne Fernandez,[14] Evelyne Fouquereau[1] and Yannick Stephan[2]
1. EA 2114 "Aging and Adult Development", University of Tours, France
2. JE 2494, University of Paris XI, France

Abstract

This is the second section of a broader study focusing on athletes' retirement decision process. A preliminary study (Fernandez, Stephan, and Fouquereau, 2006) dealt with the reasons which lead athletes to end their career and provided a new tool for assessing the pattern of these reasons, namely a self-report questionnaire called the Athletes' Retirement Decision Inventory based on the Push Pull Anti-push Anti-pull theoretical framework. This questionnaire provides a comprehensive view of how athletes fluctuate between Push, Pull, Anti-push and Anti-pull factors when they decide to end their career. The first objective of the present study was to extend this earlier work by examining the relationship between a number of personal characteristics (chronological age, gender, marital status, family status and subjective health) and the four ARDI subscales. The second goal was to identify the relative contribution of the four factors (Push, Pull, Anti-push and Anti-pull) in athletes' intention to retire. About 190 competitive athletes participated in this study. The results of standard multiple-regression analyses revealed first that the personal characteristic variables had no effect on the pattern of reasons for retirement measured by the ARDI. Secondly, the results of a sequential regression analysis indicated a relationship between the ARDI and the athletes' intention to retire; the four subscales of the ARDI predicted the athletes' intention to retire more accurately than the socio-demographic variables typically studied in the literature, with the Pull subscale emerging as the most predictive. The present study highlights the importance of how the future is perceived in the retirement decision

14 Correspondence concerning this chapter should be adressed to Anne Fernandez, Université François Rabelais, EA 2114 "Vieillissement et Développement Adulte", Département de Psychologie, 3 rue des Tanneurs, BP 4103, F-37041 Tours, Cedex 1, France. Tel: 33 (0)2-47-36-65-54, Fax: 33 (0)2-47-36-64-84, E-mail address: anne.fernandez@univ-tours.fr.

process. This finding should allow the development of specific career transition programs for athletes in which career counsellors do not confine their interview to exploring the present situation, but systematically enlarge it to analysing how the future is perceived.

It can be hoped that future studies will continue to investigate the possibilities offered by this tool for a better understanding of the athletes' retirement process.

Keywords: *Athletes' Retirement Decision Inventory (ARDI), Push Pull Anti-Push Anti-Pull, Athletes' Sports Career Termination, Retirement Decision Process.*

Introduction

Career transitions and career decision-making have become a crucial topic in sports psychology. This field of research has led to numerous studies over the last decade, with increasing interest from both researchers and career counsellors. The extant research has mainly focused on the career termination process of athletes, and more specifically on its causes and consequences (for a review, see Alfermann and Stambulova, 2007). The strong connection between the causes of retirement and how athletes adapt to it has indeed been widely demonstrated (eg., Alfermann, Stambulova, and Zemaityte, 2004; Taylor and Ogilvie, 2001). For example, several studies have shown that voluntary career termination is linked to better adaptation to retirement, while forced withdrawal from elite sport is linked to greater difficulties in managing this period (Alfermann, 2000; Webb, Nasco, Riley, and Headrick, 1998; Werthner and Orlick, 1986). The present study falls within this research area, and is based on the use of a new tool, the Athletes' Retirement Decision Inventory (ARDI; Fernandez, Stephan, and Fouquereau, 2006), whose aim is to assess the pattern of reasons which lead competitive athletes to end their career and which can be used by professional counsellors helping athletes prepare for retirement.

Before describing this scale and its specific features, a brief outline of the background to its development will be given. In the research area of reasons for sports career termination, several studies have been carried out aimed at gaining a better understanding of retirement from sports, and a number of researchers have attempted to provide exhaustive lists of these reasons. For example, Werthner and Orlick's study (1986) described seven factors that might be involved in the transition from sport: (a) A new focus, which covers an alternative to sports participation, (b) A sense of accomplishment, whereby the athlete feels that his/her goals have been reached, (c) Problems with coaches, (d) Injuries/health problems, (e) Politics/sport-association problems, (f) Financial difficulties, and (g) Support of family and friends. Swain (1991) showed that many athletes retire because they want to pursue positive alternatives such as family relationships and job opportunities. Many athletes also retire because of a desire to discover new activities and new focuses in their lives, and to seek out new challenges and sources of satisfaction in other areas of life (Stephan, Bilard, Ninot, and Delignières, 2003). Taylor and Ogilvie (1994) proposed four main causal factors for terminating an athletic career: age, deselection, consequences of an injury, and free choice (1994). Lavallee, Grove, and Gordon (1997) found that work/study commitments, loss of motivation, the politics of sport, decreased performance, finance and decreased enjoyment were the main causes for retirement. Finally, some researchers have tried to make this research area clearer by classifying the reasons for retirement according to several factors, for example (a) voluntary versus involuntary (Alfermann, 2000; Crook and Robertson, 1991; Taylor and Ogilvie, 2001; Webb et al., 1998), (b) planned versus unplanned (Alfermann et al., 2004), (c) athletic versus non-athletic (Cecić Erpič, Wylleman, and Zupančič, 2004).

However, these classifications have recently been called into question. For example, Kerr and Dacyshyn (2000) demonstrated that the distinction between freely chosen (voluntary) and forced (involuntary) retirement is not always clear because of the diversity and nature of the potential factors which determine why athletes retire. More broadly, Alfermann (2000) highlighted the complexity of these causes, and emphasized that the decision to retire from elite sport is rarely based on a single cause, but rather on a combination of a variety of factors inside and outside the sports domain. Moreover, professional counsellors are frequently confronted with athletes whose reasoning and decision-making fluctuates between different types of reasons.

Summarising the potential reasons why athletes end their careers, far from having a single cause, these are numerous and varied, with an interaction and balance between numerous factors. On the one hand, some athletes are pushed toward retirement (e.g., injury), while others desire to pursue their sports career because they still feel able to perform or are attached to the competitive athlete's social status. On the other hand, some are pulled to retirement (e.g., to spend more time with their family), while others are afraid of the uncertainty of the post-sports life or of feeling unable to succeed in a new socio-professional setting.

While these empirical reports do not correspond to any theoretical framework in the sports literature, within the general decision-making area of research, they fit the *push pull anti-push anti-pull* framework, which derives mainly from the general retirement literature (e.g., Feldman, 1994; Hanisch, 1994; Reitzes, Mutran, and Fernandez, 1998), and also from research into cross-cultural migration (Mullet, Dej, Lemaire, Raïff, and Barthorpe, 2000). Push factors have been defined as negative considerations, such as poor health or dislike of one's job, which induce older workers to retire (Shultz, Morton, and Weckerle, 1998), whereas pull factors are typically positive considerations, such as the desire to pursue leisure interests or voluntary activities, that attract older workers toward retirement (Shultz et al., 1998). In their study, Mullet et al. (2000) conceptualised the anti-push factor as attachment to the present situation, and anti-pull factors as the costs and risks perceived in the future situation.

In 2006, our aim was to develop a self-report instrument based on this *push pull anti-push anti-pull* theoretical framework, which had never been used in the specific area of sports career termination, but which we believed could provide a suitable explanation of the retirement decision process. Traditional questionnaire construction methodology was used to develop the ARDI (Fernandez et al., 2006) which is now usable, having a good psychometric basis, with good internal consistency, accounting for a sufficient proportion of the overall variance, and showing a clearly interpretable four-factor solution corresponding to the four theoretically relevant categories. The whole questionnaire consists of 39 items directly related to the four dimensions, rated on a 10-point Likert-type scale. The instrument is self-scored.

In terms of specific factors, the Anti-pull factor includes 15 items dealing with the overall risk and cost aspects of the post-career life. It corresponds to concern about life after ending the sports career, including items such as "To be afraid of not being able to adapt to another job". The Cronbach's alpha for this factor was .90.

The Pull factor contains 12 items expressing positive thinking about life after the end of the sports career such as "Can fulfil other projects". The Cronbach's alpha for this factor was .88.

The Anti-push factor is measured by 6 items corresponding to attachment to the sports career, expressing positive assessments of the athlete's present life such as "I still enjoy participating in my sport". The Cronbach's alpha for this factor was .76.

Finally, the Push factor expresses negative considerations about the athlete's present life and consists of 6 items expressing the negative aspects of the athlete's present situation that could induce him/her to end the sports career, such as "I am in conflict with my manager or coach". The Cronbach's alpha for this factor was .87.

In summary, the ARDI can help account for the overall complex process of deciding to retire from sport by showing for example how an athlete can be both pulled to retirement by the desire to discover new opportunities, and at the same time be afraid of feeling useless without sport (Anti-pull factor). Conversely, athletes can be pushed toward retirement because of deselection, and at the same time feel convinced that they can still perform (Anti-push factor). Identification of these new dimensions can be very useful for professional counsellors who advise top-level athletes in their preparation for retirement. They can accurately diagnose the importance of each factor in the decision to retire and consequently design more targeted counselling strategies.

The objective of the present study was to propose a preliminary use of the ARDI. More specifically, we pursued two main objectives: a) to examine the relationship between several personal characteristics and the ARDI in order to establish a tentative pattern of determinants based on the four ARDI dimensions, and b) to identify the relative contribution of different ARDI factors in the athlete's intention to retire.

To our knowledge, this research is the first to use the ARDI, and is thus by nature an exploratory study. Taking a traditional exploratory step, we first decided to examine the relationship between certain personal characteristics of athletes and the ARDI, retaining standard variables used in the literature, namely chronological age, gender, marital status and family status. Several of these variables had been studied in Fernandez et al.'s 2006 research, from which certain hypotheses can be drawn. In contrast, other variables have never been assessed through their link with the ARDI, and in these cases, no hypotheses can be formulated. This is the case for chronological age, family status and subjective health. Although age has received considerable research attention in the retirement process field (e.g., Cunningham, Sagas, and Ashley, 2001; Henkens, 1999; Smith and Moen, 2004), no study has specifically examined its relationship with the four ARDI subscales. Regarding family status, previous research, for example that of Turner, Bailey and Scott (1994), examined the relationship between the number and age of dependent children and retirement planning and attitude. Their results indicated that respondents with young children expressed negative attitudes toward retirement. Health status has often been identified as one of the main causes for career termination. Injury and its potential consecutive decline in sports performance, and the feeling of no longer having one's physical and psychological capabilities, have indeed been shown to be crucial in the retirement process (e.g., Cecić Erpič et al., 2004; Drawer and Fuller, 2002; Taylor and Ogilvie, 1994). However, since the relationships between these variables and the four ARDI subscales have never been explored, no specific hypotheses can be suggested. On the other hand, the relationship between gender and ARDI was examined in the original study (Fernandez et al., 2006), results from the MANOVA revealing a non-significant difference between men and women on the four ARDI subscales. It could thus be expected that this variable would have no effect on the four ARDI subscales. The effect of marital status was also examined in the earlier study, the results revealing a significant difference between single and non-single athletes, the latter feeling more insecure about their post-retirement future. Consequently, an effect of this variable could be expected on ARDI.

The second objective of the present study was to examine the relationship between the four ARDI subscales and the intention to retire. Even though the effects of specific variables, such as age, injury, deselection etc., have already been studied in the decision to retire, the role of combined reasons as classified in the ARDI have never been evaluated. Our second goal was thus to identify the relative weight of the four ARDI factors in athletes' intentions to end their careers. Since there is no literature dealing directly with the link between the ARDI and the intention to retire, no specific hypothesis has been formulated.

Method

Participants

A total of 193 competitive athletes (142 males, 51 females) from a number of French sports clubs were recruited for this study. Ages ranged from 20 to 48 years ($M = 26.15$, $SD = 5.47$). They had been competing in their sport for an average of 9 years ($SD = 6.97$) and intended to end their career within an average of 6 years ($SD = 4.23$). They were recruited from various individual (44%) and team sports (56%).

Measures

Each participant completed a questionnaire with three sections. The first part concerned demographic information (age, gender, marital and family status) and personal characteristics such as subjective health which was assessed by a single item on a Likert-type scale ranging from 1 (*poor*) to 6 (*excellent*).

The second part consisted of the 39 items of the ARDI, rated on a Likert-type scale ranging from 1 (*not important at all*) to 10 (*very important*).

The third part was comprised of sports career questions relating to the sport involved (individual vs. team), the number of years spent in competitive sport, and the time estimated before retirement. Finally, a single item measured the intention to end the career: "Overall, I feel ready to end my sports career", with responses given on a 10-point rating scale ranging from 1 (*not at all*) to 10 (*absolutely*).

Procedure

Most questionnaires were distributed by coaches, and the other participants were contacted by mail via address lists of sports federations or by personal contact. Each volunteer athlete completed the questionnaire individually and was asked not to put his/her name on it to ensure anonymity and confidentiality of the responses. There was no time limit.

In total, 480 questionnaires were distributed, of which 217 were returned (return rate of about 45%) with 193 that could be used in the data analyses.

Results

Data Screening

Following the evaluation of assumptions results, the variables were transformed to reduce skewness, reduce the number of outliers, and improve the normality, linearity, and homoscedasticity of residuals (Tabachnik and Fidell, 2006). A square root transformation was used on the chronological age variable. A logarithmic transformation was used on the measure of subjective health. A reflect and square root transformation was used on the measures of Pull and Anti-push subscales. Two outliers were identified by application of a p < .001 criterion for Mahalanobis distance, $\chi^2_{(5)} = 20.515$. These two cases were excluded and analyses were conducted on the remaining 191 cases. Finally, multicollinearity screening showed that all variables were entered in the equation without violating the default value for tolerance.

Relationships between the Four ARDI Subscales and Individual Characteristics

To assess the relationship between each ARDI factor and a number of individual characteristics, multiple regression analyses were conducted with the four ARDI subscales as dependent variables and four demographic variables (age, gender, marital status and family status) and one variable relating to subjective health as independent variables.

Since the ARDI is a new tool, no previous studies have investigated the predictors of each subscale, and thus no theoretical considerations were available to determine the order of entry of the independent variables. A series of standard multiple regressions was thus conducted. Separate analyses were performed for the four ARDI subscales.

First, a regression analysis of the Anti-pull subscale on the five independent variables (chronological age, gender, marital status, family status and subjective health) was carried out. Table 1 presents the correlations between the variables, the unstandardized regression coefficients (B), the standardized regression coefficients (β), the t statistics, the variance inflation factor (VIF), and R, R^2, and adjusted R^2 after entry of all five independent variables. R for regression was not significantly different from zero, $F(5, 182) = 2.14$, ns, with $R^2 = .05$. The five independent variables did not contribute significantly to regression.

Table 1. Standard Multiple Regression of the Anti-pull subscale on Chronological age, Gender, Marital status, Family status and Subjective Health

Variables	Anti-pull (DV)	Chronological age	Gender	Marital status	Family status	B	β	t	VIF
Chronological age	-.15					-.07	-.23	-2.10	1.85
Gender	-.04	.04				-.15	-.04	-.51	1.01
Marital status	.12	-.48**	-.02			.59	.16	1.77	1.70
Family status	.01	.66**	.03	-.63		1.04	.24	2.21	2.13
Subjective health	-.04	.13	.03	-.09	.04	-.02	-.01	-.12	1.02
						$R^2 = .05$ Adjusted $R^2 = .03$ $R = .23$			

Note. Gender was coded 1 (*male*) and 0 (*female*). Marital status was coded 1 (*single*) and 0 (*not single*). Family status was coded 1 (*with children*) and 0 (*without children*).
** $p < .001$.

Table 2. Standard Multiple Regression of the Pull subscale on Chronological age, Gender, Marital status, Family status and Subjective Health

Independent variable	B	β	t
Chronological age	-.01	-.10	-1.01
Gender	-.06	-.07	-.91
Marital status	.08	.10	1.07
Family status	.01	.01	.12
Subjective health	.05	.10	1.37
	$R^2 = .04$ Adjusted $R^2 = .01$ $R = .19$		

Note. Gender was coded 1 (*male*) and 0 (*female*). Marital status was coded 1 (*single*) and 0 (*not single*). Family status was coded 1 (*with children*) and 0 (*without children*).

A second standard multiple regression was performed between the Pull subscale as the dependent variable and chronological age, gender, marital status, family status, and subjective health as independent variables. Table 2 shows the results of this analysis. The effects for the five independent variables were not significant, $F(5, 180) = 1.37$, ns, $R^2 = .04$.

A regression analysis of the Anti-push subscale scores on the five independent variables (chronological age, gender, marital status, family status and subjective health) was then conducted. The results shown in Table 3 reveal a non-significant effect of the five variables, $F(5, 184) = 1.79$, *ns*, $R^2 = .05$.

Finally, the effects of chronological age, gender, marital status, family status and subjective health on the Push subscale were tested. Table 4 shows the results of this analysis. R for regression was not significantly different from zero, $F(5, 181) = 2.15$, *ns*, with $R^2 = .05$. The five independent variables did not contribute significantly to regression.

Table 3. Standard Multiple Regression of the Anti-push subscale on Chronological age, Gender, Marital status, Family status and Subjective Health

Independent variable	B	β	t
Chronological age	-.02	.21	2.17
Gender	-.12	-.11	-1.51
Marital status	.03	.03	.34
Family status	-.23	-.20	-1.81
Subjective health	-.04	-.07	-.97
$R^2 = .05$			
Adjusted $R^2 = .02$			
$R = .22$			

Note. Gender was coded 1 (*male*) and 0 (*female*). Marital status was coded 1 (*single*) and 0 (*not single*). Family status was coded 1 (*with children*) and 0 (*without children*).

Table 4. Standard Multiple Regression of the Push subscale on Chronological age, Gender, Marital status, Family status and Subjective Health

Independent variable	B	β	t
Chronological age	-.12	-.23	-2.20
Gender	.56	.11	1.61
Marital status	.06	.01	.15
Family status	.58	.20	2.16
Subjective health	-.07	-.07	-.35
$R^2 = .05$			
Adjusted $R^2 = .04$			
$R = .23$			

Note. Gender was coded 1 (*male*) and 0 (*female*). Marital status was coded 1 (*single*) and 0 (*not single*). Family status was coded 1 (*with children*) and 0 (*without children*).

Relationships between the Four ARDI Subscales and the Intention to End the Career

The second objective was to determine which variables contribute significantly to predicting the intention to end the career, and particularly to identifying the relative weight of different ARDI subscales in athletes' intention to retire. A sequential regression analysis was thus conducted to determine whether the information added by the ARDI improved prediction of the intention to end the career. Since the age variable is often stated as one of the most important causes for terminating a sports career (Cecić Erpič et al., 2004), it was presumed to be causally prior, and thus given higher priority in the analysis. This variable was thus entered first in order to see how well the intention to end the career could be predicted from the other predictors while holding initial differences in age constant. Secondly, the three demographic variables (gender, marital status and family status) and subjective health were entered. Finally, at the third step, the four ARDI subscales were entered in block. Results are summarized in Table 5.

At the end of each step, R was significantly different from zero. The significance of the bivariate relationship between age and intention to end the career was assessed at the end of step 1, $F(1, 181) = 37.34$, $p < .001$. The bivariate correlation was .41, accounting for 17% of the variance. After step 2, with the three demographic variables and subjective health, $F(5, 177) = 9.76$, $p < .001$, $R^2 = .21$. Increment in R^2 at this step was .04, $\Delta F(4, 173) = 2.55$, ns. Thus, addition of the three demographic variables and subjective health in the equation did not reliably improve the R^2. At the third step, with ARDI subscales added to prediction of intention to end the career by age, $R^2 = .31$, $F(9, 173) = 8.60$, $p < .001$. Addition of the ARDI subscales to the equation resulted in a significant increment in R^2, $\Delta R^2 = .09$, $\Delta F(4, 173) = 5.81$, $p < .001$, with an effect of Anti-pull subscale ($\beta = -.24$, $p < .001$) and of Pull subscale ($\beta = .21$, $p < .01$).

This pattern of results suggests that the most important predictor in the variability of intention to end the career is age. Neither the other socio-demographic variables, nor subjective health improved prediction. In contrast, the ARDI subscales contributed significantly to predicting the intention to end the career.

Table 5. Sequential Regression of the Intention to end the career on Chronological age, Gender, Marital status, Family status, Subjective Health and the four ARDI subscales

Variables	B	β	R	R^2	ΔR^2	ΔF
Step 1						
Chronological age	.24**	.41**	.41**	.17**		
Step 2						
Gender	-1.07	-.15				
Marital status	-.25	-.04				
Family status	-1.69	-.21				
Subjective health	.06	.00	.46	.21	.04	2.55
Step 3						
Anti-pull subscale	-.45**	-.24**				
Pull subscale	1.70*	.21*				
Anti-push subscale	-.88	-.13				
Push subscale	-.07	-.05	.56**	.31**	.09**	5.81**

Note. Gender was coded 1 (*male*) and 0 (*female*). Marital status was coded 1 (*single*) and 0 (*not single*). Family status was coded 1 (*with children*) and 0 (*without children*).
*$p < .01$. **$p < .001$.

Conclusion

The present study provides preliminary findings regarding an initial use of the ARDI, which is a new tool for investigating the retirement decision process of athletes. Overall, the purpose was to examine the relationship between the ARDI and several variables. More specifically, the aim was twofold: a) to look closely at the effects of several personal characteristics on the ARDI, and b) to identify the relative weight of the four ARDI subscales in athletes' intention to retire.

Regarding our first objective, results of the regression analyses revealed that the personal characteristic variables of chronological age, gender, marital status, family status and subjective health had no effect on the pattern of reasons for retirement measured by the ARDI. These results provide support for previous studies examining the relationship between personal characteristics and the decision to retire. Several studies have shown the weak impact of personal characteristics on the retirement process. For example, Turner et al. (1994) found no significant effect of gender, marital status, income, perceived health or number of children in particular on retirement planning behaviours and attitude toward retirement. Similarly, in the more specific field of athletes' career termination, Alfermann and Stambulova (2007) assessed major empirical findings which revealed many similarities and only minor differences between men and women's reasons for retiring. Results of the present study not only support but extend these findings, showing that observations made about single reasons for retirement are also valid for structured categories of reasons. In sum, the cognitive processes by which athletes fluctuate between Push, Pull, Anti-push and Anti-pull factors are not determined by the personal characteristics studied in this research. To understand better the factors intervening in the dynamic cognitive balance between Push, Pull, Anti-push and Anti-pull factors, future research should look beyond the investigation of socio-demographic variables as determinants of the ARDI, and explore the impact of social psychological variables. For example, individual and social resources of athletes could be included, since these variables have already been shown to be significant in the career transition process for athletes, particularly the possibility of a link between the social support network and career transition needs (e.g., Lavallee, 2006; Martin and Dodder, 1993; Stephan et al., 2003; Webb et al., 1998). More broadly, it should be noted that these variables form part of the four major sets of factors identified by Schlossberg, Waters and Goodman (1995) in their well-known transition model, "the 4 S System". This model proposes the variables of Situation, Self, Support and Strategies to understand how individuals cope with transition. Another promising line of investigation to understand what determines the four ARDI components is to include variables directly linked to sports practice, such as athletic identity or type of sport (individual vs. collective), which have been shown to be important in the retirement process (eg., Cecić Erpič et al., 2004; Torregrosa, Boixádos, and Cruz, 2004).

Regarding our second objective, the results indicate a relationship between the ARDI and the athletes' intention to retire, the four subscales of the ARDI predicting the athletes' intention to retire better than the socio-demographic variables typically studied in the literature. Furthermore, the Pull subscale appears to be the most predictive, which is consistent with the findings of the previous study which developed this tool. The Anti-pull and Pull factors were shown to differentiate groups best. The present study highlights the importance of how the future is viewed in the retirement decision process. This point should help develop specific career transition programs for athletes, in which career counsellors do not confine their investigation to exploring the present situation, but systematically enlarge it to analysing how the future is perceived.

These preliminary findings provide an illustration of the use of the ARDI, emphasizing the importance of having a specific tool to improve understanding of the retirement process of athletes. It can be hoped that future studies will continue to investigate the possibilities offered by this tool. For example, it could be used in a longitudinal study to provide an in-depth analysis of how athletes fluctuate between the four ARDI subscales during the retirement decision-making process, that is to say, whether the importance of each of the four ARDI subscales varies according to the time of the retirement process, and whether this fluctuation depends on external or internal factors. Another line of research could be to enlarge the use of this tool to delineate more precisely the most important psychological correlates in the reasons to retire, which is an important area of future research.

Authors Notes

The authors express their sincere gratitude to the EA 2114 for supporting this project. They would also like to acknowledge the students for their participation in the data collection for this study.

References

Alfermann, D. (2000). Causes and consequences of sport career termination. In D. Lavallee and P. Wylleman (Eds.), *Career transitions in sport: International perspectives* (pp.45-58). Morgantown, WV: Fitness Information Technology.

Alfermann, D., and Stambulova, N. (2007). Career transitions and career termination. In G. Tenenbaum and R. C. Eklund (Eds.), *Handbook of sport psychology* (3rd ed., pp. 712-736). New York: Wiley.

Alfermann, D., Stambulova, N., and Zemaityte, A. (2004). Reactions to sport career termination: A cross-national comparison of German, Lithuanian, and Russian athletes. *Psychology of Sport and Exercise, 5*(1), 61-75.

Cecić Erpič, S. C., Wylleman, P., and Zupančič, M. (2004). The effect of athletic and non-athletic factors on the sports career termination process. *Psychology of Sport and Exercice, 5*, 45-59.

Crook, J. M., and Robertson, S. E. (1991). Transitions out of elite sport. *International Journal of Sport Psychology, 22*, 115-127.

Cunningham, G. B., Sagas, M., and Ashley, F. B. (2001). Occupational commitment and intent to leave the coaching profession. *International Review for the Sociology of Sport, 36*(2), 131-148.

Drawer, S., and Fuller, C. W. (2002). Perceptions of retired professional soccer players about the provision of support services before and after retirement. *British Journal of Sports Medicine, 36,* 33-38.

Feldman, D. C. (1994). The decision to retire early: A review and conceptualization. *Academy of Management Review, 19*(2), 285-311.

Fernandez, A., Stephan, Y., and Fouquereau, E. (2006). Assessing reasons for sports career termination: Development of the Athletes' Retirement Decision Inventory (ARDI). *Psychology of Sport and Exercise, 7*(4), 407-421.

Hanisch, K. A. (1994). Reasons people retire and their relation to attitudinal and behavioral correlates in retirement. *Journal of Vocational Behavior, 45,* 1-16.

Henkens, K. (1999). Retirement intentions and spousal support: A multi-actor approach. *Journal of Gerontology: Social Sciences, 54B,* S63-S73.

Kerr, G., and Dacyshyn, A. (2000). The retirement experiences of female elite gymnasts. *Journal of Applied Sport Psychology, 12,* 115-133.

Lavallee, D. (2006). Career awareness, career planning, and career transition needs among sports coaches. *Journal of Career Development, 33*(1), 66-79.

Lavallee, D., Grove, J. R., and Gordon, S. (1997). The causes of career termination from sport and their relationship to post-retirement adjustment among elite-amateur athletes in Australia. *Australian Psychologist, 32,* 131-135.

Martin, D. E., and Dodder, R. A. (1993). A path analytic examination of sport termination. *International Review for the Sociology of Sport, 28*(1), 75-88.

Mullet, E., Dej, V., Lemaire, I., Raïff, P., and Barthorpe, J. (2000). Studying, working, and living in another EU country: French youth's point of view. *European Psychologist, 5*(3), 216-227.

Reitzes, D. C., and Mutran, E. J., and Fernandez, M. E. (1998). The decision to retire: A career perspective. *Social Science Quarterly, 79*(3), 607-619.

Schlossberg, N., Waters, E. B., and Goodman, J. (1995). *Counseling adults in transition. Linking practice with theory* (2nd ed.). New York, NY: Springer Publishing Company.

Shultz, K. S., Morton, K. R., and Weckerle, J. R. (1998). The influence of Push and Pull factors on involuntary early retirees' retirement decision and adjustment. *Journal of Vocational Behavior, 53,* 45-57.

Smith, D. B., and Moen, P. (2004). Retirement satisfaction for retirees and their spouses. Do gender and the retirement decision-making process matter? *Journal of Family Issues, 25*(2), 262-285.

Stephan, Y., Bilard, J., Ninot, G., and Delignières, D. (2003). Repercussions of transition out of elite sport on subjective well-being: A one-year study. *Journal of Applied Sport Psychology, 15,* 354-371.

Swain, D. A. (1991). Withdrawal from sport and Schlossberg's model of transitions. *Sociology of Sport Journal, 8*(2), 152-160.

Tabachnick, B. G., and Fidell, L. S. (2006). *Using multivariate statistics* (5th ed.). Boston, MA: Allyn and Bacon.

Taylor, J. and Ogilvie, B. C. (1994). A conceptual model of adaptation to retirement among athletes. *Journal of Applied Sport Psychology, 6,* 1-20.

Taylor, J., and Ogilvie, B. C. (2001). Career termination among athletes. In R. N. Singer, H. A. Hausenblas, and C. M. Janelle (Eds.), *Handbook of sport psychology* (2nd ed., pp. 672-691). New York: Wiley.

Torregrosa, M., Boixadós, M., and Cruz, J. (2004). Elite athletes' image of retirement: The way to relocation in sport. *Psychology of Sport and Exercise,5*(1), 35-43.

Turner, M. J., Bailey, W. C., and Scott, J. P. (1994). Factors influencing attitude toward retirement and retirement planning among midlife university employees. *The Journal of Applied Gerontology, 13*(2), 143-156.

Webb, W. M., Nasco, S. A., Riley, S., and Headrick, B. (1998). Athlete identity and reactions to retirement from sports. *Journal of Sport Behavior, 21,* 338-362.

Werthner, P., and Orlick, T. (1986). Retirement experiences of successful Olympic athletes. *International Journal of Sport Psychology, 17,* 337-363.

In: Sport and Exercise Psychology Research Advances   ISBN: 978-1-60456-157-9
Editors: M. P. Simmons, L. A. Foster, pp. 221-234   © 2008 Nova Science Publishers, Inc.

Chapter X

Gender Differences in Perceived Effort

Jasmin C. Hutchinson[1] and Gershon Tenenbaum[2]

Oxford College of Emory University, Oxford, GA. USA[1]
Florida State University, Tallahassee, FL. USA[2]

Abstract

Two studies were conducted pertaining to gender differences in perceived physical effort. In the first study male (n = 7) and female (n = 8) volunteer participants (*M* age = 24.33, *SD* = 3.30) rated nine perceived effort sensations, arranged into three sensation clusters (sensory-discriminative, motivational-affective and cognitive-evaluative sensations), at regular intervals during a sustained handgrip-squeezing task. Female participants were found to report significantly higher ratings of physical and affective sensations, but significantly lower ratings of motivational sensations, than males. Females in this study were also found to report significantly lower perceived self-efficacy during the handgrip task than males. Several theories have attempted to explain gender differences in the perception of physical effort. Psychosocial theories consider socialization factors that encourage physical robustness among men, and the expression of distress among women, as important contributors to gender differences in effort perception. An alternative to this assumption is the suggestion that gender differences in athletic experience may account for observed gender differences in perceived effort and self-efficacy.

A follow-up study examined gender differences in perceived effort in male and female participants with similar athletic experience and current physical activity participation. Participants completed two exertive tasks: a sustained handgrip-squeezing task (n = 35) and a sustained cycle task (n = 13). As in the previous study three dimensions of physical effort (sensory-discriminative, motivational-affective and cognitive-evaluative sensations) were measured at regular intervals during the two tasks. Results of this study indicated no significant differences between male and female participants on any of the sensation dimensions. Additionally, males and female participants did not differ significantly on either physical or task-specific measures of self-efficacy. Based upon these findings it is concluded that previously observed gender differences in effort perception are likely due to pre-existing gender differences in athletic experience, rather than socialization factors.

Introduction

The majority of research on perceived effort has been carried out with males (Koltyn, O'Connor and Morgan, 1991), and in those investigations where females have been included in the sampling process, it has been assumed or implied that males and females perceive effort in a similar manner (Mihevic, 1978). However, some studies have reported that males and females may perceive effort differently. Females have been found to display significantly higher ratings of ratings of perceived exertion (RPE) than males at both absolute (Noble, Maresh, and Ritchie, 1981; O'Connor, Raglin and Morgan, 1996) and relative power outputs (Goss, Robertson, DaSilva, et al., 2003; Koltyn et al., 1991). In contrast, other studies have not supported a gender effect in perceived effort (Green, Crews, Bosak and Peveler, 2003; Pincivero, Campy, and Coelho, 2003; Pincivero, Coelho and Erikson, 2000; Robertson, Moyna, Sward et al., 2000). Clearly, studies that examine gender differences in perception of effort are equivocal in that some investigators have reported gender differences while others failed in revealing gender effects. Conflicting evidence makes it difficult to draw any firm conclusions regarding the role gender has in perceptions of effort during exercise. The current study is aimed at expanding the inquiry of gender differences in perceived effort by examining its effect on perceptions of several dimensions of physical effort during sustained exercise.

Several components of physical effort, grouped into three dimensions, are incorporated in the current study. Previous research questioned the validity and representativeness of Borg's (1998) "gestalt concept" of exertion and the traditional single-item measure of perceived exertion (see Hutchinson, 2004, and Hutchinson and Tenenbaum, 2006 for details). Thus, the current study examined perceived effort using three dimensions of effort - sensory-discriminative, motivational-affective and cognitive-evaluative. These perceived effort dimensions were derived from Gate-Control Theory (GCT: Melzack and Wall, 1965). GCT was the first comprehensive theory of pain to account for the capability of emotional and cognitive factors to regulate the perception of pain (Pinel, 1990). GCT postulated that in each dorsal horn of the spinal cord there is a gate-like mechanism which inhibits or facilitates the flow of afferent impulses into the spinal cord before it evokes pain perception and response. Signals from the brain are capable of activating these neural gating circuits. Thus, the brain is not simply a passive receiver of pain information, but an active system that filters, selects and modulates inputs. According to GCT, pain has three distinct dimensions: sensory-discriminative dimension, involving the location, quality, and intensity of the painful sensation; cognitive-evaluative dimension, involving appraisal of the meaning of the experience; and affective-motivational dimension, involving the emotional response and the motivation to avoid harm (Melzack and Casey, 1968). Although originally developed as theory of pain perception, GCT offers significant potential for explaining and understanding the modulation of physical effort perception. Tenenbaum, Fogarty, Stewart, et al. (1999) developed a discomfort questionnaire to elicit the feelings and thoughts of people engaged in running activities. The questionnaire consisted of 32 items divided into eight correlated subscales: proprioceptive symptoms, leg symptoms, respiratory difficulties, dryness and heat, head or stomach symptoms, mental toughness, disorientation, and task completion thoughts. These eight categories were subsequently collapsed into three dimensions suggested by Gate Control Theory: sensory-discriminative, motivational-affective, and cognitive-evaluative (see Tenenbaum et al., 1999).

Since sensory-discriminative and cognitive-evaluative sensations are more closely tied to physiological input (Noble and Robertson, 1996) females were expected to report higher ratings for these sensations. Motivational-affective sensations, in contrast, are not affected merely by physical load, and are more closely linked to perceived ability and will to invest effort in the task (Bandura, 1997). Therefore males were expected to rate motivational-affective sensations more strongly than females.

This study also sought to examine possible gender differences in self-efficacy for a physically demanding task. Self-efficacy has been conceptualized as "confidence in one's ability to behave in such a way as to produce a desirable outcome for a given task" (Bandura, 1997). Self-efficacy theory predicts that higher self-efficacy is associated with less perception of effort in coping with a challenging task. According to this theory, efficacious individuals may make better use of the skills they acquire, or may immerse themselves more fully in the task so that perceptions of effort are reduced regardless of ability level (Bandura, 1997). It has previously been demonstrated that males are significantly more self-efficacious than females for a sustained exertive task (McAuley, Courneya and Lettunich, 1991). Based upon this it was expected that females would exhibit lower self-efficacy than males when confronted with physically demanding conditions.

Method of Study One

Participants

Fifteen university students (7 male, 8 female) volunteered to participate in this study. Participants had no known physical or psychological disabilities, and were between 19-29 years of age ($M = 24.33$, $SD = 3.30$).

Instrumentation

During testing participants responded verbally to several Likert-type scales, which measured two areas of interest: self-efficacy and effort perceptions. Immediately following testing participants completed several manipulation check questions.

Self-efficacy. Self-efficacy during the task (state self-efficacy) was measured on a scale ranging from 0 ("not confident at all") to 100 ("extremely confident"). Because state constructs change over time, self-efficacy was measured at 15-second intervals during the task by asking, "How confident are you in your ability to tolerate this task for the next 15 seconds?" Potential response biases were minimized by having the self-efficacy judgments recorded privately rather than given publicly, and by informing participants that their responses would remain confidential.

Effort perceptions. Nine different effort sensations were measured at regular intervals during the task. The different sensations reflected three different dimensions of symptoms: (a) sensory-discriminative, (b) motivational-affective and (c) cognitive-evaluative. The sensory-discriminative dimension is comprised of muscle aches, pain and fatigue; the motivational-affective dimension is comprised of concentration, determination and mental toughness; and the cognitive-evaluative dimension is comprised of effort, exertion and task aversion. Effort sensations were measured by verbal report on a 10-point scale ranging from 0 ("nothing") to 10 ("extremely strong"). This scale and the corresponding effort sensations were displayed to participants throughout the exertive tasks.

Manipulation check. This scale measured participants' commitment to and effort investment in the task. Participants reported their commitment and investment on a 5-point scale ranging from 1 ("completely uncommitted / very little effort") to 5 ("very highly committed" / "a large amount of effort") at the conclusion of each trial. Since it has been theorized that task-specific commitment/determination, and the effort one is ready to invest in and tolerate while experiencing exertion, may affect coping and persisting behaviors (Tenenbaum, 2001) participants who indicate that they were not willing to invest effort in the task were excluded from the analysis.

Handgrip dynamometer. Handgrip capacity in the dominant arm was measured using a calibrated Lafayette™ handgrip dynamometer Model 78010 (Lafayette Instrument Company, Lafayette, Indiana). The testing range for this dynamometer is 0-100kg.

Procedure

Participants were exposed to the sensation of physical effort via a sustained isometric contraction using a calibrated handgrip dynamometer. Participants were instructed to squeeze the dynamometer at 25% of their previously established maximum grip for as long as they possibly could. During the task participants were asked to vocally express their current perception of each sensation based upon a 0-10 scale. Perceptions were given at 15-second intervals, when prompted by the examiner, until the task was terminated.

Statistical Analysis

Data were analyzed using SPSS Statistical Software version 11.0 (SPSS Inc. Chicago, IL). A repeated measures (RM) multivariate analysis of variance (MANOVA) was employed with time intervals (15 sec) nested within three sensation variables, nested within three dimensions (i.e., sensory-discriminative, motivational-affective and cognitive-evaluative) as repeated factors. The level of statistical significance was set at $p \leq .05$.

Results of Study One

Manipulation Check

Participants displayed very high ratings for the three manipulation check questions, indicating they were committed to the task. Means and standard deviations (SDs) were 4.14 (.53), 3.58 (.90), and 4.23 (.78) for questions pertaining to task commitment, perceived task tolerance and effort investment respectively.

Main Findings

Perceived Effort. Results of a RM MANOVA revealed a significant dimension by gender effect, F (2,20) =3.27, p < .05, which is shown in Figure 1.

Males reported higher values for motivational-affective sensations (M=6.59, SD=.61) than females (M=5.73, SD=.61), effect size (ES) = 0.58, whereas females reported higher values for sensory-discriminative (M=4.45, SD=.49) (ES = 0.75) and cognitive-evaluative dimensions (M=5.69, SD=.57) (ES= 050) than males (M=3.34, SD=.49) and (M=5.03, SD=.57) respectively.

Self-Efficacy. The RM MANOVA revealed a significant gender effect for self-efficacy, F (1,6) = 7.66, p < .05, and a significant time by gender interaction effect for self-efficacy, F (7,42) = 3.70, p < .001. These effects are represented in Figure 2 and 3 respectively.

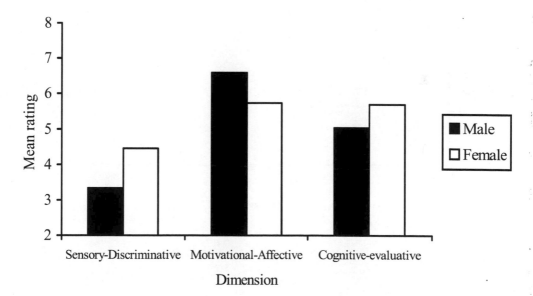

Figure 1. Mean values for sensory-discriminative, motivational-affective and cognitive-evaluative sensations by gender.

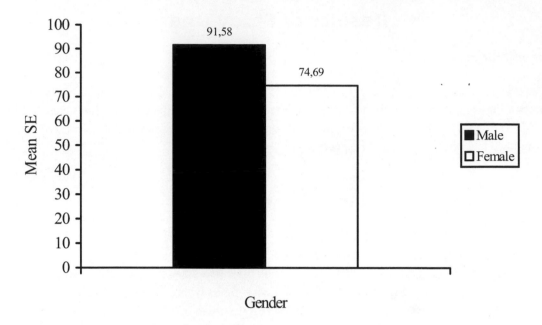

Figure 2. Mean values for self-efficacy by gender.

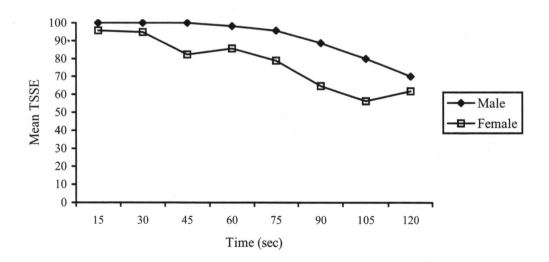

Figure 3. Time by gender interaction effect for task-specific self-efficacy.

Discussion of Study One

The main aim of this study was to examine differences in perceived effort between male and female participants in a handgrip-squeezing task. Three dimensions of perceived effort sensations (sensory-discriminative, motivational-affective and cognitive-evaluative) were measured at regular intervals during the exertive task. It was hypothesized that females would rate the task as more effortful than males; specifically females were expected to rate sensory-discriminative and cognitive-evaluative sensations higher than males. Results of a RM MANOVA revealed that females had significantly higher ratings for sensory-discriminative and cognitive-evaluative sensations, and significantly lower ratings for motivational-affective sensations, supporting the study's hypotheses. It has been suggested that socialization practices encouraging physical robustness among men (Bendelow, 1993), and the expression of distress among women (Lyons and Sullivan, 1998) contribute to gender difference in effort perception.

A further aim of the current study was to compare self-efficacy between male and female participants during a physically demanding task. Self-efficacy in this study was found to differ significantly between males and females, with males having higher self-efficacy on average, and higher sustained self-efficacy during the handgrip task. Similar findings were reported in middle aged adults by McAuley et al. (1991) who concluded that apparent efficacy differences between males and females were a function of physical, social, and cultural influences specific to a particular age range (over 45 years). However, participants in the current study were all of college age. A more likely explanation, stemming from self-efficacy theory, is that females tend to rate themselves lower in self-efficacy for skills and tasks that are stereotypically male activities. For example, women generally judge themselves to be less efficacious for scientific occupations than do men; however these differences disappear when women judge their efficacy to perform the same scientific activities when the activities are placed in the context of everyday activities (Matsui and Tsukamoto, 1991). Thus, it may be the case that females perceive exercise and exertion as a typically masculine domain, which would account for the observed gender difference in self-efficacy in both this current study and that of McAuley et al. (1991). Self-efficacy has been shown to be a cognitive mediator of associations between gender and pain perception (Jackson, Iezzi, Gunderson, Nagasaka, and Fritch, 2002). It is likely that this is also true for the related area of effort perception.

An alternative to this 'gender-appropriateness hypothesis' is the suggestion that gender differences in athletic experience may account for observed gender differences in perceived effort. It has been suggested that since males typically have more athletic experience than females, it is possible that observed gender differences in perceived effort are due to differences in athletic experience, rather than socialization factors (Winborn, Meyers, and Mulling, 1988). Athletic experience has previously been shown to account for a substantial amount of perceived effort variance (Tenenbaum et al., 1999), and must be taken into account in future studies. Morgan (2001) has argued that failure to match male and female participants on training state and physical fitness is a confounding variable affecting many studies regarding the influence of gender on perceptions of effort during exercise. Hence it is not always possible to assert that fitness differences were not responsible for the alleged gender difference in perceived effort.

Study Two

Findings from the previous study indicated that males and females perceive effort differently during a sustained handgrip task. However, it has been noted that a confounding variable that affects many studies pertaining to gender differences in effort perception is the failure to carefully match males and females on the state of training and physical fitness (Morgan, 2001). The second study extends the findings of the previous study by (a) comparing male and female participants' perceptions of effort in both an isometric handgrip task and a stationary cycling task, and (b) comparing male and female participants with similar athletic training backgrounds and levels of fitness.

It was hypothesized that, with similar levels of athletic experience, males and females would not differ in their ratings of perceived effort sensations. It was also expected that there would be no difference between males and females' reported self-efficacy for either the handgrip task or the cycle task

Method of Study Two

Participants

For the handgrip task 35 volunteer participants (21 males and 14 females) were recruited from university undergraduate and graduate classes. Participants had a mean age of 23.65 (SD=3.23) years. Thirteen of these participants (seven males and six females) also volunteered to participate in the cycle task. These participants had a mean age of 26.85 (SD=4.91) years. Participants in both tasks had no known physical or psychological disabilities that interfered with the purpose of the study.

Instrumentation

Manipulation Check. The same manipulation check used in Study One was used in the current study.

Effort Perception. Based upon the results of the first study, one sensation was selected as representative of each dimension, so a total of three sensations were assessed in Study Two. Muscle aches, determination, and effort were identified as best representing the sensory-discriminative, motivational-affective and cognitive-evaluative respectively. As in the first study, effort sensations were measured by verbal report on a 10-point scale ranging from 0 ("nothing") to 10 ("extremely strong"). Verbal ratings were given at regular intervals, when prompted by the examiner until the task was terminated. Sensations and corresponding 10-point scales were displayed to participants for the duration of the task.

Self-efficacy. This second study incorporated two self-efficacy measures - physical self-efficacy and task-specific self-efficacy. Physical self-efficacy (PSE) refers to one's appraisal of his or her ability to perform successfully in physical activities (Jackson et al., 2002), while task-specific self-efficacy (TSSE) is a domain specific measure of self-efficacy. PSE was measured using the Physical Self-Efficacy Scale (Ryckman, Robbins, Thornton, and Cantrell, 1982). The PSE scale consists of a 10-item Perceived Physical Ability (PPA) subscale and a 12-item Physical Self-Presentation Confidence (PSPC) subscale. The scores on the two subscales are summed together into an overall physical self-efficacy score. Higher values on the PSE indicate a stronger sense of physical self-efficacy. Cronbach's alpha coefficients of internal consistency have been reported at .85 for PPA, .74 for PSPC, and .80 for PSE. Test-retest reliability has been reported at .85 for PPA, .69 for PSPC, and .80 for PSE (Ryckman et al., 1982).

A two-item scale was created by the authors to measure TSSE. The items, rated on a 10-point scale from 0 ("very low") to 10 ("very high"), assessed participants' degree of certainty they would be able to perform the experimental task successfully. Self-efficacy measurement should be specific both to the situation in which the behavior occurs and level of challenge in that situation (Bandura, 2001). Self-efficacy appraisals need to reflect the level of difficulty individuals believe they can surmount because if there are no obstacles to overcome, the activity is easily performable and everyone has uniformly high self-efficacy for it. Accordingly, two items were included for TSSE, reflecting gradations of task-specific efficacy.

Athletic Experience. Participants' history of exercise participation (years), and frequency (days per week), intensity (0-10), and duration (minutes per session) of current training was measured via a self-report questionnaire.

Handgrip dynamometer. The same dynamometer used in Study One was used in the current study.

Aerobic Testing. Aerobic exercise testing was conducted using a Monark 828e mechanically braked cycle ergometer (Monark Exercise AB, Vansbro, Sweden). Heart rate (HR) data was collected using a Vantage XL Polar HR Monitor (Polar Electro, Finland). Maximal oxygen uptake and gas exchange measures were computed using 30-second breath averaging on a Parvo Medics TrueMax 2400 Metabolic Measurement System (Parvo Medics Inc., Sandy, UT).

Procedure

Two exertive tasks were performed in this study: an isometric handgrip task and a stationary cycling task. For the handgrip task, as in the previous study, participants were instructed to squeeze the dynamometer at 25% of their previously established maximum grip for as long as they possibly could. During the task participants were asked to vocally express their current perception of each sensation based upon a 0-10 scale. Perceptions were given at 15-second intervals, when prompted by the examiner, until the task was terminated. For the cycle task, maximal oxygen uptake (VO_2 max) was first obtained using a continuous cycling protocol. One week later participants returned to cycle for five minutes at 50% VO_2 max for a further five minutes at 70% VO_2 and then to volitional fatigue at 90% VO_2 max. A target HR equivalent to the prescribed % VO_2 max was determined by plotting HR responses during the VO_2 max test as a function of corresponding VO_2 responses. During testing, exercise intensity was adjusted by the examiner until the target HR (± 3 bpm) was achieved, ensuring that the prescribed relative metabolic rate was maintained. As in Study One, participants were asked to vocally express their current perception of each sensation based upon a 0-10 scale. Perceptions were given at 30-second intervals, when prompted by the examiner, until the task was terminated.

Statistical Analysis

Data were analyzed using SPSS Statistical Software version 11.0 (SPSS Inc. Chicago, IL). A RM MANOVA was employed with time intervals (30 sec) nested within three sensation variables as repeated factors. The level of statistical significance was set at $p \leq .05$.

Results of Study Two

Manipulation Check

Participants displayed very high ratings for the three manipulation check questions, indicating they were dedicated to the task. Means and SDs were 4.32 (.89), 3.88 (.98), and 4.47 (.83) for questions pertaining to task commitment, perceived task tolerance and effort investment, respectively.

Training Intensity

Participants reported duration and intensity of current training and history of participation in rigorous physical exercise. Males and females reported similar levels of training frequency, (M = 5.22 days, SD = .97; M = 4.88 days, SD = .78), intensity (M = 7.25, SD = 1.03; M = 7.25, SD = .70), duration (M = 53.75 mins, SD = 12.17; M = 55.63 mins, SD = 10.16), and history (M = 8.63 years, SD = 1.06; M = 7.88 years, SD = 1.81) respectively. Consequently, athletic experience did not differ significantly between males and females, thus, the study's aim of controlling for the possible confounding effect of training status and athletic experience was achieved.

Self-Efficacy

Both male and female participants displayed very high physical and task-specific self-efficacy for the handgrip task (see Table 1.)

Self-efficacy did not differ significantly between males and females; therefore the possible confounding effect of self-efficacy was eliminated in this study.

Table 1. Mean Values for Physical Self-Efficacy (PSE) and Task-Specific Self-Efficacy (TSSE) in the Handgrip and Cycle Task

	Males	Females
Handgrip Task		
PSE	98.7	92.9
TSSE	15.5	14.8
Cycle Task		
PSE	102.4	98.8
TSSE	17.4	15.0

Main Findings

It was hypothesized that with similar levels of athletic experience, males and females would not differ in their ratings of perceived effort sensations. The RM MANOVA indicated no significant effect for gender in either the handgrip task, $F (2,60) =.24$, $p =.79$, $\eta^2 = .04$, or the cycle task, $F (2,18) =.004$, $p =.99$, $\eta^2 =.00$. There was also no gender by sensation by time interaction effect for either the handgrip task, $F (14, 420) =.78$, $p = .69$, $\eta^2 = .03$, or the cycle task, $F (58,522) =.51$, $p = .99$, $\eta^2= .05$. Consequently, the study's hypothesis was fully supported in both the handgrip and cycle task.

Discussion of Study Two

This study aimed to extend the findings of a previous study pertaining to gender differences in effort perception. More specifically, this study examined gender differences in perceived effort in a handgrip-squeezing task and a stationary cycle task in male and female participants with comparable athletic experience. Based upon Winborn et al's (1988) athletic experience hypothesis, it was expected that there would be no difference in effort perception between male and female participants. Results revealed no significant differences in effort perception between male and female participants for either the handgrip task or the cycle task. Thus, the study's hypothesis was fully supported in both tasks. Based upon these findings, it is concluded that gender differences in perceived effort are not apparent when controlling for underlying differences in athletic experience. Furthermore, participants in this study did not differ on measures of physical and task-specific self-efficacy, indicating that self-efficacy for physical tasks is also affected by athletic experience.

Conclusion

Studies examining gender differences in perception of effort are equivocal in that some investigators have reported gender differences while others have not. Conflicting evidence has made it difficult to draw any firm conclusions regarding the influence of gender on perceptions of effort during exercise. The current investigation intended to further the understanding of gender differences in perceived effort by examining the influence of gender on perceptions of several dimensions of effort during sustained exercise. In the first study males and females were found to differ significantly in their perceptions of effort during a sustained handgrip-task. Females were found to experience sensory-discriminative and cognitive-evaluative sensations more intensely, while males reported higher ratings of motivational-affective sensations. Males were also found to possess significantly higher levels of self-efficacy for the handgrip task than females. These findings were evaluated in the light of various psychosocial theories, including the gender-appropriateness hypothesis (Matsui and Tsukamoto, 1991), the athletic experience hypothesis (Winborn et al., 1988), and self-efficacy theory (Bandura, 1977). It was concluded that while gender differences were found to exist in the perception of physical effort, this effect might have been a function of gender differences in self-efficacy and athletic experience.

A second study was conducted in which males and females with similar athletic experience were compared on three dimensions of perceived effort – sensory-discriminative, motivational-affective and cognitive-evaluative – during two physically demanding tasks, an isometric handgrip task and a stationary cycle task. Results revealed no significant effect for gender in either of the two tasks. Thus, it can be concluded that the underlying processes governing the monitoring and integration of sensory cues during exercise do not differ in males and females. It is likely that gender differences in other factors, such as physical fitness, task familiarity, or perceived self-efficacy, have led to erroneous conclusions in previous studies where gender differences in perceived effort have been reported.

References

Bandura, A. (1977). Self-efficacy: Toward a unifying theory of behavior change. *Psychological Review*, *84*, 191-215.

Bandura, A. (1997). *Self-efficacy: The exercise of control*. New York: Freeman.

Bandura, A. (2001). Guide for constructing self-efficacy scales. In G.V. Caprara (Ed.), *La valutazione dell 'autoeffcacia* [The assessment of self-efficacy] (pp. 15-37) Trento, Italy: Erickson.

Bendelow, G. (1993). Pain perceptions, emotion and gender. *Sociology of Health and Illness 15*(3), 273-294.

Borg, G. (1998). *Borg's perceived exertion and pain scales*. Champaign, IL: Human Kinetics.

Goss, F., Robertson, R., DaSilva, S., Suminski, R., Kang, J., and Metz, K. (2003). Ratings of perceived exertion and energy expenditure during light to moderate activity. *Perceptual and Motor Skills, 96*, 739-747.

Green, J.M., Crews, T.R., Bosak, A.M., and Peveler, W.W. (2003). Overall and differentiated ratings of perceived exertion at the respiratory compensation threshold: Effects of gender and mode. *European Journal of Applied Physiology, 89*, 445-450.

Hutchinson, J.C. (2004). *Psychological factors in perceived and sustained effort*. Unpublished doctoral dissertation, Florida State University, Tallahassee, FL, USA.

Hutchinson, J.C. and Tenenbaum, G (2006). Perceived effort – can it be considered gestalt? *Psychology of Sport and Exercise, 7(5),* 463-476.

Jackson, T., Iezzi, T., Gunderson, J., Nagasaka, T., and Fritch, A. (2002). Gender differences in pain perception: the mediating role of self-efficacy beliefs. *Sex Roles, 47,* 561-568.

Lyons, R., and Sullivan, M. (1998). Curbing loss in illness and disability: A relationship perspective. In J. H. Harvey (Ed.), *Perspectives on personal and interpersonal loss* (pp. 137-152). New York: Taylor and Francis.

Koltyn, K.F., O'Connor, P.J., and Morgan, W.P. (1991). Perception of effort in female and male competitive swimmers. *International Journal of Sports Medicine, 12(4),* 427-429.

Matsui, T., and Tsukamoto, S. (1991). Relation between career self-efficacy measures based upon occupational titles and Holland codes and model environments: A methodological contribution. *Journal of Vocational Behavior, 38,* 78-91.

McAuley, E., Courneya, K.S., and Lettunich, J. (1991). Effects of acute and long-term exercise of self-efficacy responses in middle-aged males and females. *Gerontologist, 31*: 534-542.

Melzack R., and Casey KL. (1968). Sensory, motivational and central control determinants of pain: A new conceptual model. In Kenshalo D, (Ed.) *The skin senses.* Springfield: Thomas.

Melzack, R., and Wall, P.D. (1965). Pain mechanisms: A new theory. *Science, 150,* 971-979.

Mihevic, P.M. (1978). Psychological influences on perceived exertion. *Medicine and Science in Sports and Exercise, 12,* 112.

Morgan, W.P. (2001). Utility of exertional perception with special reference to underwater exercise. *International Journal of Sport Psychology, 32*(2), 137-161.

Noble, B.J., Maresh, C.M., and Ritchey, M. (1981). Comparison of exercise sensations between females and males. In J. Borms, M. Hebbelinck, and A. Venerando (Eds) *Women and sports: A historical, biological, physiological and sports medicine approach* (pp.175-179). Basel: Karger.

Noble, B.J., and Robertson, R.J. (1996). *Perceived Exertion.* Champaign, IL: Human Kinetics.

O'Connor, P.J., J.S. Raglin and W.P. Morgan (1996). Psychometric correlates of perception during arm ergometry in males and females. *International Journal of Sports Medicine, 17*(6), 462-466.

Pincivero, D.M., Campy, R.M., Coelho, A.J. (2003). Knee flexor torque and perceived exertion: a gender and reliability analysis. *Medicine and Science in Sports and Exercise, 35*(10), 1720-1726.

Pincivero, D.M., Coelho, A.J., and Erikson, W.H. (2000). Perceived exertion during isometric quadriceps contraction: A comparison between men and women. *Journal of Sports Medicine and Physical Fitness, 40,* 319-326.

Pinel, J.P.J. (1990). *Biopsychology.* Boston, MA: Allyn and Bacon.

Robertson, R.J., Moyna, N.M., Sward, K.L., Millich, N.B., Goss, F.L., and Thompson, P.D. (2000). Gender comparison of RPE at absolute and relative physiological criteria. *Medicine and Science in Sports and Exercise, 32*(12), 2120-2129.

Ryckman, R.M., Robbins, M.A., Thornton, B., and Cantrell, P. (1982). Development and validation of a physical self-efficacy scale. *Journal of Personality and Social Psychology, 42*(5), 891-900.

Tenenbaum, G. (2001). A social-cognitive perspective of perceived exertion and exertion tolerance. In R.N. Singer, H. Hausenblas, and C. Janelle (Eds.), *Handbook of sport psychology* (pp. 810-820). New York, NY: Wiley and Sons.

Tenenbaum, G., Fogarty, G., Stewart, E., Calcagnini, N., Kirker, B., Thorn, G., and Christensen, S. (1999). Perceived discomfort in running: Scale development and theoretical considerations. *Journal of Sport Sciences, 17*, 183-196.

Winborn, M.D., Meyers, A.W., and Mulling, C. (1988). The effects of gender and experience on perceived exertion. *Journal of Sport and Exercise Psychology, 10*, 22-31.

In: Sport and Exercise Psychology Research Advances   ISBN: 978-1-60456-157-9
Editors: M. P. Simmons, L. A. Foster, pp. 235-249   © 2008 Nova Science Publishers, Inc.

Chapter XI

The Use of Salivary Cortisol for Measuring Stress Experienced by Athletes in the Laboratory and Field Settings

Yvonne Yuan and Polina Cheng
Hong Kong Sports Institute, Hong Kong, China

Abstract

The purposes of the study in this chapter were to evaluate the use of salivary cortisol to measure stress experienced by athletes and to study the relationship between pre-competitions stress and personality of athletes. Sixteen swimmers representing Hong Kong in regional and international competition were recruited for the study. In the laboratory, swimmers were instructed to perform a mental arithmetic test and its purpose is to arouse the participant's stress level. They were then being led through the diaphragmatic breathing technique to help them relax. The stress levels of the swimmers at pre-arousal, post-arousal, and post-relaxation were monitored by salivary cortisol, skin conductance, respiratory rate, shortened State Trait Anxiety Inventory (STAI-6), and self-reported subjective score. Changes in salivary cortisol agreed with changes in all other stress measurements (skin conductance, respiratory rate, STAI and subjective stress score). Salivary cortisol is a possible parameter to be used for monitoring stress level of athletes. The pre-competition stress experienced by the swimmers was also measured at a local competition. Athletes were instructed to provide a saliva sample for cortisol measurement, to complete the Competitive State Anxiety Inventory-2 (CSAI-2) and a subjective stress scale 30-60 minutes prior to their respective competition event. The average of saliva cortisol levels as obtained on three rest days were used as baseline for comparison. Salivary cortisol as obtained prior to competition although was higher than that obtained on the rest days, the difference was not statistically significant. It seems that the competition under study was not stressful enough to the swimmers. Attempt was also made to study whether pre-competitive stress correlated to individual's personality (sensation seeking and coping skill). No significant correlation between pre-competition stress and personality was identified in the study.

Introduction

Stress is an inherent aspect of sports competition. Stress can be regarded as a complex psychophysiological process (Pfister and Muir, 1992) often resulting in emotional, cognitive and physiological changes to the internal milieu of the sports person. In order to better understand the relation between stress and performance in sport, athletes' psychological, physiological and biochemical responses during and prior to competitions have been studied (Filaire et al., 1999; Filaire et al., 2001; McKay et al., 1997). In important competitions, many athletes do not perform as well as that during practice. Being able to monitor psychological stress and understand it better will provide feedback to athletes and help sport psychologist to tackle the problem.

Serum cortisol level is an indicator of stress experienced by the body. Both psychological stress (Sutton and Casey, 1975) and physical stress (Kuoppasalmi et al., 1980) can induce an increase in serum cortisol level. However, the procedure of obtaining blood samples is already a stress that can potentially induce an increase in cortisol level. It is therefore not practical to use serum cortisol level to assess psychological stress experienced by athletes, especially, prior to competition. The advance in technology allows measurement of cortisol in saliva. This non-invasive and stress-free method provides a practical solution to the problem. Numerous studies have used saliva cortisol to measure stress (Fibiger, Evans, Singer, 1986; Kirschbaum, Wüst, and Hellhammer, 1992; Pawlow and Jones, 2002). However, its application in the sport settings is relatively limited. The preliminary studies on the biochemical assessment of pre-competition stress found that salivary cortisol level was elevated prior to competition when compared to that prior to practice (McKay et al., 1997; Passelergue et al., 1995).

Various psychological inventories have been used to measure stress and anxiety of athletes. The Competitive State Anxiety Inventory-2 (CSAI-2) (Martins et al., 1990) has been used to measure pre-competition anxiety of athletes. Filaire et al. (2001) asked a group of judo athletes to complete the CSAI-2 prior to two competitions at different levels and found that cognitive anxiety and somatic anxiety were higher in interregional championships compared to regional championships whereas self-confidence was significantly lower.

Stress experienced by athletes in a competition depends on various personality traits. Among those, the present study will examine how sensation seeking and coping skill affect pre-competition stress of an athlete.

Sensation seeking was found to be a stress-resiliency factor. The low sensation seekers reported poorer stress management coping skills (Smith et al., 1992). It is therefore hypothesized that the low sensation seekers will experience higher stress prior to competition when compared to the high sensation seekers. The Brief Sensation Seeking Scale (BSSS) developed by Hoyle's group (Hoyle et al., 2002) will be used in this study to measure level of sensation seeking of athletes. It is an abbreviated and revised eight-item form of the measure. The BSSS includes two items representing each aspect of sensation seeking, namely 'experience seeking', 'boredom susceptibility', 'thrill and adventure seeking', and 'disinhibition'.

According to the Catastrophe model, performance is the result of the interaction of arousal and cognitive anxiety, the capacity of the athlete to manage or control cognitive state anxiety and the control of the situation (coping) will determine if the athlete can perform well during a competition (Han, 1996; Hardy L, 1990). Cresswell and Hodge (2004) found that confidence and coping with adversity are positively related. It is therefore interesting to understand how athletes cope with the competitive stress by using the Athletic Coping Skill Inventory in a competition situation.

In view of the significant effect of stress to the performance of athletes during competition, various interventions have been used to help the athletes to relax prior to competition. Breathing therapy, which often rapidly results in physiological relaxation, (Schwartz, 1995) has been widely used by practitioners for reducing physiological tension and arousal. Although there is no universal agreement on how breathing therapy works, possible explanations include altered CO_2 and altered O_2 levels, cognitive changes, and cortical and subcortical changes (Schwartz, 1995). Furthermore, breathing therapy procedures require voluntary actions and thus a diversion from other cognitive activity such as anxious and angry thoughts (Schwartz, 1995). Efficacy of deep diaphragmatic breathing has been evaluated by self-reported anxiety, (Biggs et al., 2003) and psychological inventory (Matsumoto and Smith, 2001). However, both studies depend on single measurement and are subjected to bias resulted from self-reporting. The efficacy of deep diaphragmatic breathing has not been studied with multiple measurements. There is a need to comprehensively evaluate this widely used intervention by using psychological inventory, physiological responses and biochemical response at the same time.

In this study, a group of swimmers' stress level was monitored by multiple measures under both laboratory setting (salivary cortisol, biofeedback and psychological inventory) and field setting (salivary cortisol and psychological inventory). One of the aims of the study is to reconfirm the suitability of using salivary cortisol to measure stress under both settings. The stress data collected, in the laboratory, by multiple methods, will also be used to study the efficacy of diaphragmatic breathing in reducing stress. Furthermore, the relation of pre-competition stress to personality traits (sensation seeking and coping skill) will be examined.

Methods

Participants

A group of 16 swimmers (3 male, 13 female; age 15.4 ± 2.5) representing Hong Kong in international and regional competitions were recruited for the study. Participants provided informed consent prior to commencing the study and participation was voluntary.

Laboratory Sessions

Each participant took part in two laboratory sessions that were conducted by a registered psychologist in a quiet room. The second session will allow the address of any possible training effects. Upon arriving the laboratory, participants were provided with a questionnaire to assess their activity in the hour prior to arrival at the experiment. The laboratory session would only be continued if the participant did not eat or exercise vigorously in the hour. The same questionnaire also required the participants to list medications they were currently taking, to screen for any medications that may alter cortisol levels. Sensors for biofeedback measurement (Procomp$^+$ (Version: Biograph 2.1), Thought Technology Ltd., Canada) were then attached to the participants. After having 10 minutes of seated rest, baseline measurements for accessing stress were collected.

Participants were then instructed to perform a mental arithmetic test and its purpose is to arouse the participant's stress level. Participants were presented with a series of single and double digit numbers and requested to add sequential numbers while retaining the sum in memory for addition to the next number presented and so on throughout the series. The test lasted for 3-5 minutes. Participants were then being led through the diaphragmatic breathing technique that aimed at helping the participants to relax.

Measurement of Stress

The stress levels of the participant at pre-arousal, post-arousal, and post-relaxation were monitored with methods listed below.

Saliva Cortisol

At pre-arousal, participants were instructed to rinse the mouth with distilled water and collection of saliva took place 10 minutes afterwards. However, rinsing was not performed before saliva collection at the post-arousal and post-relaxation collections. Saliva samples for the determination of cortisol were expectorated through a straw into a container. Samples collected during the laboratory sessions were stored at −20 deg C until being analyzed.

After thawing, the containers with saliva samples were centrifuged at 3000 rpm for 15 minutes resulting in a clear, watery supernatant. Cortisol levels were determined by a competitive immunoassay (Salimetrics Cortisol Kit, cat. no. 1-3002/1-3012, USA). The lower detection limit of this assay is < 0.003 µg/dl. Intra- and inter-assay variations at 1 and 0.1 µg/dl ranged from 3.35 to 6.41%.

Skin Conductance and Respiratory Rate

Procomp$^+$ biofeedback system ((Version: Biograph 2.1), Thought Technology Ltd., Canada) was used to record the stress level of the participants. Skin conductance sensor was attached to the 2nd and 3rd fingers of the left hand and respiration sensor (in the form of an elastic belt with Velcro) was attached to the abdominal.

Shortened State Trait Anxiety Inventory (Stai-6)

The shortened form of the state scale of the Spielberger State-Trait Anxiety Inventory used in this study consists of six items. Marteau and Bekker (1992) have studied this shortened form and found that its reliability and validity are acceptable.

Self-Reported Subjective Stress Scale

Participants were also asked to rate their subjective stress level with a ten-point Likert scale with 1 corresponds to 'very relax' and 10 corresponds to 'very tense'.

Personality

To evaluate the participants' personality, participants were required to complete two questionnaires at home in their own leisure time. The Brief Sensation Seeking Scale (BSSS) (Hoyle et al, 2002) consisted of eight items and participants were required to response to each on a five-point scales labeled, 'strongly disagree', 'disagree', 'neither disagree nor agree', 'agree', and 'strongly agree'. The Athletic Coping Skills Inventory-28 (ACSI-28) (Smith, et al., 1995) consists of 28 items measured on a four-point scale ranging from 'almost never' to 'almost always'. Subscales of the ACSI-28 include: Coping with Adversity, Peaking under Pressure, Goal Setting/Mental Preparation, Concentration, Freedom from Worry, Confidence/Achievement Motivation, and Coachability.

Competition Day and Resting Data

A local event – XLVIII Festival of Sport – Long Course Swimming Time Trial - was selected for the study. Athletes were instructed to provide a saliva sample, to complete the Competitive State Anxiety Inventory-2 (CSAI-2) and a subjective stress scale (Likert scale 1-10) 30-60 minutes prior to their respective competition event. All selected event took place from 9:30 – 12:00 of the day. Instructions were explained, and researchers ensured that all instructions were completely understood.

The CSAI-2 assesses two components of state anxiety - cognitive worry and somatic anxiety, and a related construct - self-confidence. The instrument contains 9 items that represent each sub-scale. Thus, each sub-scale has a range from 9 to 36. Higher scores on cognitive and somatic anxiety indicate higher levels of anxiety whereas higher scores on self-confidence sub-scale correspond to higher levels of self-confidence (Martens et al. 1990; McKay et al. 1997).

In order to eliminate the circadian effect on the saliva cortisol level, all participants were required to provide resting saliva samples on three rest days. Resting samples were collected at the same time of the day as that on the competition day. The average of these three cortisol readings was used as the baseline for comparison. Participants were instructed to collect the resting samples only on days that do not have stressful events (e.g. examination) and absent of mouth wounds. Samples were only collected if participants have not taken any alcoholic drinks 24 hours before, have not brush the teeth three hours before, have not eaten and performed vigorous exercise one hour before.

Participants were instructed to rinse their mouth with distilled water and have 10-minutes seated rest before collecting their saliva with a labeled container on the competition day and the rest days. Samples collected were kept refrigerated until transferred to freezer at −20 deg C for storage before analysis.

Statistical Analysis

SPSS (version 10.0) was used for all statistical analysis. To investigate the possible training effect on the second laboratory session and the effect of intervention, a 2 x 3 (Laboratory x Intervention) multivariate repeated measures analysis of variance was conducted. Both factors are repeated measures.

Follow-up tests included five repeated measure 2 x 3 ANOVAs for each of the stress measurements, namely salivary cortisol, subjective feeling, STAI, skin conductance, and respiratory rate. In cases of insignificant interaction between the factors were found, the main effect of each factor was followed-up with repeated contrast.

In order to investigate effect of intervention on each of the stress measurement during laboratory 1, a multivariate MANOVA with intervention (x3) as repeated measure was conducted on data obtained from laboratory 1. The same test was also performed on data obtained at laboratory 2.

Bivariate correlation was performed between changes in the stress measurements during the laboratory sessions. All changes in stress measurements due to intervention (mental arithmetic test and diaphragmatic breathing) from both laboratory sessions were pooled together for analysis.

Data obtained from the competition day were used to investigate any possible correlation between psychological traits (sensation seeking and coping skills) and stress experienced before competition (CSAI, subjective feeling, increase in salivary cortisol relative to that on rest day). In view of the limited number of participants in the study, non-parametric test, namely Spearman's rank correlation, was used in the correlation study.

Statistical significance was set at .05. A smaller p value (.005) was used for the follow-up tests, taking into consideration Bonferroni's correction.

Results

Data obtained in the laboratory sessions were used to evaluate effects of mental arithmetic test (stress) and diaphragmatic breathing (relaxation) on stress experienced by the participants. The same data were also used to compare different means of measuring stress level.

The multivariate repeated measures ANOVA performed on the stress measurements obtained at the laboratory sessions, returned with significant interaction ($F = 8.388, p = .015$) between laboratory and intervention. Interpretation of the main effects was therefore inappropriate.

Table 1 summarized results of the five 2 x 3 (Laboratory x Intervention) repeated measures ANOVA for each of the stress measurements. Apart from the subjective feeling, all the other stress measurements returned with insignificant interaction between the factors. Table 2 included a summary of the main effects of the factors as identified from each stress measurement. Significant main effect of intervention can be identified from all stress measurements. The only exception was subjective feeling, the significant interaction as specified previously deemed the interpretation of main effects inappropriate. All the stress measurements were found to be independent on the laboratory session.

Table 1. Result of five 2 x 3 ANOVAs (Laboratory x Intervention) for each of the stress measurements

1.1 Salivary cortisol

Source of variation	df	SS	MS	F	Sig.
Laboratory	1	4.01×10^{-3}	4.01×10^{-3}	5.82	.030
Intervention	2	3.95×10^{-3}	1.97×10^{-3}	11.46	.000
Interaction	2	4.40×10^{-5}	2.20×10^{-5}	.186	.831

1.2 Skin conductance

Source of variation	df	SS	MS	F	Sig.
Laboratory	1	2.01	2.01	.711	.412
Intervention	2	71.44	35.72	32.29	.000
Interaction	2	.549	.274	.956	.396

1.3 Respiratory rate

Source of variation	df	SS	MS	F	Sig.
Laboratory	1	117.13	117.13	10.93	.005
Intervention	2	1221.32	610.66	28.94	.000
Interaction	2	34.20	17.10	1.24	.291

Table 1. Continued.

1.4 STAI

Source of variation	df	SS	MS	F	Sig.
Laboratory	1	1.50	1.50	.605	.449
Intervention	2	1147.02	573.51	65.51	.000
Interaction	2	2.31	1.156	.433	.583

1.5 Subjective stress score

Source of variation	df	SS	MS	F	Sig.
Laboratory	1	.94	.94	.849	.371
Intervention	2	272.41	136.21	83.95	.000
Interaction	2	2.72	1.36	3.60	.040

Table 2. Main effects of the five 2 x 3 ANOVAs (Laboratory x Intervention) for each of the stress measurement

Stress measurements	p value of main effect	
	Laboratory	Intervention
Salivary cortisol	.030	.000*
Skin conductance	.412	.000*
Respiratory rate	.005	.000*
STAI	.449	.000*
Subjective stress score	Not applicable	Not applicable

*Significant at $p = .005$ level.

In order to determine effect of intervention on the stress measurements in each of the laboratory session, two MANOVAs with intervention (x3) as repeated measures were conducted. Results of these two MANOVAs and the follow-up tests were provided in Table 3. For laboratory 1, all stress measurements were significantly affected by intervention. It is similar for Laboratory 2, with salivary cortisol as the only exception.

Table 4 provides the descriptive statistics (means and standard deviations) of the stress measurements obtained at both laboratory sessions. Significant differences identified were obtained from follow up tests performed on the measurements. During Laboratory 1, salivary cortisol significantly increased from .088 ± .034 µg/dl at baseline to .095 ± .034 µg/dl after mental arithmetic test (stress) and decreased to .078 ± .032 µg/dl after diaphragmatic breathing (relax). Similar trend can be found in the salivary cortisol levels obtained at Laboratory 2 (baseline: .099 ± .031 µg/dl, stress: .114 ± .042 µg/dl, relax: .096 ± .035 µg/dl), however the increase after stress was not statistically significant. In both laboratory sessions, skin conductance was significantly increased after mental arithmetic test and than significantly decreased after breathing exercise. Respiration rate in both sessions tended to increase after mental arithmetic test and decrease after breathing exercise. However, in Laboratory 1, the increase after stress was not significant (baseline: 15.4 ± 4.3 /min; stress:

20.3 ± 8.2 /min). STAI scores in both laboratory sessions were significantly reduced from baseline after mental arithmetic test and than significantly increased after relaxation. Subjective stress scores in both laboratory sessions were significantly increased after mental arithmetic test and significantly decreased after breathing exercise.

Although the mean saliva cortisol as obtained prior to the competition (.261 ± .171 µg/dl) was higher than that obtained on the rest days (.172 ± .245 µg/dl), paired t-test suggested that the difference is not statistically significant ($p = .195$).

Table 5 summarized the correlation between the changes of various stress measurements as obtained in the laboratory sessions. The change in salivary cortisol was positively correlated to the changes in skin conductance (r = .619) and subjective stress score (r = .513). It is also negatively correlated to change in STAI (r = - .430). The change in STAI is negatively correlated to the changes of all other stress measurements, namely salivary cortisol (r = - .430), skin conductance (r = - .710), respiratory rate (r = - .616), and subjective stress score (r = - .933).

In order to study the relationship among various stress measurements obtained prior to the competition and personality (coping and BSSS) of the corresponding athletes, Spearman's rank correlation was performed. The only significant correlation was between pre-competition CSAI2-somatic and pre-competition subjective stress, (rho = .616, $p = .025$). No significant correlation between pre-competition stress measurement and personality trait was identified.

Table 3. Result of two MANOVAs and their follow-up tests with intervention (x3) as repeated measure

		Laboratory 1		Laboratory 2	
		F	p	F	p
		Multivariate test			
		15.59	.000*	11.13	.000*
		Univariate tests			
	Salivary cortisol	16.17	.000**	4.30	.024
	Skin conductance	38.83	.000**	25.62	.000**
Measures	Respiratory rate	16.13	.000**	22.03	.000**
	STAI	54.25	.000**	44.46	.000**
	Subjective stress score	57.24	.000**	72.88	.000**

*Significant at $p = .05$ level.
** Significant at $p = .005$ level.

Discussion

One of the aims of the study is to reconfirm the suitability of using salivary cortisol for measuring stress under laboratory and field settings. The use of salivary cortisol for measuring stress although has been used for a long time, its application to athletes is relatively new. It is therefore important to evaluate its possible application before it can be widely recommended for athletes.

Table 4. Changes in stress measurement at the laboratory sessions

		Laboratory 1			Laboratory 2		
		Baseline	Stress	Relax	Baseline	Stress	Relax
Salivary cortisol	Mean	.088	.095*	.078**	.099	.114	.096**
(µg/dl)	SD	.034	.034	.032	.031	.042	.035
Skin conductance	Mean	2.65	4.85*	3.74**	2.56	4.59*	3.25**
(mV)	SD	1.83	2.13	2.39	1.94	2.25	2.49
Respiratory rate	Mean	15.4	20.3	10.2**	13.7	16.5*	9.1**
(/min)	SD	4.3	8.2	3.2	3.8	4.9	2.2
STAI	Mean	5.3	-1.4*	6.0**	4.9	-1.9*	6.2**
		Baseline	Stress	Relax	Baseline	Stress	Relax
	SD	2.0	2.7	2.4	3.2	2.8	2.5
Subjective stress	Mean	3.6	6.5*	3.0**	3.0	6.8*	2.7**
score	SD	1.4	1.2	1.4	1.5	1.1	1.1

* Significant difference (p = .005) between baseline and stress.
** Significant difference (p = .005) between stress and relax.

Table 5. Correlation of changes in stress measurements during the laboratory sessions

	Salivary cortisol	Skin conductance	Respiratory rate	STAI	Subjective stress score
Salivary cortisol		r = .619*	r = .315	r = - .430*	r = .513*
		p = .000	p = .011	p = .000	p = .000
Skin conductance			r = .691*	r = - .710*	r = .790*
			p = .000	p = .000	p = .000
Respiratory rate				r = - .616*	r = .701*
				p = .000	p = .000
STAI					r = - .933*
					p = .000

* Significant correlation at p = .005 level.

The efficacy of diaphragmatic breathing has not been evaluated by multiple measures. The present study using physiological, biochemical, and psychological measurements to evaluate the effect of diaphragmatic breathing in helping athletes to relax from the stress generated from mental arithmetic test.

The data collected were also used to evaluate possible correlation between personality and the pre-competition stress experienced by athletes. It is hypothesized that the high sensation seekers and athletes with better coping skill are less likely to experienced stress before competition.

Table 4 listed the various stress measures at baseline, after mental arithmetic test, and after diaphragmatic breathing. Comparison of these data between the two laboratory sessions provided a chance to look for any possible training effect on the second session. If training effect does exist participants in the second laboratory session should experience less stress after the mental arithmetic test and felt more relax after the diaphragmatic breathing. Salivary cortisol was significantly increased and then decreased by mental arithmetic test and diaphragmatic breathing respectively in laboratory 1 and yet the changes were not significant in laboratory 2. The less obvious changes in the stress measures in the second laboratory session were also observed in skin conductance and respiratory rate. However, changes in STAI and subjective stress score were found to be more obvious in the second laboratory session. Data obtained in the present study suggested that physiological measurements (salivary cortisol, skin conductance, and respiratory rate) did exhibit a training effect in the second laboratory session. However, psychological measurements (STAI and subjective stress score) did not. Is it because the physiological measurements are more subjective and therefore a preferable means for measuring stress? More studies will be needed to confirm the finding.

When the changes in stress measurements in each of laboratory sessions were studied independently, data collected suggested that most of the stress measurements were sensitive to the interventions (mental arithmetic test and diaphragmatic breathing).

In laboratory 1, all stress measurements increased after mental arithmetic test and decreased after diaphragmatic breathing. The only exception was respiratory rate. Although the mean respiratory rate increased after mental arithmetic test, the difference was made insignificant because of the relatively large SD. In laboratory 2, the same observation can be obtained. However, the exception was salivary cortisol in the second laboratory session.

As mentioned previously, this is one of the very first studies to use multiple measures to study stress experienced in the laboratory settings. Changes in stress measurements as induced by interventions (mental arithmetic test and diaphragmatic breathing) were pooled together for comparison. Among all the stress measurements used in the study, only STAI score decreases in response to stress. All other stress measurements (salivary cortisol, skin conductance, respiratory rate, subjective stress score) increase with increase in stress. According to Table 5, all the correlation coefficients between pairs of stress measurements were positive, except those associated with STAI. These findings are in line with the expected trend. It seems that the stress measurements being used in the study are agreeing with each other. The only exception was that the correlation between salivary cortisol and respiratory rate was not significant. The present study reconfirms the suitability of salivary cortisol as a measure of stress experienced by athletes. Other studies have used salivary cortisol to monitor stress experienced by athletes under various conditions. Akimoto et al. (2003) used salivary cortisol to evaluate effect of acupuncture on a group of female soccer players during a competition period. Filaire, et al. (1999) demonstrated an increased in pre-competition salivary cortisol among handball and volleyball players when compared to that obtained from sedentary people.

Data collected in the laboratory sessions also provided a chance to evaluate efficacy of diaphragmatic breathing on reducing stress. Previous studies only used single measurement on self-reported anxiety (Biggs et al., 2003) and psychological inventory (Matsumoto and

Smith, 2001) to evaluate the efficacy. The multiple measurements, including both self-reported and physiological measurements, used in the present study will provide valuable information to the literature. All the stress measurements, used in the present study, were found significantly reduced after diaphragmatic breathing (Table 4). Our findings strongly supported that diaphragmatic breathing are effective in reducing stress induced by mental arithmetic test under laboratory setting.

The second part of the study was conducted under field settings. Despite the fact that previous studies (Haneishi et al., 2007; McKay et al., 1997; Passelergue et al., 1995) have found that saliva cortisol was elevated prior to competition when compared to that prior to practice, no significant difference between pre-competition saliva cortisol and rest day saliva cortisol can be identified in the present study. It seems that the competition selected in this study is not stressful enough as perceived by the participants.

The participants' pre-competition stress (saliva cortisol, CSAI-2 scores, and subjective stress score) was also compared to their personality (coping and sensation seeking). Previous study (Smith et al., 1992) suggested that low sensation seekers tend to have poorer stress management coping skills and, therefore, may experience higher stress prior to competition, whereas, athletes with better coping skills should be able to manage or control stress and anxiety prior to competition. Numerous studies have supported the contention that there is correlation between trait and state characteristics of individuals (Gould, Petlichkoff, and Weinberg, 1984; Martin and Gill, 1991; Psychountaki and Zervas, 2000; Vealey, 1986). However, due to the limited sample size, no significant correlation between stress experienced prior to competition and personality (sensation seeking and coping) of corresponding athletes was identified. Further studies with much larger sample size are suggested so as to confirm the relationship between personality and pre-competition stress of athletes. The information will be valuable to coaches and sport psychologists in helping athletes to cope with stress prior to competition.

Acknowledgment

This research was supported by the Hong Kong Sports Institute Research Grant.

References

Adlercreutz, H., Harkonen, M., Kuoppasalmi, K., Naveri, H., Huhtaniemi, I., Tikkanen, H., Remes, K., Dessypris, A., Karvonen, J., 1986. Effect of training on plasma anabolic and catabolic steroid hormones and their response during physical exercise. International *Journal of Sports Medicine* 7 Suppl 1, 27-28.

Akimoto, T., Nakahori, C., Aizawa, K., Kimura, F., Fukubayashi, T., and Kono, I., 2003. Acupuncture and responses of immunologic and endocrine markers during competition. *Medicine and Science in Sports and Exercise* 35(8), 1296-1302.

Biggs, Q.M., Kelly, K.S., Toney, J.D., 2003. The effects of deep diaphragmatic breathing and focused attention on dental anxiety in a private practice setting. *Journal of Dental Hygiene* 77, 105-113.

Cresswell, S., Hodge, K., 2004. Coping skills: role of trait sport confidence and trait anxiety. *Perceptual and Motor Skills* 98,433-438.

Fibiger, W., Evans, O., Singer, G., 1986. Hormonal responses to a graded mental workload. *European Journal of Applied Physiology* 55, 339-343.

Filaire, E., Le Scanff, C., Duche, P., Lac, G.., 1999. The relationship between salivary adrenocortical hormones changes and personality in elite female athletes during handball and volleyball competition. Research Quarterly for Exercise and Sport 70(3), 297-302.

Filaire, E., Sagnol, M., Ferrand, C., Maso, F., Lac, G., 2001. Psychophysiological stress in judo athletes during competitions. *Journal of Sports Medicine and Physical Fitness* 41, 263-268.

Fry, R.W., Morton, A.R., Garcia-Webb, P., Crawford, G.P., Keast, D., 1992. Biological responses to overload training in endurance sports. *European Journal of Applied Physiology and Occupational Physiology* 64, 335-344.

Gould, D., Petlichkoff, L., Weinberg, R.S., 1984. Antecedents, of temporal changes n, and relationshipd between CSAI-2 subcomponenets. *Journal of Sport Psychology* 6, 289-304.

Hakkinen, K., Pakarinen, A., Alen, M., Kauhanen, H., Komi, P.V., 1987. Relationships between training volume, physical performance capacity, and serum hormone concentrations during prolonged training in elite weight lifters. *International Journal of Sports Medicine* 8 Suppl 1, 61-65.

Han, M.W., 1996. Psychological· profiles of Korean elite judoists. *American Journal of Sports Medicine* 24, S67-S71.

Haneishi, K., Fry, A.C., Moore, C.A., Schilling, B.K., Li, Y., and Fry, M.D., 2007. Cortisol and stress responses during a game and practice in female collegiate soccer players. *The Journal of Strength and Conditioning Research* 21(2), 583-588.

Hardy, L., 1990. Catastrophe model of performance in sport, in: Jones, J.G., Hardy, L. (Eds.), Stress in Performance in Sport. Chichester, England: Wiley, pp 81-106.

Hoyle, R.H., Stephenson, M.T., Palmgreen, P., Lorch, E.P., Donohew, R.L., 2002. Reliability and validity of a brief measure of sensation seeking. Personality and Individual Differences 32, 401-414.

Kirschbaum, C., Hellhammer, D.H., 1989. Salivary cortisol in psychobiological research: An overview. *Neuropsychobiology* 22, 150-169.

Kirschbaum, C., Wust, S., and Hellhammer, D., 1992. Consistent sex differences in cortisol responses to psychological stress. *Psychosomatic Medicine* 54, 648-657.

Kuoppasalmi, K., Naveri, H., Harkonen, M., Adlercreutz, H., 1980. Plasma cortisol, androstenedione, testosterone and luteinizing hormone in running exercise of different intensities. *Scandinavian Journal of Clinical and Laboratory Investigation* 40, 403-409.

Leung, W., Chan, P., Bosgoed, F., Lehmann, K., Renneberg, I., Lehmann, M., Renneberg, R., 2003. One-step quantitative cortisol dipstick with proportional reading. *Journal of Immunological Methods* 281, 109-118.

Martin, J.J., Gill, D.L., 1991. The relationships among competitive orientation sport-confidence, self-efficacy, anxiety, and performance. *Journal of Sport and Exercise Psychology* 13, 149-159.

Marteau, T.M., Bekker, H., 1992. The development of a six-item short-form of the state scale of the Spielberger State-Trait Anxiety Inventory (STAI). *British Journal of Clinical Psychology* 31 (Pt 3), 301-306.

Martins, R., Vealay, R., Burton, D., 1990. Competitive anxiety in sport. Champaign, IL: Human Kinetics.

Matsumoto, M., Smith, J.C., 2001. Progressive muscle relaxation, breathing exercises, and ABC relaxation theory. *Journal of Clinical Psychology* 57, 1551-1557.

McKay, J.M., Selig, S.E., Carlson, J.S., Morris, T., 1997. Psychophysiological stress in elite golfers during practice and competition. *Australian Journal of Science and Medicine in Sport* 29, 55-61.

Mizuki, Y., Kajimura, N., Kai, S., Suetsugi, M., Ushijima, I., Yamada, M., 1992. Differential responses to mental stress in high and low anxious normal humans assessed by frontal midline theta activity. *International Journal of Psychophysiology* 12, 169-178.

Obminski, Z., Stupnicki. R., 1997. Comparison of the testosterone-to-cortisol ratio values obtained from hormonal assays in saliva and serum. *Journal of Sports Medicine and Physical Fitness* 37, 50-55.

Passelergue, P., Robert, A., Lac, G., 1995. Salivary cortisol and testosterone variations during an official and a simulated weight-lifting competition. *International Journal of Sports Medicine* 16, 298-303.

Pawlow, L. and Jones, G.E., 2002. The impact of abbreviated progressive muscle relaxation on salivary cortisol. *Biological Psychology* 60, 1-16.

Pfister, H.P., Muir, J.L., 1992. Arousal and stress: a consideration of theorical approaches, in: Pfister, H.P. (Ed.), Stress effects on central and peripheral systems. Australian Academic Press, Australia, pp 1-15.

Psychountaki, M., Zervas, Y., 2000. Competitive worries, sport confidence, and performance ratings for young swimmers. Perceptual and Motor Skills 91, 87-94.

Schwartz, M.S., 1995. Breathing therapies, in: Schwartz, M.S. (Ed.), Biofeedback: a practitioner's guide, Guilford Press, New York, pp 248-287.

Smith, R.E., Ptacek, J.T., Smoll, F.L., 1992. Sensation seeking, stress, and adolescent injuries: a test of stress-buffering, risk-taking, and coping skills hypotheses. *Journal of Personality and Social Psychology* 62, 1016-1024.

Stone, M.H., Keith, R.E., Kearney, J.T., Fleck, S.J., Wilson, G.D., Triplett, N.T., 1991. Overtraining: A review of the signs, symptoms and possible causes. *Journal of Applied Sport Science Research* 5, 35-50.

Sutton, J.R., Casey, J.H., 1975. The adrenocortical response to competitive athletics in veteran athletes. *Journal of Clinical Endocrinology and Metabolism* 40, 135-138.

Urhausen, A., Kindermann, W., 1992. Biochemical monitoring of training. *Clinical Journal of Sport Medicine* 2, 52-61.

Urhausen, A., Gabriel, H., Kindermann, W., 1995. Blood hormones as markers of training stress and overtraining. *Sports Medicine* 20, 251-276.

Urhausen, A., Gabriel, H.H., Kindermann, W., 1998. Impaired pituitary hormonal response to exhaustive exercise in overtrained endurance athletes. *Medicine and Science in Sports and Exercise* 30, 407-414.

van Dusseldorp, M., Smits, P., Lenders, J.W., Temme, L., Thien, T., Katan, M.B., 1992. Effects of coffee on cardiovascular responses to stress: a 14-week controlled trial. *Psychosomatic Medicine* 54, 344-353.

Vealey, R., 1986. Conceptualization of sport-confidence and competitive orientation: preliminary investigation and instrument development. *Journal of Sport Psychology* 8, 221-246.

In: Sport and Exercise Psychology Research Advances
Editors: M. P. Simmons, L. A. Foster, pp. 251-292

ISBN: 978-1-60456-157-9
2008 Nova Science Publishers, Inc.

Chapter XII

Overview of the Use of Skeletal Muscle Markers for Damage Detection in Sportspeople

Antonio Martínez-Amat[2], Fidel Hita[2], Fernando Rodríguez-Serrano[2], José Carlos Prados[1], Juan Antonio Marchal[1], Houria Boulaiz[1], Octavio Caba[2], Raúl Ortiz[1], Consolación Melguizo[1], Delfín Galiano[3], Celia Vélez[2], Macarena Perán[2], Esmeralda Carrillo[1], and Antonia Aránega[1]

[1] Biopathology and Medicine Regenerative Institute (IBIMER),
Department of Human Anatomy and Embryology, Faculty of Medicine, University of
Granada, Granada E-18071, Spain
[2] Department of Health Sciences, University of Jaén, Jaén E-23071, Spain
[3] Department of Physiology, Anatomy and Cellular Biology, University of Pablo de
Olavide, Sevilla E- 41013, Spain

Abstract

Muscle injuries are one of the most common traumas in sports and can be produced by intense or even moderate physical activity, especially eccentric exercise. It has been suggested that the immediate effects associated with muscle injury are mechanical, largely caused by the excessive tension to which muscle sarcomeres are subjected. Intense physical exercise induces muscle fiber lesions, whose severity depends on the duration and characteristics of the exercise, the training stage at which the sportsperson is found, and the presence of dietary or muscular (agonist/antagonist) imbalance. Although eccentric exercise has undoubted biomechanical and bioenergetic benefits, its intense or only occasional practice can produce structural and functional alterations of the muscles involved.

Immunoassay is the most widely used approach in clinical biochemistry to identify and quantify molecules and offers high sensitivity and specificity. Although some debate remains, it is generally considered that the detection of proteins bound to intracellular structures (mitochondria, nucleus, etc.), even in small amounts, usually indicates necrosis.

The molecular diagnosis of muscle damage is largely based on measurement of the plasma activity of different sarcoplasmatic enzymes (creatine kinase [CK] and lactate dehydrogenase [LDH]). These enzymes are normally strictly intracellular, and their increased activity in plasma reflects their escape via membrane structures.

Although the direct demonstration of muscle damage is histological, in practice the diagnosis is largely based on the measurement of plasma enzyme concentrations. Thus, the diagnosis can be supported by the combined measurement of biological and clinical parameters, e.g., plasma LDH activity, myoglobin, malondialdehyde (MDA), leukocyte count and changes in muscle parameters.

The diagnosis of exercise-induced muscle lesions by the measurement of markers remains controversial. Thus, the presence in plasma of increased CK activity and MDA levels reflects only muscle overload and offers low specificity and sensitivity as a muscle damage marker.

Increasing attention has been focused on the clinical relevance of the detection in plasma of cellular proteins released after tissue injury, commonly referred to as biochemical markers. The detection of α-actin and myosin molecules, closely related to muscle contraction, is of special interest and requires a reliable technique that offers high sensitivity and specificity. The aim is to be able to detect biochemical markers quickly and with high accuracy, especially when clinical and analytical findings fail to deliver an unequivocal diagnosis. The sensitivity of Western blot and the biological material used (serum obtained by a simple extraction of blood without need for biopsy) offer two major advantages for the study of skeletal muscle damage.

1. Introduction

Three key questions must be addressed in reviewing the diagnosis of skeletal muscle damage in the sports arena. Are there any reliable, sensitive and reproducible markers of muscle injury? Can variations in these biological markers be correlated with the severity of histological injuries? Are increases in these markers associated with overtraining or to a specific sports injury?

It is known that intense physical exercise induces muscle fiber injuries and that their severity depends on the duration of the exercise, its characteristics, and the training phase of the sportsperson (Asp et al., 1996).

Clinical assessment of muscle injuries in exercise is problematic. These structural injuries, with highly variable severity and prognosis, can be characterized by the remaining pain in muscle masses and sometimes by a sensation of persistent heaviness of the inferior limbs (Ebbeling et al., 1989). However, the clinical expression of this condition is not specific and its impact in sports remains very difficult to evaluate (Bigard et al., 2001).

Histologically, it has been observed that muscle edema appears after physical exercise and contributes to muscle cell damage (Komulainen et al., 1994; Vaananen et al. 1997), probably by increasing the cellular volume and therefore stretching and subsequently rupturing the cellular membrane (Komulainen et al., 1995). Komulainen also reported ultrastructural changes, e.g., disruption of Z lines of the sarcomere, loss of myofibrillar architecture and enlarged subsarcolemmal areas. Other authors have proposed that sarcomeres are joined by desmin filaments that attach different Z discs and also connect with the sarcolemma, stabilizing the membrane in mechanical stress. However, eccentric exercise can result in loss of these desmin filaments (Koh, 2002). If the muscle is studied at some hours after the physical exercise, typical inflammation-induced changes can appear (leukocyte infiltration, etc.), in addition to the mechanical damage described above.

Over the past few decades, it has been proposed that physical exercise produces an increase in free radical production by the exercised muscle groups (Wierzba et al., 2006; Das, 2006; Kostaropoulos et al., 2006; Jackson, 2005; Bailey et al., 2004; McArdle et al., 2001; McArdle et al.,1995; McArdle et al.,1999). Although it has not been definitively demonstrated that these free radicals are related to the muscle damage associated with physical exercise, available evidence points in this direction.

The most widely used biochemical indicator to evaluate muscle damage has been muscle-specific enzyme activity in plasma, especially that of creatine-kinase (CK) or lactate-dehydrogenase (LDH) (Brancaccio, 2007; Marcora, 2007; Hirose et al., 2004; Kim et al., 2007; Kobayashi et al., 2007; Apple et al., 1988;) Other less frequently applied markers include GOT (Glutamyl oxaloacetic transaminase), myoglobin, and carbonic anhydrase III. Various authors have described the relationship between the release of muscle enzymes and the amount of muscle damage produced by sports exercise (Appley et al., 1988; Friden et al., 1983; Janssen et al., 1989).

The most highly regarded marker at the present time is the troponin complex, especially T and I troponin cardiac isoforms (cTnT and cTnI) (Wu et al., 2004; Bertrand et al., 2000; Werf et al., 2003). Numerous immunoassays have been commercialized using different monoclonal antibodies. According to published data, both troponins show the same sensitivity and specificity for detecting myocardial damage and for indicating the prognosis in acute coronary syndrome (ACS) (Clark and Payne, 2007; Achar et al., 2005; Olatidoye et al., 1998; Collinson et al., 2001; Ottani et al., 1999; Bertrand et al., 2002).

If troponins are not available, the best alternative is CK-MM, which is less specific but remains valuable. Other proposed markers, e.g., total CK, LDH, and GOT (AST), cannot be recommended (Alpert et al., 2000). When an early diagnosis is essential, CK-MM plus myoglobin can be used, subsequently confirming the result with the use of a more specific indicator (troponins).

In the physical activity setting and with the application of biotechnology in sports performance, the development of molecular biology has made a striking contribution to the field of skeletal muscle damage markers. Monoclonal antibodies represent a powerful and valuable diagnostic tool. Molecular biology techniques can be used to directly detect specific molecules of actin (Aránega et al., 1999; Martínez-Amat et al., 2005, Martínez-Amat et al., 2007, Velez et al., 2000) and myosin, proteins closely related to muscle contraction (Korn et al., 1982). A highly sensitive and reliable technology (Creagh et al., 1998) is required to rapidly detect proteins that indicate muscle damage, especially in some clinically complex situations. This technology would allow a significant reduction in the negative effects of sports activity. An effective marker is vital to correctly establish effort thresholds in sports training.

The quantitative and qualitative detection of proteins can be very relevant for highly qualified sportsmen undergoing training for a specific discipline (Booth et al., 2002), where a maximum adjustment of training programs is vital to achieving an optimal performance and to accomplishing rehabilitation programs (Jin et al., 2000).

2. Functional and Structural Anatomy of the Skeletal Muscle

Broadly speaking, around 40% of the organism is constituted by skeletal muscle, and a further 10% corresponds to smooth muscle and cardiac muscle (Epstein et al., 1998). These different types of muscle share many contractile characteristics, but our interest here is in skeletal muscle function.

2.1. Skeletal Muscle Fibers

There are three types of skeletal muscle fiber: red, white and intermediate.

Red fibers are abundant in red muscles, have a small diameter, and contain a large amount of myoglobin. They possess numerous mitochondria arranged in rows between myofibrils and in clusters below the plasmatic membrane. Red muscles contract relatively slowly, therefore it is assumed that red fibers are slow fibers, with a slower nerve impulse conduction (50 - 80 m/s) (Carroll et al., 2004).

White fibers, present in white muscles, have a larger diameter, a smaller amount of myoglobin, and fewer mitochondria arranged between myofibrils at band I level. The Z line is thinner in white than in red fibers. White or fast fibers are less excitable but have a higher nerve impulse conduction velocity (70 - 110 m/s).

Intermediate fibers display intermediate characteristics between the other two types but have a more similar appearance to red fibers and are more abundant in red muscles. The number of mitochondria is similar to that in red fibers, but the Z line is thinner, as in white fibers. They run parallel to heavy filaments and end at the level of band H, which contains only heavy filaments.

2.1.1. Slow-Contraction and Fast-Contraction Muscle Fibers:

All muscle fibers are not the same. A skeletal muscle contains two main types of fibers: slow contraction fibers (slow-twitch, ST) and fast contraction fibers (fast-twitch, FT). Most classifications refer to these fiber types as ST red Type I and FT white type II. The color difference derives from the higher myoglobin content of red fibers.

ST fibers need approximately 110 ms to reach their maximum tension when stimulated, whereas FT fibers can reach their maximum tension in around 50 ms (Brooke et al., 1970). FT fibers are further classified into two sub-classes, FTa (Fast-Oxidative) and FTb (Fast-Glycolytic). A third FT fiber subtype, FTc, has also been identified.

The most significant differences between FTa, FTb, and FTc fibers have not been established, but FTa fibers are believed to be the most frequently mobilized. ST fibers are mobilized more frequently than all FTa fibers, and FTc fibers are used less frequently. Taking average percentages from published data (Brooke et al., 1970), most muscles have on average around 25% FTa fibers and 50% ST fibers; the remaining 25% of fibers are mainly FTb fibers, with FTc fibers representing only 1-3% of the muscle. Little is known about FTc fibers, which will not be further discussed in this review.

As mentioned above, skeletal muscles differ in the percentage of ST and FT fibers. In general, muscles in the upper and lower extremities of an individual have a similar fiber composition. Various studies have demonstrated that individuals with a predominance of ST fibers in their leg muscles will probably also have a high percentage of ST fibers in their arm muscles, and a similar relationship has been observed for FT fibers. However, there are some exceptions. Thus, the soleus muscle (at the back of the lower leg) is almost entirely composed of ST fibers.

2.1.2. Types of Fibers and Physical Exercise.

Given the differences between ST (red) and FT (white) fibers, they might be expected to have different functions in the physically active individual (Buchthal et al., 1970).

ST fibers. Generally, ST fibers have a higher aerobic resistance (in presence of oxygen). ST fibers are very efficient in producing adenosine triphosphate (ATP) from the oxidation of carbohydrates and fats (Figure 1). ATP is required to produce the energy needed for muscular action and relaxation. While oxidation lasts, ST fibers continue to produce ATP, allowing the fibers to remain active. The capacity to maintain muscle activity during a prolonged period of time, i.e., muscle resistance, explains the high aerobic resistance of ST fibers. For this reason, ST fibers are more frequently mobilized during low-intensity resistance exercise, e.g., marathon running or non-competitive swimming.

FT fibers, FT fibers have relatively poor aerobic resistance and are more adapted to perform in anaerobic conditions (without oxygen) compared with ST fibers (Buchthal et al., 1970; Nakagawa and Hattori, 2002). Hence, they produce ATP *via* anaerobic routes not oxidation processes (Figure 1).

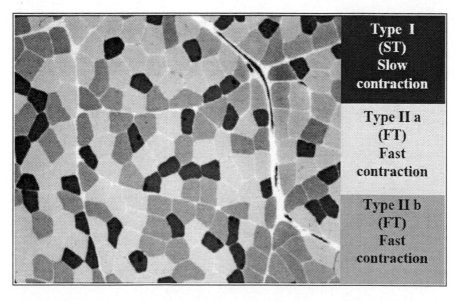

Figure 1. A photomicrograph showing Slow Contraction (ST) and Fast Contraction (FT) muscle fibers.

FTa motor units generate considerably more strength compared with ST motor units, but they are readily exhausted because of their limited resistance capacity. Hence, FTa fibers appear to be used in high-intensity low-resistance sports, e.g., sprinting. Although the length of FTb fibers has not been established it appears that they are not easily activated by the nervous system. They are mainly used in highly explosive tests rather than in normal low-intensity activities (Buchthal et al., 1970).

3. Mechanism of the Muscle Contraction

Many characteristics of muscle contraction can be demonstrated by the instantaneous electrical excitation of the nerve of a muscle or by a short electrical stimulus through the muscle, leading to a single, immediate split-second contraction (Martin et al., 1998).

Interaction between actin and myosin produces a coherent contractile force that turns chemical energy into mechanical work. The energy required for muscle contraction derives from the hydrolysis of ATP to ADP and inorganic phosphate (Pi). Nevertheless, no major difference in ATP levels is found between a resting and actively contracted muscle because of the presence of a very efficient ATP-regeneration warehouse in the cytoplasm of every muscle cell. High levels are observed of phosphocreatine (another active phosphate compound) and creatine-kinase, an enzyme that participates in the reaction between phosphocreatine and ADP, generating creatine and ATP (Bessman et al., 1981). Thus, although the contractile apparatus consumes ATP after a rapid increase in muscle activity, it is the intracellular phosphocreatine that decreases. Therefore, the phosphocreatine reserve provides ATP with energy, acting as a battery, and is recharged when the muscle is resting from the ATP generated via cellular oxidation.

ATP hydrolysis during muscle contraction is a direct consequence of interaction between myosin and actin. Myosin can also act alone as an enzyme able to hydrolyze ATP (ATPase).

The rate-limiting step is not the initial binding of ATP to myosin or the hydrolysis, since both are extremely fast, but rather the release of ATP hydrolysis products (ADP and inorganic phosphate, Pi). These form a non-covalent complex within the myosin molecule, stopping the binding and subsequent hydrolysis of more ATP. Actin strongly enhances the rate of ATP hydrolysis by myosin. In presence of actin, each myosin molecule hydrolyzes 5-10 ATP molecules per second, similar to the rate in the contracted muscle. Myosin ATPase stimulation by actin filaments reflects the physical association between them. This association does not affect the step in which myosin produces ATP hydrolysis, but actin causes a faster ADP and Pi release from the myosin molecule, freeing it to bind to another ATP molecule and initiate the reaction (Adelstein et al., 1980; Hartshorne et al., 1982; Stein and Decker, 1998).

ATP hydrolysis and binding with actin both take place in the globular head of myosin. Each of the two separated heads (due to myosin breakage by papain) has around 120 Da and is known as sub-fragment 1 of myosin (S1 Fragment). Because these heads preserve all of the ATPase activity and the actin-binding, they can be used to study the interaction between myosin and actin.

Thick and thin filaments slide past each other, producing the mechanical force for the muscle contraction. The following molecular mechanism has been described by various authors (Ford et al., 1977; Eisenberg et al., 1980) a myosin head, carrier of previous ATP hydrolysis products (ADP and Pi), moves from its position in the thick filament to the immediate proximity of a neighboring subunit of actin. This movement is thought to occur by chance diffusion and requires the flexibility with which the myosin molecule is endowed by its "hinge" zones. When myosin binds with actin, ADP and Pi are released from the myosin head, causing the myosin to incline and push the remainder of the thick filament. Then, a new molecule of ATP is bound to the top of the myosin and again separates it from the actin filament. Hydrolysis of the bound ATP rapidly relaxes the myosin head to its original conformation, preparing it for a second cycle (Huxley et al., 1983) (Figure 2).

3.1. Stimulation of Muscle Contraction: The Role of Calcium

The basic substance that stimulates the contraction is not ATP (generally found in myofibrils) but Ca^{2+}. In order to understand how muscle contraction regulates calcium, we must examine the molecular structure of the thin filament in more detail.

A thin filament, like that found in striated muscle, is more than a simple F-actin polymer. There are four more proteins that are essential for the contractile function of thin filaments. One of these proteins is tropomyosin, a fibrous protein that appears in the form of elongated dimers throughout or near the furrow of the F-actin helix. Three small proteins are bound to this molecule, designated troponins I, C and T. The presence of tropomyosins and troponins inhibits the binding of myosin heads to actin unless there are concentrations of calcium of approximately 10-5 M. In the resting muscle, calcium concentrations are around 10-7 M, therefore new cross-bridges cannot be formed (Martin et al., 1998; Moss et al., 2004).

Entry of Ca^{2+} stimulates the contraction, with the ion binding to troponin C and giving rise to a reordering of the troponin-tropomyosin complex. This movement gives actin new available sites for binding with myosin heads (Figure 3). The explanation of this contraction-activating entry of calcium into myofibrils can be found in a more detailed observation of the muscle cell. Within the cell, each myofibril is surrounded by the sarcoplasmic reticulum formed by membranous tubules. In resting muscles, the concentration of Ca^{2+} in myofibrils is approximately 10-7 M, whereas the concentration in the lumen of the sarcoplasmic reticulum can be 10000-fold higher. Motor nerve impulses depolarize the sarcoplasmic reticulum membrane, opening the Ca^{2+} channels and releasing calcium from within the myofibrils, stimulating the contraction. The signal is quickly transmitted to the whole sarcoplasmic reticulum of a myofibril *via* T-tubules (Rayment et al., 1994; Gommans et al., 2002).

However, although a sudden change in Ca^{2+} concentration is the signal for muscle contraction, it does not produce sufficient energy.

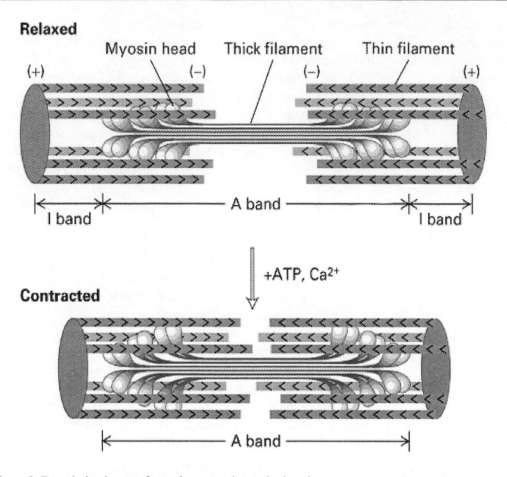

Figure 2. Descriptive image of muscle contraction and relaxation.

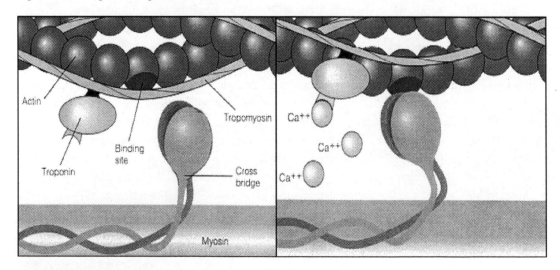

Figure 3. Regulation of muscle contraction by calcium.

3.2. Effectiveness of Muscle Contraction

The effectiveness of a machine or an engine is the percentage of contributed energy that is transformed into work and not into heat. The percentage of energy given to the muscle (the chemical energy of nutrients) that can be converted into work is below 25%, , even under optimal conditions, with the remainder becoming heat.

The reason for this low effectiveness is that half of the energy obtained from nutrients is lost during the ATP formation process, with only 40-45% of the energy of the ATP subsequently converted into work (Clarkson and Hubal, 2002) (Figure 4).

Maximum effectiveness is only obtained when the muscle is contracted at a moderate velocity. If there is a slow muscle contraction or no movement, large amounts of maintenance heat are released despite little work being done, reducing the effectiveness. Likewise, if the contraction is too fast, a large amount of the energy is used to overcome the viscosity friction within the muscle itself, which also reduces the contractile performance. In general, maximum effectiveness is reached when the contraction is at around 30% the maximum velocity (Epstein et al., 1998).

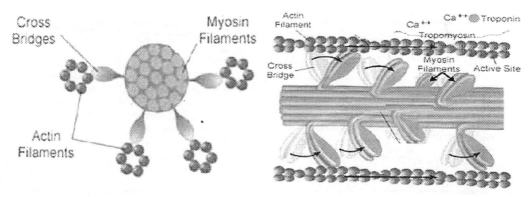

Figure 4. Molecular mechanism of muscle contraction.

3.3. Types of Muscle Contraction

Types of muscle contraction or action are traditionally given the prefix "iso-" (meaning equal), as in isotonic (constant muscle tension), isometric (constant muscle length) and isokinetic (constant velocity movement). In addition, movement can be produced under concentric (muscle shortening) or eccentric (muscle extension) conditions (Johnson et al., 1976).

Isometric means "equal length", and this state is only observed when the muscle is relaxed. In fact, it is not the muscle length but the angle of the articulation that remains constant. An isometric contraction can be more precisely defined as a muscle contraction in the absence of external movement or change in the angle of the articulation. It takes place when the force produced by a muscle is exactly balanced by the resistance imposed on it, with no movement taking place. Although not incorrect, the term isometric could be replaced by the word static without losing any scientific rigor (Table 1).

Isotonic: this term should mostly be avoided, since is virtually impossible for the muscle tension to remain continuous while there is movement. Constant tension is only possible during a movement of short amplitude under very slow or semi-isometric conditions for a limited time (because fatigue quickly reduces the tension). Whenever a movement takes place, muscle tension increases or diminishes, since acceleration or deceleration is always present and can activate a stretching reflex.

Isokinetic: This term is often used inappropriately, because it is impossible to produce a complete muscle contraction at a constant velocity. Any movement involves a certain degree of acceleration (first two laws of Newton); therefore a constant velocity is not possible in a muscle that is contracted from a resting state to which it then returns. Constant velocity can only be produced during part of the movement (Table 1).

A concentric muscle contraction refers to a muscle action that produces a force to overcome a load. Work during concentric contraction has been described as positive (Doyle et al., 1993).

Table 1. Characteristics of different types of contractile activity

	EXCENTRIC	ISOMETRIC	CONCENTRIC
MUSCLE MOVEMENT	Extension	Estatic	Shortening
MECHANIC FORCES	High	Low	Low
ELECTRIC ACTIVITY	Low	High	High
METABOLIC COST	Low	High	High
TENDENCY TO INDUCE MUSCULAR PAIN	High	Low	Low
TENDENCY TO INDUCE FATIGUE	High	Low	Low
TENDENCY TO INDUCE PAIN	High	Low	Low

An eccentric contraction indicates a muscle action in which the muscular force yields to an imposed load. Work during eccentric contraction is considered negative (Sven et al., 1998).

This classification is important, because exercises are classified according to the predominant type of contraction, and it has been observed that more oxidative damage is produced by eccentric than by concentric exercise (Armstrong et al., 1991; Proske and Morgan, 2001; Gleeson et al., 2003).

A little-considered factor in relation to eccentric muscle contraction is that the muscle tension in any complete movement is lower in the eccentric than in the isometric or concentric phase (Friden et al., 1983). However, eccentric activity is generally identified as the main cause of muscle damage (Whitehead et al., 1998). It is true that a maximum eccentric contraction can generate muscle tension that is 30-40% higher than that produced by concentric or isometric contraction. Nevertheless, this degree of tension does not occur during the eccentric phase in normal sports activities (Sven et al., 1998).

4. Muscle Damage

Over-training is a frequent reason for consulting a Sports Medicine specialist. It is usually caused by a large training load that is poorly tolerated by the organism (Fry et al., 1991). The consequences of this inadequate planning of training are sometimes exacerbated by other factors (Kenttä et al., 1998). Symptoms are non-specific, polymorphic, and deceptive, and progression of the condition is slow. However, since the severity of effects is highly dependent on the delay before treatment is applied, an early diagnosis is of great importance (Kenttä et al., 1998) (Figure 5).

The search for muscle injury biological markers has been closely related to the diagnosis of overtraining.

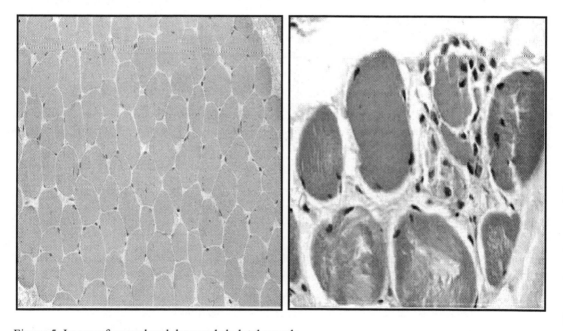

Figure 5. Image of normal and damaged skeletal muscle.

However, the relationship between cellular injuries induced by a single or repeated exercise and overtraining is not yet clear, and attention must be paid to recent and emerging experimental data.

Research into the relationship between muscle injuries due to exercise and those due to overtraining must first address the availability of reliable, sensitive and reproducible markers of injured muscle fibers.

4.1. Characteristics of Exercise-Induced Muscle Damage

Intense physical exercise induces muscle fiber injuries and, as already stated, their severity depends on the duration of the exercise, its characteristics, and the training phase of the sportsperson (Asp et al., 1996).

The nature of the muscle contraction influences the severity of injuries. Repeated muscle contractions and eccentric contractions are the cause of persistent and widespread diffuse pains. Dynamic exercises that involve eccentric contractions are a risk factor for muscle injury (Fry et al., 1991).

Clinical evaluation of exercise-induced muscle injuries is not easy. Structural injuries, whose severity and prognosis are highly variable, are characterized by the remaining muscle pain and a persistent feeling of heaviness of lower limbs (Stupka et al., 2001).

The clinical expression of this condition is non-specific; therefore it is very difficult to assess its impact in sports activities.

Exercise-related muscle injuries are characterized by discontinuous pains, muscle tension, movement restriction, performance decrease, and the appearance of muscle enzymes in blood (Kuipers, 1993). Biological diagnosis of these injuries remains difficult due to the lack of specificity, sensitivity, or reproducibility of currently used parameters (Figure 5). At a histological level, severe exercise-induced muscle injuries appear in early stages as structural injuries localized in the cytoskeleton and myofibrils (Yu and Thornell, 2002).

Under electronic and light microscopy, these injuries appear as clear spaces erasing sarcomeres, reminiscent of the rupture of fiber protein structures, including desmin and laminin. These injuries, which are initially limited to the sarcomeres, progress rapidly, producing an inflammatory reaction that gives rise to the tissue repair process (Vijayan et al., 1998). In the most severe cases, damaged cells undergo cell death and are replaced by recently formed fibers from satellite cells.

The origin and mechanism of these injuries are poorly defined (Kuipers, 1993) but three main hypotheses have been proposed, defending their mechanical, metabolic or vascular etiology.

The prevailing hypothesis proposes their physical origin, based on the damage to cellular structures produced by mechanical tensions. As stated above, muscle injuries mainly occur after the practice of exercise with a major eccentric component. However, with eccentric contraction, the peak force corresponds to a greater muscle length than that related to actin-myosin bridges (MacCully and Faulkner, 1986). Therefore, excessive force on each actin-myosin bridge could originate physical exercise-induced injuries. A further hypothesis is based on observations of a wide heterogeneity in the length of sarcomeres length in every eccentric contraction. Some sarcomeres would be stretched beyond the resistance of the elastic structures of the fibers, causing sarcolemma disruption. Alteration of the sarcomere structure is often the origin of these injuries (Ogilvie et al., 1988).

Some unloading physical activities have also been associated with muscle injuries (Hartobagyi and Denahan, 1989). Although these injuries are less severe, this has led to hypotheses that attribute the development of exercise-related injuries to non-mechanical factors.

4.2. Early Inflammatory Reaction

These initial injuries are followed by a group of events in which free radicals and calcium play an essential role. Membrane structure alterations produce an increase in intracellular calcium concentration, followed by disruption of muscle relaxation and an accumulation of mitochondrial calcium (Duan et al., 1990). The mitochondrial function is profoundly altered, leading to an alteration in ATP synthesis. This rupture of ATP synthesis affects the operation of TPA ionic pumps, which restricts the egress of sodium and leads to edema of the injured fibers. Finally, the increase in intracellular calcium produces an activation of the proteolytic system, e.g., the 2-phospholipase or calpaine system. The latter is a non-lysosomal protease involved in the development of physical exercise-related injuries (Belcastro et al., 1998).

The initial injury is followed by a local inflammatory situation, essential for the first stage of organic tissue repair (Tiidus, 1998; Stauber and Smith, 1998).

The production of reactive oxygen species (ROS) is one of the factors that trigger the inflammatory reaction. Moreover, the initial production of free radicals, caused by the increase in mitochondrial oxygen consumption, activates messengers that attract neutrophil cells, increasing vascular permeability and thereby contributing to the infiltration of damaged tissue by these cells. Once the intense exercise finishes, there is an emigration of neutrophils to the muscle. The local production of free radicals is maintained and extended, because these neutrophil leukocytes can be the direct cause of reactive oxygen production (Jaeschke, 1995). Hence, ROS play a fundamental role in the origin and development of organic post-inflammatory reaction (Atalay et al., 1996).

At a histological level, this is translated into histomorphological alterations that cause muscle decay, with the characteristic appearance of clusters of mononuclear cells that at some point invaded muscle fibers (Bigard et al., 1997).

4.3. Satellite Cells

These represent the only potentially myogenic cells in adult age (Plaghki, 1985). The ontogenic origin of satellite cells is worthy of mention. In the course of development, muscle fibers are formed by the fusion of myoblasts, producing myotubes. After their innervation, these myotubes acquire the characteristics of mature muscle fiber. Myotubes appear in two successive waves in the embryo. Primitive myogenic cells appear during muscle histogenesis and migrate to form first-generation myotubes (Cordon et al., 1990). Other myoblastic cells remain in the skeletal muscle and merge with first- or second-generation muscle fibers (Allen and Rankin, 1990), or form quiescent cells, designated satellite cells.

These cells appear in all striated muscle types except for the myocardium and are located in fibers between sarcolemma and basement membrane. They are remarkably resistant to biochemical or physical aggressions and are quickly activated when an injury occurs. These quiescent cells activate a reaction characterized by an increase in nucleus volume and DNA synthesis (Bodine-Fowler, 1994) due to the action of local growth factors (bFGF, insulin-like growth factors [IGFs] or transforming growth factor-β [TGF-β]) (Hurme and Kalimo, 1992).

There is a multiplication of satellite cells, which at least partially explains the large number of nuclei derived from damaged fibers (Jacobs et al., 1995) (Figure 6).

After the disappearance of cellular remains from damaged fibers, the rejuvenation process begins beneath the basement membrane, which generally remains intact. Satellite cells represent the main source of myogenic cells, which will guarantee muscle rejuvenation (Snow, 1977).

In addition, satellite cells near the injury appear to cause the formation of new muscle fibers and, under these circumstances, the activity of distant satellite cells are not of major importance (Schultz, 1985). It is generally considered that muscle rejuvenation processes in adult mammals reproduce the different cellular events that take place during myogenesis (Plaghki, 1985). Many myogenic factors (e.g., myoD, myf5, and myf6) are expressed during rejuvenation, participating in the maturation of new muscle fibers (Miller, 1991).

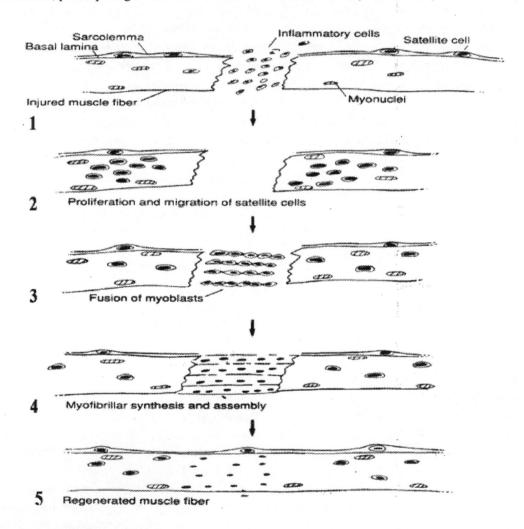

Figure 6. Muscle regeneration process.

4.4. The Origin of Muscle Injuries

As stated above, there are three main hypotheses:

The first hypothesis is linked to a failure of oxidative processes in ATP synthesis. Exercise of long duration causes an alteration of the mitochondrial function, leading to a failure in the ATP-dependent ionic pumps of the sarcoplasmatic reticulum and to a defect in the egress of calcium from the cell. The rise in intracellular calcium levels would be the cause of structural injuries, probably by activation of calcium-dependent proteases (Belcastro et al., 1998). Nevertheless, this hypothesis is controversial, since the most important and widespread injuries are observed during eccentric-type exercises, which use less energy (Cheung et al., 2003).

The second hypothesis is related to the increased production of free radicals during exercise (Jenkins, 1988). The increase in oxygen consumption is translated into an increased production of reactive species, e.g., reactive oxygen, free radicals, or superoxides (Sen, 1995). Under normal conditions, the free radicals are inactivated by defense systems (enzymes), e.g., superoxide-dismutase and glutathione-peroxidase.

Physical exercise is known to produce an increase in the production of hydrogen peroxidase and the hydroxyl radical (Or' Neil et al., 1996). In these circumstances, anti-ROS defense systems are overcome and the unstable reactivated species react with large structural molecules, e.g., membrane lipids or some proteins. This fast reaction causes injuries to the phospholipid structures of the membrane by peroxidation (Jenkins, 1988). The permeability of the membrane disrupts the ionic gradient compatible with cellular function, and all of this will have a special influence on calcium, whose intracellular increase will activate the calcium-dependent protease system. This disturbance of the intracellular calcium homeostasis may explain findings in fatigued muscle. Nevertheless, numerous technical difficulties have impeded a clear confirmation of this hypothesis to date.

Finally, a hypothesis has been proposed that attributes muscle injuries to microcirculation changes. In fact, it has been clearly demonstrated that injuries to the capillary network are secondary to myofibril alterations (Peeze-Binkhorst et al., 1989). However, the vascular hypothesis cannot explain the development of muscle injuries in the exercise other than the increase in temperature of the muscle (Armstrong et al., 1991).

A further question has been raised in recent years, related to the phenomenon of apoptosis in exercise-related muscle injuries (Carraro and Franceschi, 1997). It has been suggested that development of an inappropriate apoptotic process may at least partly explain muscle injuries caused by intense physical exercise. Apoptosis (or programmed cell death) results from the application of a complex biochemical program that induces cell death. In the normal state, this biochemical program is strictly controlled to guarantee the replacement of dead cells without affecting the cell structure of the tissue. There is experimental evidence that post-exercise muscle injuries in defective mice with dystrophy (Duchenne Muscular Dystrophy model) are due to the apoptotic process (Sandri et al., 1995). It remains an open question whether the mechanisms underlying exercise-related muscle injuries involve acceleration of the apoptotic process or have a metabolic or purely mechanic origin.

4.5. Relationship between Muscle Injuries and Overtraining

The relationship between exercise-induced muscle injuries and overtraining can appear to be easily assessable. Nevertheless, recent investigations suggest that injuries induced by repeated physical exercise may have major consequences in the clinical expression of overtraining. These relationships are more difficult to define.

Overtraining. Faced by situations of variable difficulty, the organism develops two types of reaction according to its state of tolerance. These reactions are characterized by the development of adaptation mechanisms or by the application of defense mechanisms within the general framework of a stressed state. The tolerance of individuals is modulated by their life experience and their psychological profile. When difficulties are intense or repeated or when the organism cannot develop adaptation mechanisms, a tension state is developed, generally of a neuroendocrinoimmune type. This state can induce a condition that may be severe, e.g., overtraining. An imbalance in training programs or an overload of sports effort may lead to development of an overtraining state (Kenttä and Hassmén, 1998). This state of intolerance to repeated exercise appears as different clinical symptoms, sometimes severe, that constitute endocrinal, metabolic, immune and/or psychiatric syndromes. Hence, physical training is translated into overtraining by the development of adaptation mechanisms or by the appearance of mismatch or dysregulation states.

Can exercise-induced muscle injuries be attributed to one of the manifestations of overtraining? The organism tolerates the practice of intense, long-lasting, and repeated exercise, e.g., long-distance running. This can induce the development of muscle injuries that cause the decay of some muscle fibers and their substitution by new fibers formed from satellite cells.

There is an individual susceptibility to variations in training programs, and subjects submitted to a marked increase in exercise do not all develop clinical manifestations of overtraining. Other factors that may explain the appearance of clinical signs of overtraining have been identified, such as monotonous training, nutritional imbalance, climate, and psychological stress, among others (Urhausen et al., 1998). High training loads can induce muscle injuries and the release of sarcoplasmatic enzymes into plasma (Kuipers and Keizer, 1988).

High-intensity training generally induces a 2 to 10-fold increase in plasmatic CK concentration compared with resting conditions (Vincent and Vincent, 1997). However, there is broad consensus that these variations in CK cannot be considered markers of overtraining, for several reasons. On one hand, because the presence of these enzymes in plasma does not faithfully reflect the magnitude or nature of post-exercise muscle injuries, and on the other hand because it is not associated with some states of overtraining that are clinically confirmed by biological signs of muscle injuries (Kuipers and Keizer, 1988) (Figure 7).

As indicated above, the lack of sensitivity and reproducibility of CK activity means that variations in this biological parameter should be interpreted with great caution. Assessment of the extent of exercise-induced injuries cannot be based on variations in this parameter, which is not specific to muscle microinjuries of this etiology. Thus, plasma CK activity can also increase after direct muscle contusions or traumas (Bigard, 2001).

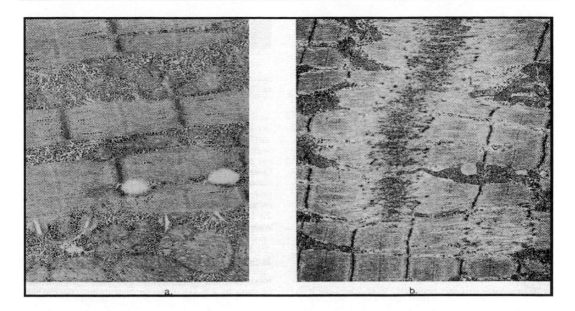

Figure 7. (a) An electron micrograph showing the normal arrangement of actin and myosin filaments and z disk configuration in the muscle of a runner before a marathon race. (b) A muscle sample taken immediately after a marathon race shows z disk streaming caused by the eccentric actions of running. Reprinted from hagerman et al. (1984).

In summary, prolonged and intense physical exercise is a cause of muscle injury, especially if there is a major eccentric component. The severity of these injuries is variable and can be detected by the simple finding of sarcoplasmatic enzymes in the blood or by degenerative injuries affecting a high percentage of muscle fibers.

4.5.1. Biochemical Modifications Produced by Overtraining

An increasing number of authors believe that the overtraining syndrome (OTS) is initiated by small alterations in the osteomuscular system, especially those that affect muscle fibers.

These types of injury are known as adaptive microinjuries and are usually produced in the muscle by eccentric and concentric contractions and in the articulations by high work volumes. The adjective "adaptive" is applied to these injuries because they are considered an inflammatory process that is eventually resolved by treatment of the microinjury (Bigard, 2001).

Besides producing stiffness, eccentric exercise reduces the maximum force of the muscle and produces low-frequency fatigue. It also produces alterations in the Z band of myofibers, mitochondria inflammation, increased intramuscular pressure, alteration of the de novo synthesis of glycogen, an increased inorganic phosphorus/ phosphocreatine ratio, and elevation of resting lactate levels (Yu and Thornell, 2002).

At any rate, various authors, including Smith, consider that muscle damage is the initial cause of OTS and also responsible for its perpetuation (Stauber and Smith, 1998).

Cytokines appear to be implicated in OTS development. Structures injured by training (muscle, connective tissue or bone) synthesize these molecules, which are responsible for coordinating different systems to promote the recovery of damaged tissues. During the acute response of the organism to training, several peripheral cell mechanisms are implicated in the contribution of energy, involving reactions associated with cytokine and hormone production.

Resistance OTS can appear as a result of successive and cumulative metabolism alterations in skeletal muscle, which become chronic during training. This process is initiated by an alteration in carbohydrate metabolism. During resistance exercises, properties of the saccharine chains of two blood glycoproteins (alpha-2 macroglobulin and alpha-1 acid glycoprotein) are decreased or modified. These glycoproteins are probably used during combustion of glycogen from the liver during exercise followed by a reduction in medium-chain fatty acids, which is related to an alteration in the synthesis of long-chain fatty acids in the liver (Bigard, 2001).

The reduction in muscle glycogen from intense training derives from the increased consumption required by the sports activity. However, it is also possible that subacute damage in fibers, caused by eccentric contractions, may reduce glucose transporter protein GLUT-4 in the muscle cell, interfering with glycogen synthesis. The decrease in muscle glycogen, besides contributing to overtraining, facilitates excessive uptake of branched chain amino acids and contributes to their oxidation in myofibers. This reduces the availability of myofibers to synthesize central neurotransmitters, which may be related to fatigue of cerebral origin.

In addition, the reduction in muscle glycogen caused by intense and prolonged exercise is related to an increased local expression of cytokines (IL-6), a decrease in glucose transporter expression, an increase in cortisol, and a reduction in insulin secretion and beta-adrenergic stimulation. Moreover, leptin has important effects on the hypothalamus and participates in regulating the hormonal metabolism of exercise and training.

Exercise-induced muscle damage and the subsequent repair process stimulate the expression of inflammatory cytokines (e.g., alpha-TNF) and stress proteins (HSP-72). During states of supercompensation and overtraining, a process similar to myopathy can be observed in skeletal muscle, with a reduction in the replacement of contractile proteins.

The last stage of overtraining concludes with the catabolism of proteins. This can imply a shift from the use of carbohydrates and fats to proteins in OTS, with release of the energy needed by muscles during prolonged aerobic exercise (Bigard, 2001).

The inflammatory process can eventually affect the liver, brain, and immune system. In the liver, systemic inflammation stimulates the synthesis of several proteins, known as acute phase proteins, which further complicates the problem. Nevertheless, in several sports (e.g., soccer), there does not appear to be an acute-phase response to training (Allen and Rankin, 1990).

Exercises that support the weight of the body, e.g., running, also cause muscle damage. Some authors have attributed some of these injuries to uric acid (Allen and Rankin, 1990).

An increase in plasma creatine phosphokinase and myoglobin is frequently observed as an expression of muscle damage after long aerobic activities, e.g., marathons. This has led some authors to consider these elevations to be a sign of overtraining in this type of exercise. Nevertheless, similar elevations can be found after acute exercise by athletes who do not suffer from OTS (Bigard, 2001).

Some athletes, mainly those involved in very long races, suffer muscle injuries with the complication of renal insufficiency, because the kidney is injured by products derived from muscle destruction (rhabdomyolysis). In other athletes, prolonged exercise (especially running) can produce digestive hemorrhages and a consequent ferropenic anemia (Skenderi et al., 2006).

5. Muscle Damage Markers

5.1. Introduction

Ideally, a biochemical marker of skeletal muscle damage should be simple to determine using a method that is available 24 hrs a day and can be as rapidly applied as are magnetic resonance or ultrasound. The optimal marker should be muscle-specific, with a high intracellular concentration that is rapidly released after injury and maintains elevated and stable blood concentrations for an extended time period. The marker should be undetectable in the serum of healthy individuals or at a very low concentration that can be clearly differentiated from the levels that are produced when the organ is damaged. It should offer high diagnostic sensitivity, especially during the first hours after the injury, and a diagnostic specificity close to 100% (Adams, 1994).

Biological diagnosis of muscle damage is essentially based on the measurement of the plasma activity of different sarcoplasmatic enzymes (CK and LDH). These enzymes are normally strictly intracellular, and an increase in their plasma activity reflects their release through membranous structures (Kayashima et al., 1995; Prou et al., 1996). Presence of products from membrane peroxidation can also be tested in expired air (ethane or pentane) or in plasma (malondialdehyde [MDA] or products derived from thiobarbituric acid [TBARs]) (Leaf et al., 1997). The plasma concentration of MHC class I fragments was measured as a better marker of muscle injury, but the tools required for this type of measurement were withdrawn from the market for technical reasons, (Koller et al., 1998). Measurement of the plasma concentration of the cardiac isoform of subunits I or T of troponin was also proposed, although it only serves to confirm that detected proteins are not of cardiac origin and does not allow assessment of the presence of muscle isoforms of contractile proteins in plasma (Bonetti et al., 1996; Clarkson and Tremblay, 1988).

Although direct demonstration of muscle damage is essentially histological, the measurement of plasmatic enzymes is the main diagnostic method in current use. Measurements of muscles and of articulation amplitude have been proposed to evaluate the functional impact of injuries (Lynn et al., 1998). However, a set of different biological and clinical parameters would be required to support the diagnosis, e.g., increase in plasma activity of LDH, myoglobin, and MDA, leukocyte count, and muscle alterations (Kayashima et al., 1995).

5.2. Classic Markers

Enzymes are proteins responsible for catalyzing chemical reactions in all tissues of the organism. They are composed of amino acid chains with a specific sequence that determines their three-dimensional structure. This structure determines the conditions of its activity and its substrate-specificity. They have been detected and identified in plasma or serum after their release from damaged cells or from intact cells undergoing various types of stress. In both situations, there is an increased permeability of the membrane. These intracellular enzymes spread from interstitial territory via lymphatic drainage to the general circulation.

Enzymes have been used as skeletal muscle and cardiac markers because their catalytic activity can be detected by means of a sensitive analytical method. This activity, assumed to be proportional to their concentration, can be quantified in a sensitive and selective manner. Among all of the enzymes that have been studied, only LDH and CPK have proven useful for the study of muscle cardiac damage.

The use of markers to diagnose exercise-related muscle injuries remains a major challenge. Thus, plasma CK and other enzymes are not related to the severity of exercise or secular pains and are markers with low specificity and sensitivity (Sorichter et al., 1997).

In 1964, the International Union of Biochemistry recommended a classification of enzymes based on the reaction they catalyze. In 1973, a new and longer version was published, in which the scientific name described the type of reaction, the substrate, the coenzyme, and the product. In addition, enzymes are designated by four numbers separated by a point and preceded by the abbreviations EC (Enzyme Commission). The first number defines the group according to the chemical reaction it catalyzes, of which there are six types. The next two numbers indicate the sub-group and sub-sub-group to which they are assigned. The last digit identifies the enzyme.

Enzymatic activity is measured in International Units per unit of volume (UI/mL, U/L...). The international unit represents the amount of enzyme that transforms one micromole of substrate in one minute under previously established standard conditions. Each analytical technique defines the unit of activity and its subunits.

5.2.1. Creatine-Kinase (CK)

Also known as ATP-Creatine-N-phosphotransferase, CK catalyzes the reversible reaction of transferring phosphate to creatine to form creatine phosphate from ATP.

Cytoplasmic CK exists in three isoenzymatic forms in tissues, designated BB (CK1), MB (CK2) and MM (CK3). They derive from the association of two subunits of 360 amino acids with a molecular weight of around 40,000 Da (Lang, 1981). Subunit M was initially isolated from muscle and subunit B from the brain (Nanji, 1983). The three CK isozymes have distinct tissue locations. In muscle, the enzyme is mainly type MM, whereas type BB predominates in other tissues, especially in brain (Takagi et al., 2001). Hybrid MB is localized in the myocardium, where it represents around 20% of the total CK activity (Ingwall et al., 1985). However, the organ-specificity of CK-MB is not 100%. Thus, CK-MB rates of >5% are observed in spleen and prostate.

The amount of CK-MB in skeletal muscle varies according to the nature of the muscle and is generally < 1% of total CK (e.g., in psoas), but the CK-MB content of the diaphragm is 2-3-fold smaller than that of the myocardium. In the skeletal muscle (where approximately 5% of CK activity is CK-MB), CK-MB activity can be increased by physiological (intense exercise) or pathological conditions (genetic or secondary myopathies) (Ohman et al., 1990; Adams, 1994). Subunits M and B can both form complexes with immunoglobulin to give rise to "macro CK" or "macrokinases" (Lee, 1994), which electrophoretically migrate between CK1 and CK2.

Macro CK type I is an immunoglobulin enzyme complex, generally BB-IgG (Jones et al, 1990). Macro CK type II is an oligomeric form of mitochondrial CK and probably constitutes a fragment of the internal membrane of the mitochondria. Mitochondrial forms of CK, known as CK Mt, can also be observed. Electrophoresis techniques can be used to separate CK into its different isoforms. Thus; three isoforms can be separated from MM isozyme (MM1, MM2, MM3) and two can be obtained from MB isozyme (MB1, MB2).

A. Total Activity Determination:

Measurement of creatine-kinase in biological media without any separation or previous purification gives the total activity of the enzyme (total CK). It is based on indirect measurement of the rate of ATP formation when the enzyme is in contact with phosphocreatine and adenosine diphosphate (ADP). Under these conditions, presence of adenylate-kinase (AK) in a biological sample also generates ATP from the ADP that has been used in the process. Therefore, AK, mainly from erythrocytes (hemolysis) or muscle interferes in the measurement of CK, leading to an overestimation and false positive results. Commercial reagents contain inhibitors, e.g., adenosine monophosphate (AMP) or diadenosine pentaphosphate (A2P5), which reduce interference from AK without completely suppressing it.

B. Results Interpretation:

The increase in CK activity is an early event, from around two hours after the end of exercise. Plasma accumulation of CK increases over time and reaches a maximum level between the fifth and ninth day (Brancaccio et al., 2007).

After isometric exercise, which is characterized by maximum contractions, blood CK levels increase after 6-8 hours and the maximum level is attained after 24 hours. with measurements > 1000 mU/ml. Graves *et al.* found that creatine-kinase MB increased by up to 50% in individuals performing maximum isometric contractions for more than 20 minutes. Nevertheless, it has not been definitively established whether the CK MB found after isometric exercise is of skeletal or myocardial muscle origin. This represents am important issue, since many recreational and work activities involve high-intensity exercise that includes isometric contractions (Clarkson et al, 1986, Fredsted et al, 2007).

In eccentric exercise, in which a large amount of force is generated, the increase of CK in blood is slower. The activity of this enzyme begins to increase on the second day after exercise, reaching maximum levels on the fifth or sixth day. A remarkable increase in CK can be observed. Thus, eccentric exercise of forearm flexors, which are small muscles, increases the amount of CK to 10000 mU/ml, with mean values of 2000 mU/milliliter (Ebbeling et al., 1989).

To date, no clear explanation has been established for the slow increase in blood CK after high-intensity eccentric exercise, especially when compared with the fast increase of this enzyme in resistance and isometric exercises. There may be a greater hypoxia in the muscles, which can, alongside other factors, increase the permeability of the membrane, allowing release from the muscle of CK and other proteins during or immediately after physical exercise (Evans and Cannon, 1991).

CK elevation after eccentric exercise also appears to respond to a progressive and slow activation of certain muscle enzymes that lead to the degradation of cellular components.

Another explanation is that CK may enter the lymphatic system before its release into the blood, and lymphatic drainage in muscle tissues is reduced by the marked accumulation of fluids.

C. CK Isoform:

The use of high-resolution separation techniques has demonstrated the heterogeneity of CK-MM and CK-MB isozymes. Unlike atypical forms, e.g., macro-CK type I (CK-BB bound to immunoglobulin) and type II (polymeric mitochondrial CK), which are rarely found in serum, CK-MM and CK-MB isoforms are present in the normal process of degradation of the enzyme and appear in all human serum samples. They are the result of posttranscriptional modifications of CK isozymes, which preserve the catalytic activity of the enzyme but differ in molecular weight and other properties (Stein and Decker, 1989).

Isozymes represent a specialized adaptation of the enzymes in different cells and tissues. CK isozymes comprise groups of monomers. There are three CK isozymes, each of which is composed of two monomers, M and B, which are grouped in dimers to constitute the functional enzyme. CK-MM (homodimer of monomer M) represents 95% of total CK and is mainly located in skeletal muscle. CK-MB (heterodimer of monomers M and B) is more abundant in myocardium, representing 20% of total CK in diseased myocardium and a smaller proportion in healthy myocardium (Ingwall et al., 1985). CK-BB, a third type of isozyme, is preferentially localized in the central nervous system and intestine (Nanji, 1983).

Hence, CK-MB constitutes the most cardio-specific isozyme of those that comprise total CK. However, a small proportion of CK-MB can also be observed in skeletal muscle, where it can be increased in certain physiological or pathological conditions (Adams et al., 1993) and even in some extramuscular diseases, e.g., certain cancers (Tsung et al., 1981). Therefore, this presence of a physiological or pathological extra-myocardial "background" of circulating catalytic CK-MB activity in plasma of healthy people limits its value to evaluate myocardial necrosis. Another important limitation of the semiologic value of CK-MB is interference from the in vivo or in vitro methods of measuring catalytic activity, which can produce an overestimation of this activity.

After tissue necrosis, $CK-MM_3$ and $CK-MB_2$ are released into plasma, where, due to carboxypeptidase action, $CK-MM_3$ is rapidly converted into $CK-MM_2$ and $CK-MM_1$ and $CK-MB_2$ is converted into $CK-MB_1$ (Perryman et al., 1984). Under normal conditions, the tissue isoforms of $CK-MM_3$ and $CK-MB_2$ are in balance with the plasma isoforms ($CK-MM_2$-$CK-MM_1$ and $CK-MB_1$) and $CK-MM_3/CK-MM_1$ and $CK-MB_2/CK-MB_1$ ratios are close to 1. Conversion from tissue isoforms into plasma isoforms is faster for $CK-MB_2$ than for $CK-MM_3$ (Figure 8).

5.2.2. Lactate Dehydrogenase (LDH).

LDH is an enzyme (EC 1.1.1.27) that catalyzes the conversion of pyruvate to L-lactate by concomitant oxidation of NADH to NAD^+. LDH is present in most human tissues, mainly in myocardium, kidney, liver, and muscle. It has a molecular weight of 134000 Dal and is constituted by the formation of a tetramer from two peptide chains, M ("Muscle") and H ("Heart").

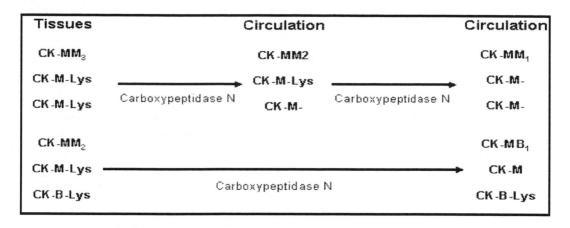

Figure 8. In vivo generation of ck-mm and ck-mb isoforms.

According to Rasmussen et al. (2002), LDH is a cytoplasmic enzyme, whereas other authors (Brandt et al., 1987; Brooks et al., 1999, Rasmussen et al., 2002) affirmed the presence of a mitochondrial LDH in muscle.

Hence, there are five isozymes that each contains four subunits:

- LDH-1 (4H) - in heart
- LDH-2 (3H1M) - in reticuloendothelial system
- LDH-3 (2H2M) - in lungs
- LDH-4 (1H3M) - in kidneys
- LDH-5 (4M) - in liver and striated muscle

The proportion of isozymes varies among tissues. Isozyme LDH1 predominates in the heart (35-70% of total LDH activity). In the liver, however, isozyme LDH5 is predominant (30-85%). Erythrocytes are rich in LDH1 and LDH2. Monomers H and M significantly differ in their amino acid composition and therefore in their kinetic structure and properties. They are probably encoded by two different genes.

In general, tissues that develop an aerobic metabolism present larger concentrations of subunits H (LDH1 and 2). Subunit H presents a greater affinity for lactate than for pyruvate (the inverse of unit M). Isozymes with a larger H content produce an increase in the concentration of pyruvate, which becomes acetyl CoA (pyruvate decarboxylase pathway) and is introduced into the Krebs cycle to generate high concentrations of ATP. Isoforms LDH1 and LDH2 predominate in the myocardium, which needs a constant supply of energy. Study of these distribution patterns allows the identification of specific tissue injuries. In the cardiac muscle, the LDH1/LDH2 ratio is usually lower than 1, at 0.5-0.75.

A. Determination of Total LDH Activity

NAD (nicotinamide adenine dinucleotide) and NADP (nicotinamide adenine dinucleotide phosphate), are enzyme cofactors widely used to measure the activity of enzymes and metabolites. When this activity is reduced, for example during an enzyme or substrate assay, NADH and NADPH show absorbances in the ultraviolet region of the spectrum, with a maximum absorbance at 340 nm.

The following reaction is used to determine LDH activity:

$$Pyruvate + NADH + H^+ — L - lactate + NAD^+$$

B. Interpretation of LDH Results

Since LDH is widely distributed, it can be increased by a multitude of causes, especially tissue destruction. Knowledge of the origin of an increase can be facilitated by determining LDH isozymes. LDH is elevated in myopathies, myocardial infarction, pulmonary infarct, cerebral hemopathy and hemolysis, vascular and systemic diseases (polyarteritis nodosa, dermatomyositis, polymyositis), and metastatic cancer.

In acute myocardial infarction, LDH begins to risc after 12-24 hours, with a peak at 2-4 days (frequently 1500-2500 units), and returns to normal values at 8-14 days (Table 2). A 5-10-fold increase can usually be found in acute hepatitis.

For the differential diagnosis of myocardial necrosis, an increase of >33% in the LDH1 fraction (alpha-HLDH, usually 50-70% of the total in myocardial infarction) is considered, with absolute values of LDH1 >140 IU and an LDH1/LDH ratio > 0.5.

Determination of the LDH in pleural effusion assists differentiation between exudate and transudate, since the former shows 60% of the value of LDH in plasma.

5.3. Time Course of Different Markers of Muscle Damage

The absence of a simple, sensitive and reproducible marker of muscle injury represents a major drawback for estimation of the severity of damage. As demonstrated in animals, there is no relationship between plasma sarcoplasmic enzyme activity and the extent of histological injuries (Van der Meulen et al., 1991). The degree of muscle injury in animals was found to increase with longer periods of exercise on a rolling carpet, although this increase was not proportional with time.

Table 2. Normal values of LDH in serum

NORMAL VALUES OF LDH IN ADULTS	115 to 225 UI/L
Levels of LDH-1	From 17 to 27 %
Levels ofLDH-2	From 27 to 37 %
Levels ofLDH-3	From 18 to 25 %
Levels ofLDH-4	From 3 to 8 %
Levels ofLDH-5	From 0 to 5 %

Moreover, the extent of injury as evaluated by CK, LDH or plasmatic aminotransferase activity is always much greater than estimated based on histological results (Evans and

Cannon, 1991). Animal experiments have also used β- glucuronidase activity as a marker of muscle damage.

An increase in CK plasma activity was even observed in rats after swimming, an exercise that did not involve muscle damage (Komulainen et al., 1995). Unexpectedly, climbing a slope produced a much smaller increase in plasma CK activity compared with swimming. These results raise doubts about the specificity and sensitivity of plasma CK activity. Although very widely used, measurement of the plasma activity of sarcoplasmic enzymes (e.g., CK or LDH) does not function well as a prognostic factor for exercise-induced muscle injuries or cell decay. No close correlation has been established between visible histological muscle injuries and the release of sarcoplasmic enzymes into plasma.

5.4. New Markers

Although many of the methods for measuring the total CK activity fulfill analytical requirements, they are not sufficiently effective to diagnose exercise-related muscle damage.

The measurement of CK activity has traditionally been considered as a biochemical marker of cardiac damage. However, the most widely used methods for CK activity measurement show interference from other kinases of different origins (e.g., adenylate kinase, increased in plasma by hemolysis), from CK isozymes (mitochondrial CKMM), or from known CK- immunoglobulin complexes (e.g., macrokinases). Because of this coexpression in skeletal and myocardial muscle, increases in serum or plasma CKMM activity can be observed when there are no signs of muscle damage using the most effective imaging methods. Hence, CK activity cannot be considered the best biochemical criterion for the diagnosis of skeletal muscle damage.

With the introduction of molecular biology into the field of physical activity and the development of biotechnology, very positive advances in muscle damage markers are being achieved. In particular, the technological and conceptual breakthrough represented by monoclonal antibodies has contributed a powerful and highly valuable diagnostic tool.

5.4.1. Troponins

Besides their formation by actin, the thin filaments of striated muscle contain two main accessory proteins that exert a regulating function, controlling the construction and rupture of cross-sectional bridges between heavy and thin filaments and producing mechanical energy. One of these proteins is troponin, a very large (78000 Da) globular protein, which was discovered by the Japanese biochemist S. Ebashi and his group in 1965.

Troponin has three subunits, TnC, TnI, and TnT, each with a specific function. Troponin C (TnC) binds to calcium ions to produce movement; it has a molecular weight of 18000 Da.

The inhibiting subunit of troponin is TnI, which has a molecular weight of 23000 Da and a specific actin-binding site. Its function consists of inhibiting the interaction of actin with the cross-bridges of the myosin head. Subunit TnI is phosphorylated by kinase phosphorylase, which is usually activated by phosphorylase b, transforming it into active phosphorylase a.

The third component of troponin, TnT, has a molecular weight of 37000 Da and binds to tropomyosin, interlocking them into a troponin-tropomyosin complex. The complete molecule of troponin has a globular shape and contains one of the subunits TnC, TnI, or TnT (Figure 9).

The release of Troponin T (TnT) is typically biphasic: the first peak appears in 50% of patients at 4 hours (versus 25% for CK), with a maximum at 12-24 hours. This first major increase corresponds with release of the tertiary complex due to myofibril damage, which subsequently degrades to free protein complex C-cTnI + cTnT, together with release of cTnT from the cytosolic pool. A second peak is observed on the fourth day, especially in reperfused patients (Mair et al., 1994) and people with coronary artery bypass grafting (CABG) (Mair et al., 1994).

The presence of cTnT in plasma is not specific for the diagnosis of ischemic heart disease. It is released in cases of cardiac insufficiency due to myocyte injury. Studies of pigs undergoing left ventricle remodeling after AMI showed cTnI and cTnT values 40-80% below normal, due to chronic loss of troponins in a damaged myocardium with inadequate capacity to re-express genes that would increase protein synthesis (Wilkinson and Grand, 1978).

The half-life of troponin is 120 minutes, although circulating protein can be detected at up to 21 days after muscle damage due to myofibril degradation (up to one week more than for CK). It presents a high organ specificity, and an elevation of its concentration in blood clearly indicates necrosis of myocardial cells. It is therefore a marker of myocardial damage.

Each troponin molecule is fixed to the thin filament by two binding sites, one specific to actin fiber and the other specific to tropomyosin fiber. The binding to tropomyosin appears to take place at a fixed point, but the formation or rupture of binding to the actin filament depends on the binding to Ca++. A troponin molecule is found at 40-nm throughout the length of a thin filament. Therefore there are one tropomyosin molecule and one troponin molecule for every seven monomers of actin G.

It is when the muscle tissue suffers damage that some of the protein components related to the contraction-relaxation process can be detected in the blood. Troponins are biochemical markers that can be used for the detection of cell damage. Subunits T, C, and I are proteins of the contractile apparatus that appear in different isoforms according to their muscle of origin. Determination of these substances with other biochemical markers opens up new possibilities for the diagnosis of different diseases, notably acute myocardial infarction (AMI).

The value of the troponin in diagnosis has been widely discussed. The classic determination was troponin T (TnT) measurement. However, it has recently been shown that troponin I (TnI) has greater sensitivity and efficacy for the diagnosis of different types of muscle damage (cardiac and skeletal muscle).

There have been numerous studies and comparisons with other parameters, including LDH isozymes, CK and its isozymes (e.g., CK-MB), myoglobin, and even with TnT itself. Comparisons revealed that TnI was the best option for the diagnosis of damage to these muscles (Stephan Sorichter et al., 1997).

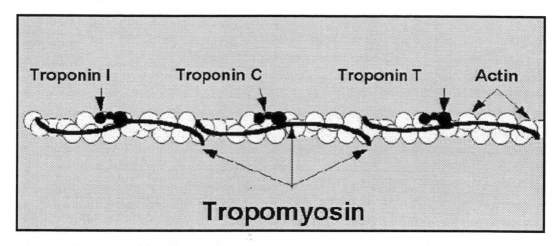

Figure 9. Schematic representation of the thin filament of myofibril of striated muscle.

A. Troponin I Isoforms as Markers of Muscle Damage

The use of antibodies that recognize TnI and the other two subunits has been proposed, since TnI has been reported to be released into the blood, sometimes free and sometimes forming a complex with the other troponin subunits. There are only three isoforms of TnI. The tissue-specific subtypes are as follows: slow-twitch skeletal muscle isoform troponin I, (sTnI); fast-twitch skeletal muscle isoform troponin I, (rTnI); and cardiac troponin I, (cTnI) (Wilkinson et al., 1978). The three isoforms are encoded by different genes and show a variability of 40% in their amino acid sequences. The cTnI has an additional residue of amino acid at its N-terminal end (Mair et al., 1994).

It has also been demonstrated that skeletal muscles do not express cTnI, either during their development phase or as a response to stimuli. Therefore, its absolute specificity for myocardial injury allows cTnI to be used to distinguish between cardiac injuries and skeletal injuries and between myocardial infarction from muscle injuries (rhabdomyolysis, polytraumatism) and from non-cardiac surgery. Troponin I has also shown elevated levels in cases of unstable angina and cardiac hydrops. cTnI is 13-fold more abundant than CK-MB in the myocardium and does not usually circulate in the blood, which is why the signal-to-noise ratio is more favorable for the detection of myocardial necrosis. Accumulated data from different studies indicate that troponin I can be detected (above levels in non-AMI samples) at 3-6 hours after the onset of chest pain. Most commercialized methods use the differential capacity of cTnI, in its free form or in a complex. In some tests, responses to the different forms of cTnI are practically equivalent, whereas in other tests they show a substantial difference.

The isoform sTnI has absolute specificity for skeletal muscle, with a wide diagnostic window, allowing diagnoses to be made early (at 2-6 hours) and late (at 24-48 hours). It also offers a high sensitivity.

The response of sTnI has been studied, comparing its concentration over time with that of CK, MB, and MHC in blood samples from different groups of athletes (Gunst et al., 1998). In general, there was a higher increase from baseline values for sTnI than for the other markers studied. Highest release levels appeared earliest for MB (mean of 2 hours), followed by sTnI (mean of 6 hours), CK (mean of 1 day), and MHC (mean of 2 days). The results of this study demonstrated that a high muscular effort, associated with the eccentric contraction or longitudinal changes that occur during the eccentric exercise, causes a rapid dissociation and/or degradation with a rapid release of sTnI.

The sTnI isoform shows an increase at 2-6 hours after the start of the exercise that produces muscle damage, with a higher response if the exercise is eccentric (Gunst et al., 1998). sTnI has a wide range as an initial marker, peaking at 24 hours and remaining elevated for at least one or two days. Unlike all other available markers, sTnI is exclusively a skeletal muscle protein. It increases quickly in plasma, and, above all, an early peak indicates alterations of the fine filament of troponin after exercise-induced muscle damage.

Finally, although use of the TnT is recommended for diagnostic tests, CK-MB and myoglobin are also useful parameters, especially for determining the phase of damage and for therapeutic decision-making. For the determination of muscle damage, TnT appears earlier than TnI but is not as specific as the latter.

5.4.2. Myosin Chains

Myosin is another protein that reversibly interacts with actin during muscle contraction. It is constituted by a heavy chain with two light chains at each end. There are two types of light chains: type 1 light chains, with a molecular weight of 29000 Da, and type 2 light chains, with a molecular weight of 24000 Da. Molecules of myosin type 1 and type 2 light chains exist in several isoforms that differ in their amino acid composition. However, specific isoforms have not been identified in the myocardium. Several monoclonal antibodies have been developed to recognize different epitopes of myosin light chain (Weeds et al., 1971). Type ß myosin heavy chain (ß-MHC) is the predominant chain in humans with healthy or damaged myocardium. Myosin, formed by ß-MHC and the light chains, is the most important structural protein of the myocardium. ß-MHC is also expressed in skeletal muscle fibers and is therefore not cardiac-specific (Harrington et al., 1984). It has been suggested that it may be useful to detect smaller myocardial damage (Hoberg et al., 1987) and to identify patients with severe coronary disease and determine their prognosis (Katus et al., 1988; Ravkilde et al., 1995).

5.4.3. Myoglobin

Myoglobin is a single-chain globular protein of 153 amino acids that is mainly found in striated muscle cells (skeletal and cardiac muscle). It represents 2% of total muscle proteins, and has the function of transporting and storing oxygen in the cell. It reversibly binds with oxygen, increasing its delivery to mitochondria and playing a major role in the aerobic metabolism of the cell. A small part is bound to structural elements of muscle cells, with the remainder localized in the cytoplasm. It does not present myocardial specificity. After tissue necrosis, myoglobin is released by muscle cells and appears in the blood sanguineous circulation and urine. Its main advantage is the speed of its elevation in blood.

Myoglobin is an early biological marker of myocardial necrosis. Its molecular weight (17800 Da) gives it a fast diffusion time, faster than other heavier molecules, e.g., CK (80000 Da) or LDH (130000 Da). Myoglobin appears in peripheral blood at two or three hours after pain onset reaches pathological levels, i.e. at 3-6 hours before the appearance of CK-MB. The maximum concentration is reached at 6-9 hours, compared with 12-19 hours for other cardiac markers. It is renally eliminated (Ohman et al., 1990; Mair et al., 1994).

6. Muscle Cell. Actin and its Importance

6.1. Introduction

Actin is one of the two most abundant muscle proteins and can represent more than 20% of total muscle cell proteins (Korn, 1982; Aránega et al., 1991). It is also one of the best preserved proteins (Hirano et al., 1987). Its generalized presence and evolutionary stability indicate the key biological importance of this protein.

Actin is also the main component of the thin filaments of muscle. It can be isolated from the tissue by high dilution in saline solutions. This treatment disperses the actin filaments into globular subunits composed of a 43 KD polypeptide (Korn, 1982) known as globular actin (G-actin). Each molecule of G-actin is closely associated with Ca2+, which stabilizes its globular configuration, and also with an ATP molecule by a noncovalent bond (Alberts et al., 1986).

6.2. Polymerization

G-actin has a low ionic force and polymerizes into filaments (F-actin) by a noncovalent and reversible bond (Grazi et al, 2004). This reaction needs physiological levels of Mg2+ (Oosawa et al, 1971). After polymerization, new additions and losses of actin monomers take place at the end of filaments until the structure reaches a stable state. The actin filament is polarized. Electron microscopy readily demonstrates the presence of these filaments together with those of myosin, which bind to F-actin at a 45°angle in absence of adenosine-triphosphate (Moore at al., 1970).

The most widely studied actin molecule is that in the thin filament of striated muscle. In this tissue, the interaction between actin and myosin is the chemical mechanism for contraction (Eisenberg, 1980). Muscle contraction is one of the most evident manifestations of the role of F-actin in eukaryotic cell motility. Important functions of actin-myosin in non-muscle cells include cell motility, cytokinesis, phagocytosis, and platelet retraction (Korn, 1982).

Actin polymerization in muscle is solely important to produce and maintain the thin filaments essential for contractile activity. Although the state of actin organization in the cell is related to the interactions of G- and F-actins with other proteins (Pollard, 1986), polymerization is a property of actin alone (Figure 10).

For this reason, it is essential to elucidate the mechanism of actin polymerization in order to understand the dynamics of the complex microfilament systems.

As already mentioned, G-actin monomers are bound to an ATP molecule by a noncovalent bond. It is hydrolyzed to adenosine diphosphate (ADP) and free inorganic phosphorus (Pi) during polymerization, in a process that involves the transitory formation of F-actin + Pi (Carlier, 1987).

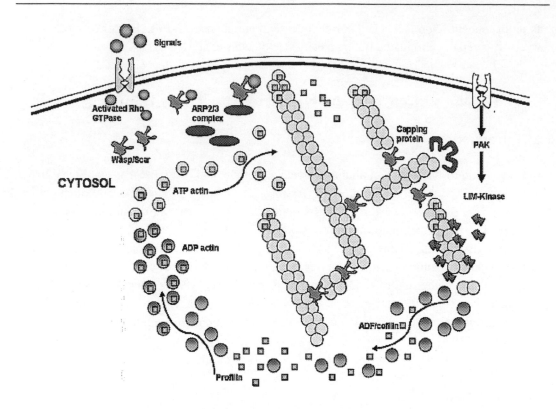

Figure 10. Schematic representation of the principal events in the actin polymerization process. Actin is an ATP-binding protein that preferentially polymerises at the end of an actin filament. Then, an actin subunit rapidly hydrolyzes its bound ATP into ADP and phosphate (Pi) and slowly releases the hydrolyzed phosphate. Some external signals are able to activate WASp/Scar proteins, which in turn activate the Arp2/3 complex. Active Arp2/3 complex binds to the side of an existing filament and nucleates new filament growth towards the cell membrane. Actin binding proteins, including capping protein, ADF/cofilin, profilin, tropomyosin, formins, and Ena/VASP. These proteins are able to modulate the actin polymerisation phenomenon, but it is not fully understood how these reaction mechanisms coordinate to organize actin filaments.

ATP is not re-synthesized, but ADP bound with G-actin, which is dissociated from the end of the filament, exchanges with ATP in solution, regenerating G-actin-ATP (Korn, 1982). Hence, polymerization and depolymerization result in a continuous hydrolysis of ATP, and actin can therefore be considered an adenosinetriphosphatase (ATPase).

Myofilament functions require ATP as a regulator of this double process (Korn, 1982). ATP modulation is parallel to F-actin formation. In an early phase of polymerization, when there is a large concentration of actin monomers, the elongation is faster than ATP hydrolysis in the filament. When this concentrations decreases, the filament elongation is shorter than ATP hydrolysis. Hence, ATP-actin and ADP-Pi-actin reach both ends of the filament. When the monomer concentration is near its critical point, the ATP-actin subunits disappear.

As result of ATP hydrolysis, the critical concentration of ATP is lower at one end of the filament than at the other. This situation may induce partial filament depolymerization. However, this depolymerization may be lower in presence of Pi, which binds with F-acti subunits to form ADP-Pi-actin. Nevertheless, this could reduce but not eliminate the difference in critical ATP concentration between the ends of the filament. Therefore, ATP and Pi levels are two potential mechanisms for regulating the dynamics of microfilaments in muscle cells (Korn et al., 1987).

6.3. Structure

Under the electron microscope, F-actin protein appears as a right-handed double helix with a crossover every 36 nm. Hanson, a pioneer in the study of actin filaments (Hanson, 1967), studied paracrystals of actin because they could be readily observed by imaging methods, using a paracrystal induced by a large concentration of Mg^{+2}.

However, images of F-actin obtained by X-ray diffraction showed a left-handed single helix, with some controversy about the orientation of the subunits (Egelman, 1985; Engelman et al., 1984).

Fowler and Aebi (Fowler and Aebi, 1983) described a model of actin filaments with a diameter of 7-8 nm, with globular subunits parallel to the longitudinal axis of the filament. Engelman and Padrón (Engelman and Padrón, 1984) constructed a model in which the diameter of actin filaments of actin was 9.5 nm and the globular subunits were perpendicular to the longitudinal axis of the filament.

The ideal model of actin filaments consists of identical subunits ordered in a helix, which would determine the symmetry of filaments. Thus, the symmetry of an ideal filament is determined by two parameters, the subunit height (2.73 nm) and the angle between subunits (167°). Various studies reported that differences between angles formed by actin subunits in different filaments are small and can vary within a filament under different conditions (DeRosier and Tilney, 1984).

Multiple efforts have been made to determine the atomic structure of actin (Kabsch et al., 1990). One of the most important studies in this respect was by Milligan (Milligan et al., 1990), who used electron microscopy and helical image processing methods to create three-dimensional maps of F-actin. Results showed that the long axis of monomers is located throughout the helix of the filament and has a maximum diameter of 95-100 A. They identified an internal and external domain in monomers, located at 26 and 17A, respectively, from the axial filament. They also locate two connections between monomers, a longitudinal connection between adjacent internal domains and a diagonal one between the internal and external domain. The authors also located the binding sites for tropomyosin and heads of myosin. They demonstrated that, in absence of Ca^{+2} and heads of myosin, tropomyosin is in the internal domain of actin, closing the contacts of the helix, and that the site of greatest binding with myosin is in the lower part of the front surface of the external domain and appears to extend, through the internal domain, near the binding site to tropomyosin.

6.4. Isoforms

In large vertebrates the cytoskeletal protein actin exists in six different isoforms that are encoded by distinct genes (Firtel, 1981). These genes are expressed with specific patterns in each tissue: two predominant isoforms in non-muscle cells (β and non-muscular γ), two in smooth muscle cells (α and smooth muscle γ), one in cardiac muscle (cardiac α) and one in skeletal muscle (skeletal α). The complexity of expression of the different isoforms has given rise to multiple suggestions about possible functional differences of actin (Bravo et al., 1981; Korn, 1982).

Myogenesis, when the cell exhibits major changes in their pattern of expression of different isoforms, is a widely used model for their localization (Minty et al., 1982; Vankerckhove et al., 1986). Biochemical and immunohistochemical methods have been used to determine whether muscle and non-muscle actin are at different localizations during myogenesis (Lin, 1986). Lubit and Schwartz (Lubit and Schwartz, 1980) used a specific antibody for non-muscle isoforms of actin and observed that it did not mark actin present in band I microfilaments of muscle fibers. Brown and coworkers (Brown et al., 1983) used an antibody that reacted with the γ actin isoform (non-muscle γ-actin and smooth muscle γ-actin) in frozen sections of mouse diaphragm. This antibody marked the periphery of mitochondria but did not mark band I of the contractile muscle apparatus. Fatigati and Murphy (Fatigati and Murphy, 1984) analyzed smooth muscle α-actin, non-muscle β-actin, smooth muscle γ-actin and non-muscle γ-actin isoforms in 15 different smooth muscles. They observed a large proportion of smooth muscle α-actin in tissue with a high degree of muscle tone, and this isoform disappeared in culture cells when their phenotype was modified from contractile to proliferative. Otey et al. (Otey et al., 1988) obtained an antibody that only recognizes the α-skeletal isoform of actin.

De Couet (De Couet, 1983) analyzed the amino acid sequence of actin in mammals and birds. They concluded that an ancestral gene of muscle actin, expressed in lower vertebrates, was duplicated before or during an early phase of evolution, generating an actin gene of smooth muscle and an actin gene of striated muscle. A second duplication gave rise to actin genes of cardiac striated actin, actin genes of striated skeletal muscle, actin genes of vascular smooth muscle, and actin genes of nonvascular smooth muscle. Hightower and Meagher (Hightower and Meagher., 1986) compared nucleotide and amino acid sequences from 20 actin genes and observed less than 3% divergence between muscle actin and cytoplasmic actin genes in large vertebrates.

To date, 183 different sequences have been described for actin, available at SwissProt. The large vertebrates have six different isoforms of actin that are encoded by different genes (Firtel, 1981). The expression pattern of these genes is specific to each tissue: α (cardiac muscle), α1 (skeletal muscle), α2 (vascular smooth muscle), α3 (intestinal smooth muscle), β (cytoplasmic) and γ (cytoplasmic). (Sheterline et al., 1995).

α actin is similar in human (Homo sapiens), mouse (Mus musculus), and chicken (Gallus gallus) (Hamada et al., 1982; Alonso, 1987; Chang et al., 1985; Von Arx et al., 1995). α actin differs from α 1 actin in four amino acids and from α 2 actin and α 3 actin in five There is greater heterogeneity between α and β actin, which differ from γ actin in 22 and 21 amino acids, respectively.

6.5. Use of A-Actin in Muscle Injury

α actin is one of the most abundant proteins present in the contractile apparatus of muscle fibers. It represents more than 20% of total proteins in the sarcomere (Korn, 1982; Aránega et al., 1991) and is the most important component of thin filaments. Its presence can be detected in the first stages of myocardial infarction by using highly sensitive immunoblotting techniques, even at one hour after onset of symptoms, and in patients with angina (Aránega et al., 1992). It shows a high specificity and sensitivity. There is no interference from muscle involvement and it shows a two-phase release pattern, being detectable at seven days after the ischemic episode (Aránega et al., 1993).

Other molecules besides troponins have demonstrated their usefulness in the diagnosis of cardiac damage, as in the case of α actin. Thus, Aránega et al. (Aránega, 1991) contributed very interesting results in favor of using α actin as a molecular marker of ischemic heart disease. Release of circulating actin α was observed in sera from patients with unstable angina (Aránega et al., 1992), showing a sensitivity of 63.6-100%. α actin was detected in only one out of twenty control sera and in only four out of thirty sera from individuals with muscle damage, similar results to findings reported for troponin (Katus et al., 1989). A two-phase release pattern was observed for α actin with one peak in the first hour and another at 50 hours after symptom onset, and it could still be detected at one week (175 h) after clinical symptoms appear. No statistically significant relationships in mean values were found among anginas of different types and no association was found with tobacco use, hypercholesterolemia, diabetes, or history of ischemic heart disease. α-actin has been also detected in the sera of patients with AMI (Aránega et al., 1993).

α-actin is an early marker released between 0 and 6 hours, as already indicated by Aránega et al., 1993. This kinetics may correspond to a fast and early release of actin from the cytoplasmic compartment, which would subsequently be accompanied by the structural component.

α actin has been detected in sera from patients with unstable angina (Aránega et al., 1992). A significant relationship has also been demonstrated between high α actin values and numerous complications (Aránega et al., 1993), giving this molecule both a diagnostic and a prognostic role in unstable angina.

7. Conclusion

According to our review of the literature, there are as yet no reliable, sensitive, and reproducible markers of muscle fiber injuries induced by intensive exercise. Therefore, diagnosis of the severity and extent of these injuries remains highly problematic. An increase in available muscle injury markers is not associated with a maximum training state. However, damaged fibers originate the release of pro-inflammatory cytokines, with consequences for the development of signs that form part of the classic clinical picture of maximum training. Repetition of intense exercise without an adequate recovery period also represents a situation of risk for the development and progression of muscle damage (Bigard, 2001).

The ideal marker must be muscle-specific with a high intracellular concentration, a rapid release after injury, and the stable persistence of a high concentration in the blood for an adequate time period. It should be undetectable in healthy individuals or present at only very low concentrations that can be clearly differentiated from its presence due to organ damage. It should also offer high diagnostic sensitivity, especially in the first few hours after the injury, and high diagnostic specificity (Adams et al., 1994).

α-actin is the most abundant molecule in the cytosolic compartment of the cell and can be detected up to 72 h after its release (Korn, 1982; Korn et al., 1987), which represents an advantage over troponin (Katus et al., 1992). Moreover, the other markers studied are released into the blood in smaller amounts after intense exercise and show a later peak in comparison with α-actin, which can be detected immediately after the exertion of maximum force. These data agree with findings by Aránega et al. (Aránega et al., 1993), who showed that α-actin is released into the blood immediately after cardiac ischemia and can therefore be detected at a very early stage.

With the above background, actin can be considered the ideal candidate to overcome the diagnostic shortcomings of other markers. Comparison of its results with those of other markers in current use could yield new information of great interest for its usefulness in the field of sports performance.

Various studies have shown that α-actin has ideal characteristics for use as a novel and more effective biochemical marker of skeletal muscle damage (Martínez-Amat et al., 2005, Martínez-Amat et al., 2007). Its ready and early detection in the sera of sportspeople is not possible with any of the commercialized markers. Further direct research is warranted to optimize the testing of α-actin in the serum or plasma of patients with skeletal muscle damage, developing equipment to allow rapid and accurate automated tests. The study of α-actin will increase our knowledge of muscle damage and contribute to the detection of muscle damage in sportspeople at risk of injury. This will represent a major advance in the control of training-related injuries in sportspeople.

References

Achar, SA; Kundu ,S; Norcross, WA. Diagnosis of acute coronary syndrome. *Am. Fam. Physician*, 2005, 72(1), 119-26

Adams, JE, Abendschein, DR, Jaffe, AS. Biochemical markers of myocardial injury: is MB creatin kinase the choice for the 1990s?. *Circulation,* 1993, 88, 750-763.

Adams, JE. Comparable detection of acute myocardial infarction by creatine kinase MB isoenzyme y cardiac troponin *I. Clin. Chem.*, 1994, 40, 1291.

Alberts, B, Bray, D, Lewis, J, Raff, M, Roberts, K, Watson, JD. El Citoesqueleto. Biología Molecular de la Célula, 1986, 587-654.

Allen, RE; Rankin, LL. Regulation of satellite cells during skeletal muscle growth and development. *Proc. Soc. Exp. Biol. Med.*, 1990, 194, 81-86.

Alonso, S. Coexpression and evolution of the two sarcomeric actin genes in vertebrates. *Biochimie*, 69, 1987, 1119-1125.

Apple, FS, Rhodes, M. Enzymatic estimation of skeletal muscle damage by analysis of changes in serum creatine kinase. *J. Appl. Physiol.*, 1988, 65, 2598-600.

Aránega, AE. Determinación por Western Blott de alfa actina en Isquemia Cardíaca. Tesis Doctoral Universidad de Granada. 1991.

Aránega, A, González, FJ, Aránega, AE, Muros, MA, Fernández, J, Vélez, C, Prados, J, Alvarez, L. Effects of fibric acid derivatives on accumulation of actin in myocardiocytes. *Int. J. Cardiol.*, 1991, 33, 47-54.

Aránega, AE, Reina, A, Vélez, C, Alvarez, L, Melguizo, C, Aránega, A. Circulating alpha-actin in angina pectoris. *J. Mol. Cell. Cardiol.,* 1992, 24, 15-22.

Aránega, AE, Reina, A, Muros, MA, Alvarez, L, Prados, J, Aránega, A. Circulating alpha-actin protein in acute myocardial infarction. *Int. J. Cardiology,* 1993, 38, 49-55.

Aránega, AE, Vélez, C, Prados, J, Melguizo, C, Marchal, JA, Arena, N, Alvarez, L, Aranega, A. Modulation of alpha actin and alpha actinin proteins in cardiomyocytes by retinoic acid during development. *Cell Tissues Organs,* 1999, 164, 82-89.

Armstrong, RB, Warren, GL, Warren, JA. Mechanisms of exerciseinduced muscle fibre injury. *Sports Med.,* 1991, 12, 184-207.

Asp, S; Daugaard, JR; Kristiansen, S; Kiens, B; Richter, EA. Eccentric exercise decreases maximal insulin action in humans: muscle and systemic effects. *J. Physiol.,* 1996, 494, 891-898.

Atalay, M; Marnila, P; Lilius, EM; Hanninen, O; Sen, CK. Glutathionedependant modulation of exhausting exercise-induced changes in neutrophil function in rats. *Eur. J. Appl. Physiol.,* 1996, 74, 342-357.

Bailey, DM; Young, IS; McEneny, J; Lawrenson, L; Kim J; Barden J; Richardson, RS. Regulation of free radical outflow from an isolated muscle bed in exercising humans. Am *J. Physiol. Heart. Circ. Physiol.,* 2004, 287(4), 689-99.

Belcastro, AN; Shewchuk, LD; Raj, DA. Exercise-induced muscle injury: a calpain hypothesis. *Mol. Cell Biochem.,,* 1998, 179, 135-145.

Bessman, SP, Geiger, PJ. Transport of energy in muscle: the phosphorylcreatine shuttle. *Science,* 1981, 211, 448-452.

Bigard, AX; Merino, D; Lienhard, F; Serrurier, B; Guezennec, CY. Muscle damage induced by running training during recovery from hindlimb suspension: the effect of dantrolene sodium. *Eur. J. Appl. Physiol.,* 1997, 76, 421-437.

Bigard, AX. Exercise-induced muscle injury and overtraining. Sci Sports, 2001, 16, 204-215.

Bodine-Fowler, S. Skeletal muscle regeneration after injury: an overview. J Voice, 1994, 8, 53-62.

Bonetti, A; Tirelli, F; Albertini, R; Monica, C; Monica, M; Tredici, G. Serum cardiac troponin T after repeated endurance exercise events. *Int. J. Sports Med.,* 1996, 17, 259-262.

Brancaccio, P; Maffulli, N; Limongelli, FM. Creatine kinase monitoring in sport medicine.*Br. Med. Bull.,* 2007,81-82, 209-30.

Brandt, RB; Laux, JE; Spainhour, SE; Kline, ES. Lactate dehydrogenase in rat mitochondria. Archives of Biochemistry and Biophysics, 1987, 259, 412-422.

Bravo, R; Fey, SJ; Larsen, PM; Celis, JE. Coexistence of three major isoactins in a single sarcoma 180 cell. *Cell,* 1981, 25, 195-202.

Brooke, MH; Kaiser, KK. Muscle fiber types: How many and Chat kina? Archives of Neurology, 1970, 23, 369-379.

Brooks, GA; Dubouchaud, H; Brow, M; Sicurello, JP; Butz, E. Role of mitochondrial lactate dehydrogenase and lactate oxidation in the intracellular lactate shuttle. *Proceedings of the National Academy of Sciences of the USA,* 1999, 96, 1129-1134.

Brown, SS; Malinoff, HL; Wicha, MS. Connectin: Cell Surface Protein That Binds Both Laminin and Actin. *Proc. Nati. Acad. Sci. USA,* 1983, 80, 5927-5930.

Buchthal, F; Schmalbruch, H. Contraction times and fiber types in intact muscle. Acta Physiologica Scandinavica, 1970, 79, 435-452.

Carlier, MF. Measurement of Pi dissociation from actin filaments following ATP hydrolysis using a linked enzyme assay. Biochem. Biophys. *Res. Commun.*, 1987, 143 (3), 1069-1075.

Carraro, U; Franceschi, C. Apoptosis of skeletal and cardiac muscles and physical exercise. Aging Clin Exp Res, 1997, 9, 19-34.

Carroll, CC; Carrithers, JA, Trappe, TA. Contractile protein concentrations in human single muscle fibers. J. Muscle Res. Cell. Motil., 2004, 25(1), 55-69.

Cheung, K; Hume, P; Maxwell, L. Delayed onset muscle soreness : treatment strategies and performance factors. Sports Med, 2003, 33, 145-164.

Clark, M, Payne, J; Elevated cardiac troponins: their significance in acute coronary syndrome and noncardiac conditions. J Okla State Med Assoc, 2006, 99(6),363-7

Clarkson, PM, Byrneswc, KM, Mccormick, IP, White, JS. Muscle soreness and serum creatine kinase activity following isometric, eccentric and concentric exercise. Int. J. Sports Med., 1986, 7, 152-165.

Clarkson, PM; Tremblay, I. Exercise-induced muscle damage, repair, and adaptations in humans. J Appl Physiol, 1988, 65, 1-5.

Clarkson, PM, Hubal, MJ. Exercise-Induce muscle damage in humans. Am. J. Phys. Med. Rehabil., 2002, 81, 52-69.

Collinson, PO, Boa, FG, Gaze, DC. Measurement of cardiac troponins. Ann. Clin. Biochem., 2002, 38 (Pt 5), 423-49

Condon, K; Silberstein, L; Blaum HM; Thompson, WJ. Development of muscle fiber types in the prenatal rat hindlimb. Dev Biol, 1990, 138, 256-274.

Das, UN. Exercise and inflammation.Eur Heart J, 2006, 27, 1385

De Couet HG. Studies on the antigenic sites of actin: a comparative study of the immunogenic crossreactivity of invertebrate actins. J Muscle Res Cell Motil. 1983 Aug; 4(4):405-27.

DeRosier, DJ; Tilney, LG. The Form and Function of Actin. Cell Muscle Motil, 1984, 5, 139-169.

Doyle, JA, Sherman, WM, Strauss, RL. Effect of eccentric and concentric exercise on muscle glycogen replenishment. Jour. Appli. Physi., 1993, 74, 1848-1855.

Duan, C; Hayes, DA; Delp, PD; Armstrong, RB. Rat skeletal muscle mitochondrial calcium and injury from downhill walking. J Appl Physiol, 1990, 68, 1241-1251.

Ebbeling, CB; Clarkson, PM. Exercise-induced muscle damage and adaptation. Sports Med, 1989, 7, 207-234.

Eisenberg, E; Hill, TL; Chen, Y. Cross-bridge model of muscle contraction. *Biophys J.,* 1980, 29, 195-227.

Engelman, EH; Padron, R. X-Ray diffraction evidence that actin is a 100 A filament. *Nature,* 1984, 307, 56-58.

Epstein, MW; Herzog, M. Theoretical Models of skeletal Muscle. New York Wiley, 1998.

Evans, WJ; Cannon, JG. The metabolic effect of exercise-induced muscle damage and rapid adaptation. *Med. Sci. Sports Exerc.,* 1991, 19, 99-127.

Fatigati, V; Murphy, RA. Actin and tropomyosin variants in smooth muscles. Dependence on tissue type. *J. Biol. Chem.,* 1984, 259, 14383-14388.

Firtel, RA. Multigene families encoding actin and tubulin. *Cell,* 1981, 24, 6-7.

Fowler, WE, Aebi, UA. Consistent Picture of the Actin Filament Related to the Orientation of the Actin Molecule. *J. Cell Biol.*, 1983, 97, 264-269.

Fredsted A; Gissel H; Madsen K; Clausen T. Causes of excitation-induced muscle cell damage in isometric contractions: mechanical stress or calcium overload? *Am. J. Physiol. Regul. Integr. Comp. Physiol.*, 2007 Jun; 292(6):R2249-58.

Friden, J; Sjøstrøm, M; Ekblom, B. Myofibrillar damage following intense eccentric exercise in man. *International Journal of Sports Medicine*, 1983, 4, 170-176.

Friden, J; Kjorell, U; Thronell, L. Delayed muscle soreness and dytoskeletal alterations: an immunocytological study in man. *Int. J. Sports Med.*, 1984, 5, 15-18.

Fry, RW; Morton, AR; Keast, D. Overtraining in athletes. *Sports Med.*, 1991, 12, 32-65.

Gleeson, N; Eston, R; Marginson,V; McHugh, M. Effects of prior concentric training on eccentric exercise induced muscle damage. *Br. J. Sports Med.,* 2003, 37(2), 119-25.

Gommans, IM; Vlak; MH; de Haan, A; Van Engelen, BG. Calcium regulation and muscle disease. *J. Muscle Res. Cell Motil.*, 2002, 23(1), 59-63.

Grazi, E; Cintio, O; Trombetta, G. On the mechanics of the actin filament: the linear relationship between stiffness and yield strength allows estimation of the yield strength of thin filament in vivo. *J. Muscle Res. Cell Motil.*, 2004, 25(1), 103-115.

Gunst, JJ; Langlois, MR; Delanghe, JK. Serum creatine kinase activity is not a reliable marker for muscle damage in conditions associated with low extracellular glutathione concentration. *Clin .Chem.,* 1998, 44, 939–943.

Hamada, H; Petrino, MG; Kakunaga, T. Molecular structure and evolutionary origin of human cardiac muscle actin gene. *Proc. Natl. Acad. Sci*, 1982, 79, 5901-5905.

Hanson, J. Axial period of actin filaments. *Nature,* 1967, 213, 353-356.

Harrington, WF; Rodgers, ME. Myosin. *Annu. Rev. Biochem.*, 1984, 53:35-73.

Hartobagyi, T; Denahan, T. Variability in creatine kinase: methodological, exercise and clinically related factors. *Int. J. Sports Med.*, 1989, 10, 69-80.

Hirano, S; Nose, A; Hatta, K; Kawakami A; Takeichi, M. Calcium-dependent cell-cell adhesion molecules (cadherins): subclass specificities and possible involvement of actin bundles. *J. Cell Biol.*, 1987, 105, 2501-2510

Hirose, L; Nosaka, K; Newton, M; Laveder, A; Kano, M; Peake, J; Suzuki, K. Changes in inflammatory mediators following eccentric exercise of the elbow flexors.*Exerc. Immunol. Rev.*, 2004, 10, 75-90.

Hoberg, E; Katus, HA; Diederich, KW. Myoglobin, creatine kinase-B isoenzyme, and myosin light chain release in patients with unstable angina pectoris. *Eur. Heart*, 1987, 8, 988-994.

Hurme, T; Kalimo, H. Activation of myogenic precursor cells after muscle injury. *Med. Sci. Sports Exerc.*, 1992, 24, 197-205.

Ingwall, JS; Kramer, MF; Fifer, MA; Lorell, BH; Shemin, R; Grossman, W. The creatine kinase system in normal and diseased human myocardium. *N. Engl. J. Med.*, 1985, 313, 1050.

Jackson, MJ. Reactive oxygen species and redox-regulation of skeletal muscle adaptations to exercise. *Philos. Trans R. Soc. Lond B. Biol .Sci.*, 2005, 360, 2285-91.

Jacobs, SCJM; Wokke, JH; Bär, PR; Bootsma, AL. Satellite cell activation after muscle damage in young and adult rats. *Anat. Rec.,* 1995, 242, 329-336.

Jaeschke, H. Mechanisms of oxidant stress-induced acute tissue injury. *Proc. Soc. Exp. Biol. Med.*, 1995, 209, 104-111.

Janssen, GME; Kuipers, H; Willems, GM; Does, RJMM; Janssen, MPE; Geurten, P. Plasma acticity of muscle enzymes. Quantification of skeletal muscle damage and relationship with metabolic variables. *Int. J. Sports Med,* 1989, 3, S160-S168.

Jenkins, RR. Free radical chemistry: relationship to exercise. *Sports Med.*, 1988, 5, 156-170.

Jin, H; Yang, R; Li, W; Lu, H; Ryan, AM; Ogasawara, AK; Van Peborgh, J; Paoni, NF. Effects of exercise training on cardiac function, gene expression, and apoptosis in rats. *Am. J. Physiol. Heart Circ. Physiol.*, 2000, 279(6), 2994-3002.

Johnson, B; Adamczyk, J; Tennos, K; Stromme, SA. Comparación of concentric and eccentric muscle training. *Med. Sci. Sports*, 1976, 8, 35-38.

Jones, DA; Jackson, MJ; Edwards, HT. Release of intracellular enzymes from an isolated mammalian skeletal muscle preparation. *Clin. Sci. Lond,* 1983, 65, 193-201.

Kabsch, W; Mannherz, HG; Suck, KD; Pai, EF; Holmes, KC. Atomic structure of the actin: Dnase I complex *Nature,* 1990, 347, 37-44.

Katus, HA; Diederich, KW; Uellner, M; Remppis, A; Schuler, G; Kubler, W. Myosin light chains release in acute myocardial infarction: non-invasive estimation of infarct size. *Cardiovasc. Res.*, 1988, 22(7), 456-63.

Katus, HA. Enzyme linked immuno assay of cardiac troponin T for the detection of acute myocardial infarction in patients. *J. Mol .Cell Cardiol.*, 1989, 21 (12), 1349-1353.

Katus, HA. Development and in vitro characterization of a new immunoassay of cardiac troponin T. *Clin. Chem.,* 1992, 38 (3), 386-393.

Kayashima; S; Ohno, H; Fujioka, T; Taniguchi, N; Nagata, N. Leucocytosis as a marker of organ damage induced by chronic strenuous exercise. *Eur. J .Appl. Physiol.*, 1995, 70, 413-420.

Kenttä, G; Hassmén, P. Overtraining and recovery. A conceptual model. *Sports Med.,* 1998, 26, 1-16.

Kim, HJ, Lee, YH; Kim, CK. Biomarkers of muscle and cartilage damage and inflammation during a 200 km run. *Eur. J. Appl. Physiol.,* 2007, 99(4), 443-7.

Kobayashi, Y; Takeuchi, T; Hosoi, T; Yoshizaki, H; Loeppky, JA. Effect of a marathon run on serum lipoproteins, creatine kinase, and lactate dehydrogenase in recreational runners. *Res. Q. Exerc. Sport,* 2005, 76(4), 450-5.

Koh, TJ. Do Small Heat Shock Proteins protects skeletal muscul from injury? *Exerc. Sport Sci. Rev.*, 2002, 30, 117-121.

Koller, A; Mair, J; Schobersberger, W; Wohlfarter, T; Haid, C; Mayr, M; Villiger, B; Frey, W; Puschendorf, B. Effects of prolonged strenuous endurance exercise on plasma myosin heavy chain fragments and other muscular proteins. *J. Sports Med. Phys. Fitness*, 1998, 38, 10-27.

Komulainen, H; Kytöla, J; Vihko, V. Running-induced muscle injury and myocellular enzyme release in rats. *J. Appl. Physiol.*, 1994, 77(5), 2299-2304.

Komulainen, J; Takala, T; Vihko, V. Does increased serum creatine kinase activity reflect exercise-induced muscle damage in rats? *Int. J. Sports Med.*, 1995, 16, 150-164.

Korn, ED. Actin polimerization and its regulation by proteins from nonmuscle cells. *Physiol. Rev.*, 1982, 62, 672-737.

Korn, ED; Carlier, MF; Pantaloni, D. Actin polymerization and ATP hydrolisis. *Science,* 1987, 238, 638-644.

Kostaropoulos, IA: Nikolaidis, MG; Jamurtas, AZ; Ikonomou, GV; Makrygiannis, V; Papadopoulos, G; Kouretas, D. Comparison of the blood redox status between long-distance and short-distance runners. *Physiol. Res.,* 2006, 55, 611-6.

Kristiansen, S; Kiens, B; Richter,EA. Exercise metabolism in human skeletal muscle exposed to prior eccentric exercise. *J. Physiol.,* 1998, 509(Pt 1), 305-13.

Kuipers, H; Keizer, HA. Overtraining in elite athletes: review and directions for future. *Sports Med.,* 1988, 6, 79-92.

Kuipers, H. Exercise-induced muscle damage. *Int. J. Sports Med.,* 1993, 15, 132-145.

Lang, H. Creatine kinase isoenzymes- patophysiology and clinical application (review). Berlin-Heidelberg-New York, 1981, 4, 1-10.

Leaf, DA; Kleinman, MT; Hamilton, M; Barstow, TJ. The effects of exercise intensity on lipid peroxidation. *Med. Sci .Sports Exerc.,* 1987, 29, 1036-1049.

Lee, KN. Relevance of macro creatine kinase type 1 and type 2 isoenzymes to laboratory and clinical data. *Clin. Chem.,* 1994, 40, 1278-1283.

Lin, JJC. Assembly of different isoforms of actin and tropomyosin into the skeletal tropomyosin-enriched microfilaments during differentiation of muscle cells in vitro. *J. Cell Biol.,* 1986, 103, 2173-2183.

Lubit, BW; Schwartz, JH. An antiactin antibody that distinguishes between cytoplasmic and skeletal muscle actins. *J. Cell Biol.,* 1980, 86, 891-897,

Lynn, R; Talbot, JA; Morgan, DL. Differences in rat skeletal muscles after incline and decline running. *J. Appl. Physiol.,* 1998, 85, 98-104.

MacCully, KK, Faulkner, JA. Characteristics of lengthening contractions associated with injury to skeletal muscle fibers. *J. Appl. Physiol.,* 1986, 61, 293-309.

Mair, J; Thome-Kromer, B; Wagner, I; Lechleitner, P; Dienstl, F; Puschendorf, B; Michel, G. Concentration time courses of troponin and myosin subunits after acute myocardial infarction. *Coron. Artery Dis.,* 1994, 5, 865-872.

Marcora, SM; Bosio, A. Effect of exercise-induced muscle damage on endurance running performance in humans. *Scand. J. Med. Sci .Sports,* 2007.

Martinez Amat A. Determinación de α-actina en deportistas de alto rendimiento como detección precoz de liberación proteica. Tesis Doctoral Universidad de Granada. 2005.

Martinez Amat A; Boulaiz H; Prados J, et al. Release of alpha-actin into serum after skeletal muscle damage. *Br. J. Sport Med.,* 2005, 39:830-834.

Martinez Amat A; Marchal Corrales JA; Rodríguez F; Prados JC; Hita F; Caba O; Carrillo E; Martin I; Aranega A. Role of α-actin in muscle damage of injured athletes in comparison with traditional markers. *Br. J. Sports Med.,* 2007, 41:442–446.

McArdle, A; Van Der Meulen, JH; Catapano, M; Symons, MC; Faulkner, JA; Jackson, MJ. Free radical activity during contraction-induced injury to the extensor digitorum longus muscles of rats. *J. Physiol.,* 1995, 487, 157P-158P.

McArdle, A; Van Der Meulen, JH; Catapano, M; Symons, MC; Faulkner, JA; Jackson, MJ. Free radical activity following contractioninduced injury to the extensor digitorum longus muscles of rats. *Free Radic. Biol. Med.,* 1999, 26(9-10), 1085-91

McArdle, A; Pattwell, D; Vasilaki, A; Griffiths, RD; Jackson, MJ. Contractile activity-induced oxidative stress: cellular origin and adaptive responses. *Am. J. Physiol.,* 2001, 280(3), C621-C627.

Miller, JB. Myoblasts, myosins, MyoDs and the diversification of muscle fibers. *Disorders,* 1991, 1, 7-17.

Milligan, RA; Whittaker, M; Safer, D. Molecular structure of F-actin and location of surface binding sites. *Nature,* 1990, 348, 217-221.

Minty, AJ; Alonso, S; Caravatti, M; Buckingham, ME. A fetal skeletal muscle actin mRNA in the mouse and its identity with cardiac actin mRNA. *Cell,* 1982, 30, 185-192.

Moss, RL; Razumova, M; Fitzsimons, DP. Myosin crossbridge activation of cardiac thin filaments: implications for myocardial function in health and disease. *Circ. Res,.*2004, 94(10), 1290-300.

Nakagawa, Y; Hattori, M. Relationship between muscle buffering capacity and fiber type during anaerobic exercise in human. *J. Physiol. Anthropol. Appl. Human Sci,* 2002, 21(2), 129-31.

Nanji, AA. Serum creatine kinase isoenzymes: a review. Muscle and Nerve, 1983, 6, 83-90.

O'neil, C; Stebbins, C; Bonigut, S; Halliwell, B; Longhurst, J. Production of hydroxyl radicals in contracting skeletal muscle of cats. *J. Appl. Physiol.,* 1996, 81, 1197-1206.

Ogilvie, RW; Armstrong, RB; Baird, KE; Bottoms, CL. Lesions in rat soleus muscle following eccentrically biased exercise. *Am. J. Anat.,* 1988, 182, 335-346.

Ohman, EM; Teo, KK; Johnson, AH; Collins, PB; Dowsett, DG; Ennis, JT; Horgan, JH. Abnormal cardiac enzyme responses after strenuous exercise: alternative diagnostic aids. *Br. Med. J. Clin. Res. Ed.,* 1990, 285 (6354), 1523-1536.

Oosawa, F; Kasai, M. Skeletal proteins. Subunits in Biological Systems. Deker New York, 1971, 261-332.

Otey, CA; Kalnoski, MH; Bulinski, JC. Immunolocalization of muscle and nonmuscle isoforms of actin in myogenic cells and adult skeletal muscle. Cell Motility and the Cytoskeleton, 1988, 9, 337-348.

Peeze-Binkhorst, FM; Kuipers, H; Tangelder, GJ; Slaaf, DW; Reneman, RS. Exercise-induced focal skeletal muscle fiber degeneration and capillary morphology. *J. Appl. Physiol.*, 1989, 66, 2857-2865.

Perryman, BH; Knoll, JD; Roberts, R. Carboxypeptidase-catalyzed hydrolysis of C-terminal lysine: Mechanism for in vivo production of multiple forms of creatin kinase in plasma. *Clin. Chem.*, 1984, 30:662-674.

Plaghki, L. Régénération et myogenèse du muscle strié. *J. Physiol.,* 1985, 80, 51-110.

Pollard, TD. *Assembly and dinamics of the actin filament system in nonmuscle cells.* J. Cell Biochem., 1986, 31 (2), 87-95.

Proske, U; Morgan, DL. Muscle damage from eccentric exercise: mechanism, mechanical signs, adaptation and clinical applications. *J. Physiol.*, 2001, 537(Pt 2):333-45.

Prou, E ; Margaritis, I ; Tessier, F ; Marini, JF. Effects of strenuous exercise on serum myosin heavy chain fragments in male athletes. *Int. J. Sports Med.,* 1996, 17, 263-277.

Rasmussen, HN; Van Hall, G; Rasmussen, UF. Lactate dehydrogenase is not a mitochondrial enzyme in human and mouse vastus lateralis muscle. *J. Physiol.,* 2002, Jun, 1, 541, 575-80.

Rayment, I; Holden, HM. The Three dimensional structure of a molecular motor. *Trenes Biochem. Sci.*, 1994, 19, 129-134.

Sandri, M; Carraro, U; Podhorska-Okolow, M; Rizzi, C; Arslan, P; Monti, D; Franceschi, C. Apoptosis, DNA damage and ubiquitin expression in normal and mdx muscle fibers after exercise. *FEBS Lett,* 1995, 373, 291-305.

Schultz, E. Satellite cell behavior during skeletal muscle growth and regeneration. *Med. Sci. Sports Exerc.*, 1995, 21, S181-6. 80

Sen, CK. Oxidants and antioxidants in exercise. *J. Appl. Physiol.*, 1995, 79, 675-686.

Sheterline P; Clayton J; Sparrow J. Actin. Protein Profile, 1995;2(1):1-103.

Skenderi KP; Kavouras SA; Anastasiou CA ; Yiannakouris N ; Matalas AL. Exertional Rhabdomyolysis during a 246-km continuous running race. *Med. Sci. Sports Exerc.,* 2006, Jun; 38(6): 1054-7.

Snow, MH. Myogenic cell formation in regenerating rat skeletal muscle injured by mincing I. A fine structural study. *Anat. Rec.*, 1977, 188, 181-199.

Sorichter, S; Mair, J; Koller, A; Gebert, W; Rama, D; Cazolari, C; Artner-Dworzak, E; Puschendorf, B. Skeletal troponin I as a marker of exercise-induced damage. *J. Appl. Physiol.*, 1997, 83, 1076-1082.

Stauber, WT; Smith, CA. Cellular responses in exertion-induced skeletal muscle injury. *Mol. Cell Biochem.*, 1998, 179, 189-196.

Stein, W; Decker, E. Post-transcritional isoforms of CK: mechanisms and possible clinical applications. Biologie Prospective, Paris: John Libbey Eurotext, 1989, 235-241.

Stupka, N; Tarnopolsky, MA; Yardley, NJ; Phillips, SM. Cellular adaptation to repeated eccentric exercise-induced muscle damage. *J. Appl. Physiol.*, 2001, 91,1669-1678.

Takagi, Y; Yasuhara, T; Gomi, K. Creatine kinase and its isozymes. Rinsho Byori, 2001, 116, 52-61.

Tiidus, PM. Radical species in inflammation and overtraining. *Can. J. Physiol .Pharm.,* 1998, 76, 533-548.

Tsung, SH. Several conditions causing elevation of serum CKMB and CKBB. *Am. J. Clin. Pathol.*, 1981, 75, 711-725.

Urhausen, A; Gabriel, HHW; Weiler, B; Kindermann, W. Ergometric and psychological findings during overtraining: a long-term folowup study in endurance athletes. *Int. J. Sports Med.*, 1998, 19, 114-120.

Vaananen, I; Mantysaari, M; Huttunen, P; Komulainen, J; Vihko, V; Komulainen, J; Vihko, V. The effects of a 4-day march on the lower extremities and hormonal balance. *Mil. Med.*, 1997, 162(2), 118-22.

Van Der Meulen, JH; Kuipers, H; Drukker, J. Relationship between exercise-induced muscle damage and enzyme release in rats. *J. Appl. Physiol.*, 1991, 71, 999-1004.

Velez, C; Aranega, AE, Marchal, JA, Melguizo, C, Prados, J; Carrillo, E; Aranega, A. Development of chick cardiomyociyes: Modulation of intermediate filaments by basic fibroblast and platelet-derived growth factors" *Cell Tissue Organs,* 2000, 167, 163-170.

Vijayan, K; Thompson, JL; Riley, DA. Sarcomere lesion damage occurs mainly in slow fibers of reloaded rat adductor longus muscles. *J. Appl. Physiol.*, 1998, 85, 1017-1023.

Vincent, HK; Vincent, KR. The effect of training status on the serum creatine kinase response, soreness and muscle function following resistance exercise.*Int. J. Sports Med.,* 1997, 18, 431-437.

Von Arx, P; Bantle, S; Soldati, T; Perriard, JC. Dominant negative effect of cytoplasmic actin isoproteins on cardiomyocyte cytoarchitecture and function. *J. Cell Biol.,* 1995, 131, 1759-1773.

Weeds, AG; Pope, B. Chemical studies on light chains from cardiac and skeletal muscle myosin. *Nature,* 1971, 234, 85-88.

Whitehead, NP; Allen, TJ; Morgan, DL; Proske, U. Damage to human muscle from eccentric exercise after training with concentric exercise. *J. Physiol.,* 1998, 512, 615-20.

Wierzba, TH; Olek, RA; Fedeli, D; Falcioni, G. Lymphocyte DNA damage in rats challenged with a single bout of strenuous exercise. *J. Physiol. Pharmacol.,* 2006, 57 Suppl 10:115-31.

Wilkinson, JM; Grand, RJA. Comparison of amino acid sequence of troponin I from different striated muscles. *Nature,* 1978, 271, 31-35.

Wu, HJ; Chen, KT; Shee, BW; Chang, HC; Huang, YJ; Yang, RS. Effects of 24 h ultra-marathon on biochemical and hematological parameters. *World J. Gastroenterol.,* 2004, 10(18), 2711-4.

Yu, JG; Thornell, LE. Desmin and actin alterations in human muscles affected by delayed onset muscle soreness: a high resolution immunocytochemical study. *Histochem. Cell Biol.,* 2002, 118, 171-179.

In: Sport and Exercise Psychology Research Advances   ISBN: 978-1-60456-157-9
Editors: M. P. Simmons, L. A. Foster, pp. 293-306   2008 Nova Science Publishers, Inc.

Chapter XIII

Longitudinal Factorial Invariance, Differential, and Latent Mean Stability of the Coping Inventory for Competitive Sports

Richard Fletcher[15]
School of Psychology
Massey University, Albany, New Zealand

Abstract

The ways in which people deal with the stresses of sports competition are called coping strategies (Lazarus and Folkman, 1984). Recently Gaudreau and Blondin (2002) developed the multidimensional Coping Inventory for Competitive Sports (CICS) and provided strong evidence using confirmatory factor analysis for the existence of ten coping strategies used in sporting competition (thought control, mental imagery, relaxation, effort expenditure, logical analysis, seeking support, venting of unpleasant emotion, mental distraction, disengagement and social withdrawal). The aims of this study were to extend the findings of Gaudreau and Blondin (2002) to test the higher-order factor structure of the CICS, and examine the structural and differential stability of the CICS over four time points. Results suggested that a two-factor higher order model of task oriented and emotional oriented coping best fitted the data. Measurement invariance was observed for all subscales. Latent growth curve models suggested subscale scores decreased over time. At the second order factor level the use of task oriented coping decreased over the 10-week season, whereas the use of emotional oriented coping remained stable.

Keywords: *Coping, factorial invariance, differential stability, sports, competition.*

15 Correspondence concerning this article should be addressed to Richard Fletcher, School of Psychology, Massey University Albany, Private Bag 102 904, North Shore Mail Centre, New Zealand. e-mail: R.B.Fletcher@massey.ac.nz.

Recent advances in methodological and statistical procedures afford psychological researchers more sophisticated methods that move beyond traditional psychometric measurement of stability or reliability. These developments allow much stronger and robust procedures for examining issues such factorial invariance as well as intraindividual stability of latent constructs over time. The replicability of latent factors, and stability of individuals' scores, across multiple time points can be examined under the structural equation modelling (SEM) umbrella (Conroy, Metzler and Hofer, 2003; Schutz, 1998; Long and Schutz, 1995). Shutz (1998) provided a comprehensive overview of the advantages of using SEM for assessing the stability of psychological traits, while Conroy et al. (2003) applied the stringent sequential approach to testing factorial invariance, a method suggested by Meredith (1993) to provide evidence for the factorial and latent mean stability of a psychological measure. One important advantage of these approaches is that the psychometric properties of a psychological measure can be assessed over time. Longitudinal measurement provides a more robust test of the factorial and individual stability of test scores than cross-sectional studies which are more widely used.

Schutz (1998), and Usala and Hertzog (1991) suggested that the SEM approach to testing measurement stability has three major advantages. Firstly, structural stability of measures can be modelled over time by examining the autoregressive coefficients of a latent variable measured at several time points. Secondly, the stability of error free latent variables can be tested, and thirdly, the temporal stability of error variance can be explained. In essence this approach to testing stability is consistent with framework of classical test theory (CTT) as it assesses the degree to which a persons "true" score, or the latent constructs, remain stable over time, and in this instance time is more than four occasions (Kenny and Campbell, 1989, Schutz, 1998).

Two aspects of stability that can be tested are differential and structural stability. Differential stability simply refers to an individual's latent score remaining consistent over time. In essence this approach is a form of intra-individual stability that assesses the degree to which an individual's score is consistent in terms of the rank ordering in a group over time. To determine differential stability using SEM one simply estimates the covariance between factors at different time points (Conroy et al, 2003). As with test retest reliability, the higher the correlation the greater the stability of the latent score.

Structural stability refers to the replicability over time of the factor loadings (Long and Schutz, 1995). The observed measures and the latent variable should, if invariance is present, remain stable over time and is termed latent factorial invariance (LFI: Marsh 1993, Usala and Herzog, 1991).

Within the SEM environment, structural stability or LFI can be tested using a series of progressively more stringent constraints (Meredith, 1993). The first level of constraint is termed *configural* factorial invariance, and merely specifies that the number and patterns of the factor loading correspond over subsequent data collections (i.e., multiwave data). As a test of invariance, this is the least demanding but provides a reasonable initial estimate (Hofer, Horn and Eber, 1997). *Weak* factorial invariance adds additional constraints so that factor loadings across different waves of data are designated to be equal. This test assesses the degree to which the factor-variable regressions over the different waves of data remain constant and provides a test of whether the magnitude as well as the pattern of loadings is invariant over testing periods. *Strong* factorial invariance sets equality constraints on the intercepts for observed variables regressions to the latent constructs over the different data waves. Essentially, this model stipulates that differences across the waves of data are at the level of the latent means rather than the level of the observed mean given that these are constrained to be equivalent. *Strict* invariance is considered to be the most stringent of the hierarchy of invariance tests, as it adds the constraint that error terms associated with the observed variables are invariant over time. This final invariance test is in many ways unrealistic as it suggests that random errors for each observed variable, across waves of data, are behaving in the same way. Clearly this is an unrealistic assumption that requires a great deal more justification if it is to be used (Byrne, 2001). Under Meredith's (1993) hierarchy of constrained invariance tests, the models are nested allowing the best fitting model to be determined using the chi-square difference test in which change in the chi-squares relative to the change in the degrees of freedom (*df*) between each model is checked against tabled values.

It is also possible to assess the degree to which the latent factors remain stable over time using latent growth models (LGM: Duncan, Duncan, Strycker, Li, and Alpert, 1999) This method describes the within-and-between-person trajectories on a latent variable both relative to initial levels with regards to changes over time. In essence, LGM's describe the how observed measures on the same individual can be used to determine the underlying latent trajectories over time (Curran and Hussong, 2003). LGMs involve specifying two latent factors: the intercept and the slope which depict changes in the behaviour over time. The intercept factor is the baseline level of the behaviour and is specified by fixing the factor loading to 1.0 for each observation of the behaviour at each time point. The slope factor is identified by fixing the factor loading for the behaviour at time one to 0.0, while the other factor loadings for the remaining time points are set to values that represent the distance between the time points (e.g., 1, 2, and 3 weeks, suggesting a linear growth trajectory). LGMs are powerful in that they provide information about correlations over time, and also about fluctuations in variance and mean values which can be positive or negative, linear or non-linear.

Over the last decade sports and exercise psychology consulting has emerged as an adjunct to athletic performance enhancement, and the availability of high quality sports specific measures of psychological functioning is critical. Often the nexus between theory and practice can be achieved by developing psychometrically valid measures that can be used in theory testing and development, as well as in practical situations. Robust methodologies are critical to this process. The majority of measures of coping used in the sporting domain have been based on variables drawn from the mainstream psychological literature and often these can lack contextual relevance to sport. Gaudreau and Blondin (2002) developed a sport specific multidimensional measure of coping based on Lazarus and Folkman's (1984) model in which coping is conceptualized as comprising both cognitive and behavioural actions that are used to regulate both internal and external situational specific demands. Using a rigorous approach to questionnaire development Gaudreau and Blondin (2002) developed the Coping Inventory for Competitive Sports (CICS) and provided strong support for the first-order factor structure of the ten subscales; thought control, mental imagery, relaxation, effort expenditure, logical analysis, seeking support, venting of unpleasant emotion, mental distraction, disengagement/resignation, and social withdrawal. While first-order factor structure of the CICS was clearly established, Gaudreau and Blondin (2002) suggested that future research should investigate its hierarchical structure and its invariance properties. Thus the aims of the present study are firstly to provide confirmatory evidence of the hierarchical factor structure of the CICS, and secondly to test the CICS's LFI by using Meredith's (1993) tests of invariance, differential stability and latent means analysis.

Method

Data were collected as part of a larger study involving 219 female athletes (mean age = 23 years: *SD* = 6.35) competing over a competitive playing season (ten weeks). Data were collected across four time periods: initial baseline, one, six and ten weeks later. All data were collected within five days of a competitive match.

Measure

The Coping Inventory for Competitive Sports (CICS: Gaudreau and Blondin, 2002) is comprised of 39 items which assess 10 coping strategies: thought control, mental imagery, relaxation, effort expenditure, logical analysis, seeking support, venting of unpleasant emotion, mental distraction, disengagement/resignation and social withdrawal. Each subscale is composed of four items except for effort expenditure which consists of three items. All items use a five-point Likert-type scale (1 = not used at all to 5 = used very much). Using confirmatory factor analytic methods Gaudreau and Blondin, (2002) reported that the 10 CICS first order-factor models provided the best fit to the data. Reliability estimates for each of the factors ranged between $\alpha = 0.67$ to $\alpha = 0.87$.

Data Analysis

All CFAs, stability models, and LGM were calculated using AMOS 4.01 (Arbuckle, 1999). Missing data was 8%, 19%, 21%, and 27% respectively for the four data collection points. A significant issue in longitudinal research is how to treat missing data. Methods such as pair-wise or list-wise deletion, or mean imputation are inappropriate to use as they tend to yield biased estimates (Little and Rubin, 1989, Wothke, 2000). Little and Rubin (1989) suggested that when analyzing repeated measures data with missing data it is necessary to consider whether data is missing completely at random (MCAR) or missing at random (MAR). The assumption is that MCAR is more restrictive in that it assumes the pattern of missing values is completely independent of the all the variables in the model. MAR, on the other hand, is less restrictive in that it assumes that the missing data may be related to other variables. Following Conroy, Metzler and Hofer's (2003) example of examining the 'missingness' of data, the number of missing waves of data were found not to be correlated (p>.05) to the total scores on the CICS at each time point. The missing data was therefore deemed to be MAR and full-information maximum likelihood estimation was used to calculate each model with missing data (see Wothke, 2000) using AMOS 4.01 (Arbuckle, 1999).

In line with Gaudreau and Blondin's (2002) suggestion, the CICS was tested for its hierarchical structure. For each time point the CICS was subjected to confirmatory factor analysis (CFA) to determine the higher order factor structure with one, two or three second-order factors. For the single second-order factor model a separate model for each time point was estimated using the items to specify each subscale which in turn identified a single second-order factor.

For the models specifying two-higher order factors the same process was adopted with thought control, mental imagery, relaxation, effort expenditure, logical analysis, and seeking support subscales specifying a task oriented coping factor (TOC), while the venting of unpleasant emotions, mental distraction, disengagement, and social withdrawal factors identified an emotional orientated coping factor (EOC).

For the second-order three factor model the TOC factor was identified as above, the EOC factor was identified using the venting of unpleasant emotions, and the third factor, avoidance oriented coping (AOC) was identified using mental distraction, disengagement, and social withdrawal. However, as EOC and AOC were found to be more highly correlated (0.58, 0.52, 0.83 and 0.77) at each successive data wave, the three factor second-order model was not pursued further.

For all analyses the goodness-of-fit statistics included the root mean error of approximation (RMSEA; Steiger, 1990) where values of <.05 are indicative of good model fit and values >.05 and <.08 indicate acceptable model fit (Browne and Cudeck, 1993); the Normed Fit Index (NFI; Bentler and Bonnet, 1980) where values >.90 indicate acceptable fit; the Tucker-Lewis index (TLI; Tucker and Lewis, 1973) where values >.90 indicate adequate fit of the model to the data; and the comparative fit index (CFI; Bentler, 1990) where values > .90 indicate adequate fit (Mulaik, James, Van Alstine, Bennett, Lind, and Stillwell, 1989).

All invariance models were calculated with covariances specified between the error terms for each observed variable across each wave of data. For example, the error term for variable one was allowed to covary between the error terms for variable one at time two etc. Similarly all latent variables were allowed to covary across the four waves of data. Allowing errors to correlate is based on the assumption that the errors are not independent within persons across time (Marsh, 1993).

To test the structural and differential stability of the SCSCI, the approaches suggested by Meridith (1993) were used. Three models (configural, weak and strong invariance) for each of the 10 subscales were calculated over the four time points to determine the degree of invariance. Models were also tested for the two higher-order factor CICS. Strict invariance was not examined as there was no justification for expecting random errors to be equal over the four waves of data (Byrne, 2001).

Configural invariance was tested by identifying factor constraints as required so that one variable-factor regression was set to 1.0 for one item in each data wave with the remaining unconstrained to take on any value. Weak invariance added the equality constraint of factor-variable regressions across data waves, and strong invariance added equality constraints to the factor variable means across data waves, to test whether factor loadings and unique means were invariant over the four waves of data. The factor means and variances were set to zero and one respectively at data wave one to allow latent means to be compared.

Two LGMs for each subscale as well as the two higher order factor models were specified: a no-growth, and a linear growth model. Strong invariance constraints, except for the correlated errors on the error terms for each observed variable, were used. Convergence problems resulted in the decision not to correlate the residuals across time points: relaxing this constraint resulted in slightly worse fit. The no-growth model identified two correlated latent factors, an intercept factor and a slope factor, using total scores for each subscale at each data wave. The covariance between the intercept and slope factors provided an indication of the average rate of change in individuals' scores over the data waves. The intercept factor loadings were all constrained to 1.00 and the slope factor loading were set to zero. To overcome identification problems the variance for the slope factor was set to 1.0 and the covariance between the intercept and slope factors was also set to 1.0 for all no-growth models. The growth model was specified in a similar way except that the factor loadings for the slope factor were set to zero at time one and 1, 6, and 10 to represent the weeks between data waves. As no identification problems were noted, the variance for the slope factor and the covariance between the two latent factors were allowed to be freely estimated.

All invariance and LGM models are considered to be nested and therefore to test the difference between each level of the models the chi-square difference test was applied (see Byrne, 2001). Because χ^2 statistic is known to be sensitive to large sample sizes, more emphasis is placed on the degree of change in the other fit indices as these provide more information about model-data fit (Conroy et. al, 2003; Byrne, 2001). Furthermore, Cheung and Rensvold (2002) have suggested a more sensitive statistic to use when examining nested models is the ▲CFI (CFI $_{constrained}$ − CFI $_{unconstrained}$) with changes ≤ .01 indicating the null hypothesis for invariance should not be rejected (Cheung and Rensvold, 2002).

Results

Table 1 shows the descriptive statistics for the ten CICS subscales and their associated estimates of reliability for each time point. The results suggest that most subscales were moderately to highly reliable over the four time points. There were, however, a few alpha reliability estimates that were low to moderate, but generally over the four time points the estimates of reliability were at or above the minimally accepted level of $\alpha = .70$ (Nunnally, 1967).

Eight separate models were calculated for the one and two second-order factor models, and their associated fit indices are shown in Tables 2 and 3 respectively. Examination of the various models suggests that the two-factor second-order model was better at describing the data as the model fit indices were consistently higher across all time points. The correlations between the two factors were small to moderate although they were statistically significantly different from zero across all time points. Reliability estimates for the TOC factor over the four time points were $\alpha = .80, .82, .77,$ and $.83$ respectively. For the EOC factor $\alpha = .71, .73, .81,$ and $.87$ for each data wave.

Table 1. Means, standard deviations, and reliability coefficients for the CICS subscales and total scores across four time points

	Time 1				Time 2				Time 3				Time 4			
	N	M	SD	α	N	M	SD	α	N	M	SD	α	N	M	SD	α
Thought Control	201	12.61	3.29	0.63	178	12.19	3.68	0.71	172	11.69	3.32	0.68	159	11.76	3.19	0.65
Mental Imagery	202	11.61	3.73	0.76	178	10.96	3.82	0.81	172	11.09	3.39	0.69	159	11.08	3.36	0.75
Relaxation	202	10.14	3.56	0.77	178	9.73	3.70	0.82	172	9.80	3.63	0.82	159	10.19	3.69	0.85
Effort Expenditure	201	10.78	2.35	0.56	178	10.39	2.65	0.72	172	10.47	2.41	0.72	159	10.33	2.23	0.56
Logical Analysis	202	11.74	3.23	0.66	178	11.32	3.36	0.71	172	10.95	3.15	0.70	159	11.33	4.22	0.51
Seeking Support	202	9.09	3.56	0.74	178	8.78	3.47	0.73	172	8.86	4.28	0.73	159	9.38	3.75	0.80
Venting unpleasant emotion	202	8.18	3.06	0.69	178	8.05	3.53	0.80	172	7.90	3.54	0.68	159	8.49	3.44	0.78
Mental Distraction	202	6.87	2.83	0.68	178	6.55	2.85	0.75	172	7.19	3.21	0.80	159	7.58	3.42	0.84
Disengagement	202	6.15	2.72	0.78	178	6.38	2.75	0.77	172	6.79	2.93	0.77	159	7.20	3.36	0.85
Social withdrawal	202	7.10	2.57	0.57	178	6.74	2.62	0.69	172	7.32	3.02	0.74	159	7.61	2.95	0.73
Total CICS	202	94.11	17.76	0.88	178	91.13	18.86	0.89	172	92.10	19.46	0.89	159	95.00	22.31	0.91

**Table 2. Fit indices for the one factor second-order model for the CSSCQ
at each time point**

Time	χ^2	df	RMSEA	TLI	CFI	PCFI
Coping Time 1	1236	692	0.06	0.96	0.96	0.87
Coping Time 2	1247	692	0.06	0.96	0.96	0.85
Coping Time 3	1534	692	0.07	0.93	0.94	0.83
Coping Time 4	1415	692	0.07	0.94	0.95	0.84

**Table 3. Fit indices for the two factor second-order model for the CSSCQ
at each time point**

Time	χ^2	df	RMSEA	TLI	CFI	PCFI	r TOC – EOC
Coping Time 1	1101	691	0.05	0.97	0.97	0.86	0.16
Coping Time 2	1092	691	0.05	0.97	0.97	0.86	0.29
Coping Time 3	1291	691	0.06	0.95	0.96	0.85	0.21
Coping Time 4	1169	691	0.06	0.96	0.96	0.85	0.41

Examination of Table 4 shows that all subscales achieved at least weak factorial invariance with four of these exhibiting strong invariance (mental imagery, relaxation, logical analysis, and venting of unpleasant emotion). Six of the subscales (thought control, effort expenditure, seeking support, mental distraction, disengagement/resignation and social withdrawal) demonstrated partial invariance.

For the effort expenditure and disengagement subscales there were problems with the with model fit, with instances of the RMSEA being zero or very close to zero and the remaining fit indices being one or close to one. In general, most if not all of the relative fit indices were >.98 for each of the separate subscale analyses. While these fit indices might suggest the models were being over-fitted, the RMSEA, which penalizes over-fitting models, suggested that the model fit was good with most RMSEA's being <.05 and nearly all below the minimally acceptable criteria of <.08 (Browne and Cudeck, 1993).

For the CICS two-factor model using the subscale score to identify the EOC and TOC factors, the absolute fit suggested that weak invariance had been achieved. Again, the small change in relative fit indices ($\blacktriangle$CFI) suggested that the model fit was still at an acceptable level to judge the strong invariance model an appropriate choice, given the stringency of the constraints placed upon it.

Adding more stringent constraints to the hierarchy of invariance for all models did result in statistically significantly decrements in absolute fit, but did not result in a sizeable decrease in the relative fit indices. Generally, the level invariance that was achieved across the various subscales suggested it was worth examining the latent growth models at the subscale level.

Table 4. Fit indices for the 10 CICS subscales, and full two factor higher-order CICS over four time points

		χ^2	df	▲ χ^2	▲ df	RMSEA	NFI	TLI	CFI	▲ CFI
Thought	Configural	123	74			0.05	0.98	0.99	0.99	
	Weak	135	83	12	9	0.05	0.98	0.98	0.99	0.00
	Strong	207	96	72*	13	0.07	0.97	0.97	0.98	-0.01
Imagery	Configural	84	74			0.02	0.99	0.99	0.99	
	Weak	99	83	15	9	0.03	0.99	0.99	0.99	0.00
	Strong	135	96	36*	13	0.04	0.98	0.99	0.99	0.00
Relaxation	Configural	94	74			0.04	0.99	0.99	0.99	
	Weak	114	83	20*	9	0.04	0.98	0.99	0.99	0.00
	Strong	148	96	34*	13	0.05	0.98	0.99	0.99	0.00
Effort	Configural	31	30			0.02	1.00	0.99	1.00	
	Weak	35	36	4	6	0.00	0.99	1.00	1.00	0.00
	Strong	86	46	51*	10	0.06	0.99	0.98	0.99	-0.01
Logic	Configural	86	74			0.03	0.99	0.99	0.99	
	Weak	93	83	7	9	0.02	0.99	0.99	0.99	0.00
	Strong	140	96	47*	13	0.05	0.98	0.99	0.99	0.00
Support	Configural	90	74			0.03	0.98	0.99	0.99	
	Weak	108	83	18*[a]	9	0.04	0.98	0.99	0.99	0.00
	Strong	234	96	126*	13	0.08	0.96	0.96	0.97	-0.02
Venting	Configural	119	74			0.05	0.98	0.98	0.99	
	Weak	136	83	17*[a]	9	0.05	0.98	0.98	0.99	0.00
	Strong	173	96	37*	13	0.06	0.97	0.98	0.99	0.00
Mental	Configural	90	74			0.03	0.98	0.99	0.99	
	Weak	106	83	16	9	0.04	0.98	0.99	0.99	0.00
	Strong	197	96	61*	13	0.07	0.96	0.97	0.98	-0.01
Disengage	Configural	77	74			0.02	0.99	0.99	0.99	
	Weak	84	83	7	9	0.01	0.98	0.99	1.00	0.01
	Strong	150	96	66*	13	0.05	0.97	0.99	0.99	-0.01
Withhold	Configural	125	74			0.06	0.98	0.98	0.99	
	Weak	156	83	31*	9	0.06	0.97	0.97	0.99	0.00
	Strong	247	96	91	13	0.09	0.95	0.96	0.97	0.02
CICS two factor model	Configural	1012	652			0.05	0.95	0.98	0.98	
	Weak	1035	676	23	24	0.05	0.95	0.98	0.98	0.00
	Strong	1117	706	82	30*	0.05	0.95	0.98	0.98	0.00

Note: * p<.05.
[a] significantly different at the p<.05 but not at p<.01.

Table 5. Differential stability estimates for the strong invariance models

	T1-T2	T2-T3	T3-T4	T1-T3	T1-T4	T2-T4
Thought	0.71	0.54	0.67	0.71	0.62	0.54
Imagery	0.80	0.73	0.72	0.67	0.60	0.59
Relaxation	0.74	0.64	0.68	0.60	0.58	0.64
Effort	0.60	0.44	0.41	0.46	0.43	0.47
Logic	0.82	0.75	0.74	0.66	0.64	0.64
Support	0.86	0.72	0.69	0.77	0.77	0.78
Venting	0.75	0.68	0.62	0.67	0.61	0.69
Mental	0.84	0.74	0.85	0.70	0.75	0.66
Disengage	0.74	0.58	0.66	0.61	0.52	0.39
Withhold	0.78	0.56	0.71	0.56	0.68	0.68
TOC	0.79	0.68	0.66	0.65	0.58	0.61
EOC	0.67	0.49	0.73	0.60	0.55	0.64

Table 5, shows the standardized differential stability estimates for the ten CICS subscales and the two second-order TOC and EOC factors. Considering that the data were collected over a ten week period the stability of the factor covariance's were moderate to large over the various time points and provided evidence for the latent stability of the CICS subscales and second-order factors.

Table 6 shows the absolute and relative fit indices for the no-growth and growth latent mean models for the subscale and the two-factor CICS. The no-growth model was used as a baseline to compare the growth model to. The result suggests that for all the subscales, except the effort expenditure and venting of unpleasant emotions, the growth models resulted in a statistically significant increase in absolute fit. For all models, the incremental fit indexes suggested good fit, however values for the RMSEA were >.08. Given these were reasonably parsimonious models, more weight should be given to the remaining comparative fit indices. The standardized covariance ($R_{\text{int-splope}}$) provided an indication as to the amount and direction of growth/change that occurred over the testing period. All subscale values were low to moderately negative suggesting that there was an overall decrease in these constructs over the 10-week competition.

Results for the two-factor CICS again suggested the growth model to fit the data better as both absolute and comparative fit was evidenced. Interestingly the $R_{\text{int-splope}}$ for TOC strategies showed that there was as a decline over the 10-week playing season, whereas EOC strategies remained fairly constant.

Discussion

The main aims of this study were to confirm the underlying factor structure of the CICS (Gaudreau and Blondin, 2002) and to determine its structural, differential and latent mean stability over four data collection periods.

Table 6. Fit indices for LGC models for no-growth and growth

		χ^2	Df	▲χ^2	▲ df	RMSEA	NFI	TLI	CFI	R-int-slope
Thought	No growth	36.8	8			0.12	0.98	0.98	0.99	
	Growth	24.1	6	12.7*	2	0.12	0.99	0.99	0.99	-0.50
Imagery	No growth	25.5	8			0.10	0.99	0.99	0.99	
	Growth	11.3	6	14.2*	2	0.06	0.99	0.99	0.99	-0.57
Relaxation	No growth	13.4	8			0.06	0.99	0.99	0.99	
	Growth	7.6	6	5.8*	2	0.04	0.99	0.99	0.99	-0.24
Effort	No growth	11.1	8			0.04	0.99	0.99	0.99	
	Growth	7.4	6	3.7	2	0.03	0.99	0.99	0.99	-0.56
Logic	No growth	23.8	8			0.01	0.98	0.99	0.99	
	Growth	15	6	8.8*	2	0.08	0.99	0.99	0.99	-0.34
Support	No growth	11.7	8			0.05	0.99	0.99	0.99	
	Growth	10.8	6	0.9	2	0.06	0.99	0.99	0.99	-0.29
Venting	No growth	7.5	8			0.00	0.99	1.0	1.0	
	Growth	5.7	6	1.8	2	0.00	0.99	0.99	.099	-0.38
Mental	No growth	42.3	8			0.14	0.97	0.97	0.98	
	Growth	18.7	6	23.6*	2	0.09	0.99	0.99	0.99	-0.06
Disengage	No growth	30.8	8			0.11	0.98	0.98	0.98	
	Growth	17	6	13.8*	2	0.09	0.99	0.99	0.99	-0.17
Withhold	No growth	23.1	8			0.09	0.99	0.99	0.99	
	Growth	13.3	6	9.8*	2	0.07	0.99	0.99	0.99	-0.11
Coping	No growth	125.6	32			0.11	0.97	0.98	0.98	
	Growth	93.8	28	31.8*	4	0.10	0.98	0.98	0.99	(TOC) -0.38
										(EOC) 0 .05

p<.05

From a methodological perspective this is a robust analyses of this measure. The results clearly show the CICS to have strong psychometric properties over 10-week period. From a practical perspective, users of the measure can have confidence that the results obtained are meaningful and interpretable and add greatly to the validity evidence for this measure.

This investigation supports the underlying factor structure of the CICS from both the first-order and second-order factor perspective. The ten factors suggested by Gaudreau and Blondin (2002) were clearly identifiable as the factor loadings and the various fit indices were high across all four time points. A comparison of the one and two higher-order factor models shows that the two factor model fits the data better. Across all four time points the two factor higher-order model consistently demonstrated the higher model-fit indices. This is not surprising as the underlying theory for the CICS is based around Lazarus and Folkman's (1984) two factor model of coping, namely task and emotional coping mechanisms.

At Time-1 and 4, however, there were some factors where the reliability was low: thought control, effort expenditure, and logical analysis. Social withdrawal while low at Time-1 did meet the minimally acceptable level of reliability over the remaining time points. While some of these alpha coefficients were low, one should remember that reliability is only a lower bound for validity, and that in the larger scheme of construct validation it is underlying structure of the measure that is of central importance. Hence the results of the CFA's are most salient. Indeed, Li (2003) suggests that where reliability and validity are in contradiction one should always give precedence to the later. From a theoretical perspective the results from the CFA's of the CICS provide strong empirical support for a robust factor structure.

The invariance of the CICS was established under Meredith's (1993) stringent hierarchical tests for all subscales given the small changes in the relative fit indices. Although the absolute fit for all models suggested a decrement in fit, especially when more stringent constraints were placed on the model, the relative fit indices did not change very much. Thus, it was concluded that the weak to strong invariance held across the subscales as the change in relative fit across the models was relatively small across all indices.

The factor structure for the CICS two-factor model (EOC and TOC scales) also showed strong consistency over 10-weeks. Again the minor changes in relative fit suggested that strong invariance had been achieved and the results demonstrate that scores for the second order model can be used with confidence over multiple testing points.

The CICS also exhibited reasonably good differential stability with most of the stability coefficients reaching acceptable standards. In other words, individual true scores over the four time points were moderately to highly stable. The higher stability coefficients were between Time-1 and 2, and although there was a decrement in some of the stability coefficients over time. These were not overly concerning, except for the effort expenditure subscale which was low throughout the four testing periods. The effort expenditure scale had only three items and thus this will impact the magnitude of reliability coefficients. A closer inspection the item wording for these three items shows that they are very similar. For example, "I applied myself by giving a consistent effort", "I gave relentless effort", and "I gave my best effort". In other words, there is item redundancy in this subscale which results in construct under- representation. More items need to be added to this subscale to fully capture the effort expenditure coping strategy.

For the two higher order factors the stability coefficients were reasonable and suggested that over a ten-week playing season were stable. The TOC scale showed slightly greater consistency over the various data waves compared to the EOC scale.

LGC modelling of the CICS suggested that the latent means were not stable over the four time periods. In fact, for all LGC models of the subscales there was a negative trend for the latent means. In other words, as the season progressed the average within-person trajectory suggested that most coping strategy usage declined slightly. At the second-order level the growth model suggested better fit. The results suggest that over a ten-week playing season these females tended to use emotional coping strategies more consistently than task based coping strategies.

Overall, this study has shown that the CICS has strong psychometric properties over a ten-week competitive playing season. Users of the CICS can have confidence interpreting either subscales scores from the ten first-order factors, or alternatively the scores from the two second-order factors. Furthermore, when examining coping over time or where an intervention is used, researchers can have confidence that the measurement properties of the CICS are robust and thus any results can be interpreted with confidence.

References

Arbuckle, J. L. (1999). *Amos 4.0 [Computer software]*. Chicago: Smallwaters.

Bentler, P. M. (1990). Comparative fit indices in structural models. *Psychological Bulletin, 107*, 238-246.

Bentler, P. M., and Bonett, D. G. (1987). This week's citation classic. Current Contents, Social and Behavioural Sciences, 19, 16.

Browne, M. W., and Cudeck, R. (1993). Alternative ways of assessing model fit. In K. A. Bollen and J. S. Long (Eds.), *Testing Structural Equation Models* (pp. 445-455). Newbury Park, CA: Sage.

Byrne, B. M. (2001). *Structural Equation Modelling with AMOS. Basic Concepts, Applications and Programming*. New Jersey: Lawrence Erlbaum Associates, Inc.

Cheung, G. W., and Rensvold, R. B. (2002). Evaluating goodness-of-fit indexes for testing measurement invariance. Structural Equation Modeling, 9, 233-255.

Conroy, D. E., Metzler, J. N., and Hofer, S. M. (2003). Factorial invariance and latent mean stability of performance failure appraisals. *Structural Equation Modelling, 10,* 401-422.

Curran, P. J., and Hussong, A. M. (2003). The use of latent trajectory models in psychopathology research. *Journal of Abnormal Psychology, 4,* 526-544.

Duncan, T. E., Duncan, S. C., Strycker, L. A., Li, F., and Alpert. A. (1999). *An introduction to latent variable growth curve modeling: Concepts, issues, and applications*. Mahwah, NJ: Lawrence Erlbaum Associates.

Gaudreau, P., and Blondin, J. P. (2002). Development of questionnaire for the assessment of coping strategies employed by athletes in competitive sport settings. *Psychology of Sport and Exercise, 3,* 1-34

Hofer, S. M., Horn, J. L., and Eber, H. W. (1997). A robust five-factor structure of the 16PF: Evidence from independent rotation and confirmatory factorial invariance procedures. *Personality and Individual Differences, 23,* 247-269.

Lazarus, R. S., and Folkman, S. (1984). *Stress appraisal and coping*. New York: Springer.

Li, H. (2003). The resolution of some paradoxes related to reliability and validity. *Journal of Educational and Behavioural Statistics, 28,* 89-95.

Little, R. J. A., and Rubin, D. B. (1989). The analysis of social science data with missing values. *Sociological Methods and Research, 18,* 292-326.

Long, B. C., and Schutz, R. W. (1995). Temporal stability and replicability of a workplace and coping model for managerial women: A multiwave panel study. *Journal of Counselling Psychology, 42,* 266-278.

Kenny, D. A., and Campbell, D. T. (1989). The measurement of stability in over-time data. *Journal of Personality, 57,* 445-481.

Marsh, H. W. (1993). Stability of individual differences in multiwave panel studies: Comparison of simplex and one-factor models. *Journal of Educational Measurement, 30,* 157-183.

Meredith, W. (1993). Measurement invariance, factor analysis and factorial invariance. *Psychometrika, 58,* 525-543.

Mulaik, S. A., James, L .R., Van Alstine, J., Bennett, N., Lind, S., and Stilwell, C. D. (1989). Evaluation of goodness-of-fit indices for structural equation models. *Psychological Bulletin, 105*, 430-445.

Nunnally, J. C. (1967). *Psychometric theory*. New York: McGraw-Hill Schutz, R. W. (1998). Assessing the stability of psychological traits and measures. In J. Duda (Ed.), *Advances in sport and exercise psychology measurement* (pp. 393-408). Morgantown, VA: Fitness Information Technology.

Schutz, R. W. (1998). Assessing the stability of psychological traits and measures. In J. L. Duda (Ed.), *Advances in sport and exercise psychology measurement* (pp. 393-408). Morgantown, WV: Fitness Information Technology.

Steiger, J. H. (1990). Structural model evaluation and modification: An interval estimation approach. *Multivariate Behavioural Research, 25*, 173-180.

Tucker, L. R., and Lewis, C. (1973). A reliability coefficient for maximum likelihood factor analysis. *Psychometrika, 38*, 1-10.

Usala, P. D., and Hertzog, C. (1991). Evidence of stability of state and trait anxiety in adults. *Journal of Personality and Social Psychology, 60*, 471-479.

Wothke, W. (2000). Longitudinal and multigroup modelling with missing data. In T. D. Little, K. U. Schanbel, and J. Baumert (Eds.), *Modelling longitudinal and multigroup data: Practical issues, applied approaches, and specific examples*. Mahwah, NJ: Lawrence Erlbaum Associates.

In: Sport and Exercise Psychology Research Advances   ISBN: 978-1-60456-157-9
Editors: M. P. Simmons, L. A. Foster, pp. 307-327   © 2008 Nova Science Publishers, Inc.

Chapter XIV

Immune and Hormonal Stress Responses to an Immersion in a Siphon Placed on the Bottom of an Alpine Cave of 700M Depth: Case Report

E. Stenner [16,2], *A. Bussani* [3], *C. Piccinini* [2] *and B. Biasioli* [2]

[1]School of Sports Medicine, Faculty of Medicine and Surgery,
University of Trieste, Italy
[2]Department of Laboratory Medicine, A.O.U, Ospedali Riuniti di Trieste, Italy
[3]Department of Biological Oceanography,
National Institute of Oceanography and Applied Geophisics, Italy

Abstract

The aim of this study was to investigate the immunological (lymphocytes and lymphocytes subset), the hypothalamus pituitary adrenocortical (cortisol) and the hypothalamus pituitary (growth hormone GH) responses to an immersion with self-contained underwater breathing apparatus (SCUBA) in an unexplored siphon, placed in a cave about 700 m under the surface. The combination of heavy and long duration exercise before (5 hours of descending) and after (13 hours of ascending) the immersion in a demanding environment, the siphon altitude (quota: 1200 m), the exercise effort during diving in cold water (cave temperature: 2°C; water temperature: 2°C), the absolute darkness, the confinement, the restrictions with the associated risk of getting stuck and the emotion for the exploration as well as the awareness that if an accident happened the situation became drastically very critical represent a unique multiple stress model that may be helpful in understanding the immune and endocrine expression of acute physiological and psychological stress. Owing to the high skill of the performance and to the enormous difficulties for carrying all the technical equipment on the bottom of this cave, only one cave-diver was tested; however this

16. Correspondence concerning this chapter should be addressed to Elisabetta Stenner, Department of Laboratory Medicine, AOU, Ospedali Riuniti di Trieste, 34100, Via Stuparich, 1, Italy. Tel: +39(0)403992064, Fax: +39(0)40272335, E-mail address: elisabetta.stenner@libero.it

subject repeated the same immersion in two different days following the same schedule. Five blood drawings were performed. 1. at 7:30 am, at the hospital (sea level), 2. 7:30 pm on the bottom of the cave (quota: 1230 m), before the siphon immersion, 3. after the immersion, 4. at the exit of the cave (quota: 1930m), 5. 24 hours after resting and we focused our attention on the pre-post immersion time interval. Moreover, blood drawings, as controls, were performed at the same resting time envisaged for the day of the experiment to minimize the specimen processing time influences and any circadian fluctuation. A marked increase in GH and cortisol hormone was measured while a dramatic decrease in the total absolute number of lymphocytes and all studied lymphocytes subpopulations (CD3+ T cells, CD4+ T helper cells, CD8+ T cytotoxic cells, CD19+ B cells and CD16+CD3- natural killer cells was found. Our data confirm that extreme physiological/psychological conditions of cave diving are stressors that are able to alter both the immune and hormonal response. In particular the marked rise of GH values during diving underlines the great intensity of cave diving effort due to the difficult route that the cave diver covered and the bulky technical equipment dressed while the rise of cortisol is likely due to the combination of emotional stress and exercise. Moreover, cold temperature, darkness and sleep deprivation could also enhance cortisol secretion. The unusual and marked drop of total absolute number of lymphocytes as well as all the lymphocytes subpopulations, just during the exercise appear dependant at least in part, to the very long duration characteristic of all the performance (spelunking and diving) and the associated effects induced by the augmented cortisol levels with respect to basal condition, in particular during the immersion. Finally it should be noted that also sleep deprivation could negatively influenced the immune response to physical exercise.

Keywords: *cave diving, immune response, stress hormones, exercise*

Introduction

Underwater caves represent a natural environment of peerless beauty which is available to only an elite of spelunkers that practice cave diving. The extraordinary variety of the scenarios that can be spotted in these places largely derives from the different spelogenetic processes that generated the cavity. Actually, there are five general types of underwater caves: lava tubes, which originated from the cooling process of lava flows; sea caves, due to the erosion of submerged rocks by sea water; coral caves, composed mainly of limestone and coral skeletons; glacier caves, usually formed at the bottom a glacier; solution caves, which originated from the erosion of limestone or dolomite, but also gypsum, marble, and even salt rocks, by fresh water. Solution caves, in particular, according to the permeability of rocks, are characterised by the presence of freshwater springs which often form a widespread and very complex hydrologic system. Siphons and sinks are typical elements of such a system: the former are areas where water flows into the underwater cave system, while the latter are openings into submerged caves. A large number of different speleothems can be seen in underwater solution caves, such as stalagmites, extending upwards from the bottom of the cave, and stalactites, hanging down from the cave ceiling; moreover other unique decorative formations contribute to render the exploration of these cavities an astonishing experience, but also a very demanding and sometimes life-threatening sport activity [Mount 1995]. In fact, even if the risk of accident is low especially for experienced spelunkers [Ashford et al. 1999], it is also true that when it happens the consequences are usually very critical: aside from the well known risks of the self-contained underwater breathing apparatus (SCUBA) diving, the lack of communications with the outside clearly results in lengthy waiting times before the arrival of the rescue team [Frankland 1975] and the transport of the injured spelunker out of the cave can take even days.

Such extreme conditions prevented from studying the physiological responses to the subterranean environment: up to date there are few works about the energetic cost [Bizzarrini et al. 2002], the muscle damage and the intravascular haemolysis [Stenner et al 2006], the red cell changes [Stenner et al 2007] and hormonal responses [Stenner et al 2007b]. However, no published data about cave diving in deep caves are available.

It is well known that acute physical and psychological stress can influence hypothalamus-pituitary adrenocortical and hypothalamus-pituitary systems [Axelrod and Reisine 1984]. In particular, high intensity [Pritzlaff et al. 1999] and long duration exercise [Godfrey et al. 2003] is associated with a marked rise of growth hormone (GH) as well as the mode and the presence or not of partial vascular occlusion combined with exercise [Takarada et al. 2000; Reeves et al. 2006]. Moreover, strenuous exercise [Scavo et al.1991; Urhausen et al. 1995] and darkness [Pritzlaff et al. 1999] are known to be a stimulus for cortisol secretion.

Also the responses of total absolute number of lymphocytes (Lym-TOT) and lymphocytes subpopulations (CD3+, CD4+, CD8+, CD19+ and CD16+CD3-) to an episode of acute exercise are highly described; it is known in fact that the exercise, especially when coupled with mental stress, is associated with a transient redistribution of immunocompetent cells. Specifically, Lym-TOT and lymphocytes subpopulations usually increase during exercise and decrease below the initial level post exercise [Pedersen and Hoffman-Goetz 2000; Nielsen 2003]. Finally, the changes observed after exercise, the so called "open window", are usually considered the basis of athletes increased risk of upper respiratory tract infections [Pedersen and Toff 2000]. Isolation and confinement (e.g. spaceflights, submarines, single-person cave isolation, diving) [Schmitt and Scaffar 1993; Shimamiya et al. 2005] as well as sleep deprivation [Heiser et al. 2000] are also stressors that can affect transitorily the immune system. Darkness, instead, through the melatonin actions [Pandi-Perumal et al. 2006] is likely to enhance both cell-mediated and humoral immunity. Lastly, whether cold temperature influences lymphocytes and lymphocytes subsets or not is still controversial [Castellani et al. 2002]. Unlike other extreme sports, in alpine cave diving these stressors are present simultaneously. These athletes in fact need to descend the cave, prepare themselves for the solo immersion, do the exploration usually in cold water and then begin the ascent, often without resting. Moreover, they move in darkness and often during the night. In conclusion, in our experiment we considered that the combination of heavy and long duration exercise before (5 hours of descending) and after (13 hours of ascending) the immersion in a demanding environment, the siphon altitude (quota: 1200 m), the exercise effort during diving in cold water (2°C), the darkness, the isolation, the restrictions with the associated risk of getting stuck, the emotion for the solitary exploration and the critical consequences if an accident happened, represent a unique multiple stress model that may be helpful in understanding the immune and hormonal responses to acute physiological and psychological stress.

To investigate these responses we used the following parameters: growth hormone (GH), cortisol, absolute number of total lymphocytes (Lym-TOT) and lymphocytes subpopulations (CD3+, CD4+, CD8+, CD19+ and CD 16+).

Methods

Subject

Owing to the high skill level required to perform this kind of cave diving exploration and to the enormous difficulties for carrying all the technical equipment for the cave diver on the bottom of this cave, only one cave-diver was tested; however this subject repeated the same immersion in two different days following the same schedule. The tested cave diver (43 years old, weight: 78 Kg, height: 182 cm) is of a long and high level experience; he usually explores cave siphons alone and goes in a deep cave at least once per month. He lives and works at sea level, he is not a night shift worker, and he generally goes to bed between 11.00 pm to 12.00 pm; at the time of the expedition he was not taking any drugs.

He volunteered for this study and provided informed consent after being taught the purpose and the method of the experiment. The local ethics committee at the University of Trieste approved the experimental protocol and during the experiment all necessary precautions were taken to insure the well-being of the athlete, in accordance with the ethical standards laid down in the 1964 Declaration of Helsinki.

Some days before the performance he underwent a preliminary medical check-up and a series of routine blood tests to ascertain that he was in good health.

Experimental Design

The experiment was carried out in winter, in a cave (Abisso Gortani: quota 1930 m, internal temperature: 2 °C) on Monte Canin, Friuli Venezia Giulia, Italy) which presents a high level of difficulty.

The first blood drawing was performed at the hospital situated at sea level (T0 - 7.30 am); then the cave diver, together with the support group, drove to the mountain (altitude: 1100 m, temperature: -4 °C) and flew by helicopter (Picture 1) to the bivouac near the entrance of the cave (altitude: 1930 m, temperature: -11 °C). Here he ate about 150 g of pasta with 50 g of meat, 50 g of bread and 50 g of cheese and, at 2:00 pm, he entered the cave (internal temperature: 2 °C) with the spelunking staff (Picture 2, 3).

About 5 hours later he reached the bottom of the cave, 700 meters below the surface (altitude: 1230 m, temperature: 2°C). Here he had his second blood drawing (T1: 7.30 pm) (Picture 4) and then began the underwater exploration (Picture 5, 6) that lasted 46 minutes. He used NITROXEANX 30 air, covered about 60 m of siphon without emerging and passed some restrictions. After the immersion he had his third blood drawing (T2: 9.30 pm) before having a snack (about 50 g of bread, 50 g of cheese, 40 g of lard and 30 g of almond brittle). About 10 hours later he exited the cave (altitude: 1930 m, temperature: -15°C), after a very long and heavy ascending, and had his fourth blood drawing (T3: 7.30 am). Finally, the last blood drawing was done (sea level) 24 hours after resting (T4: 7.30 am).

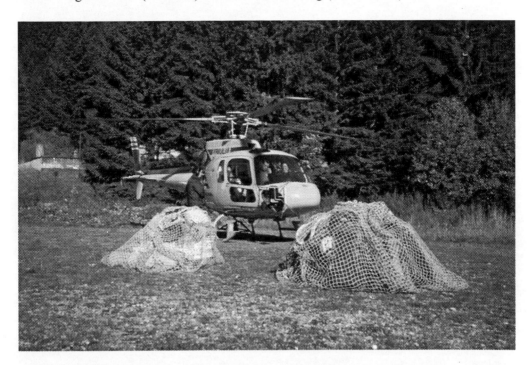

Picture 1. Helicopter taking off to the bivouac with all the equipment.

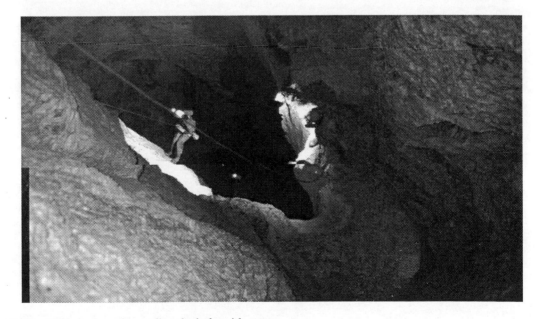

Picture 2. Spelunkers descending the hole with ropes.

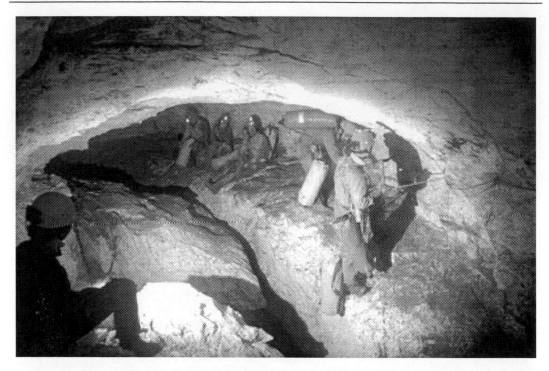

Picture 3. Short recovery during the descending .

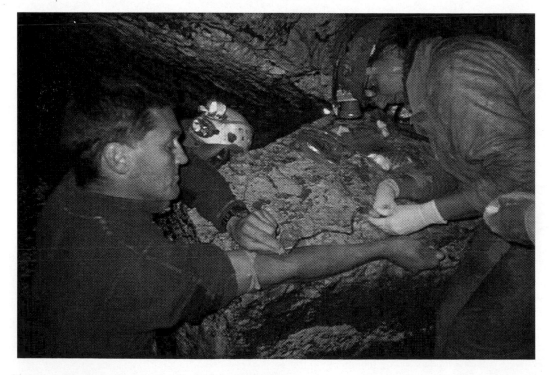

Picture 4. Blood drawing before the siphon immersion .

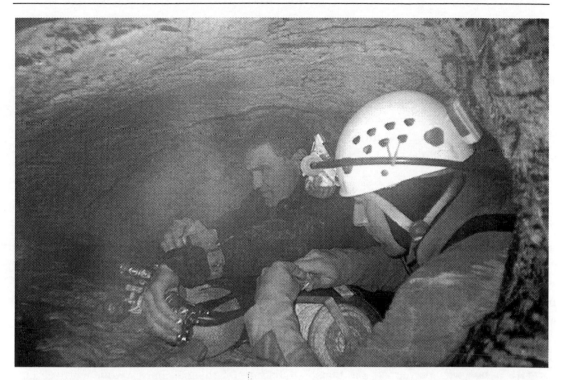

Picture 5. Check up of all the cave diver equipment.

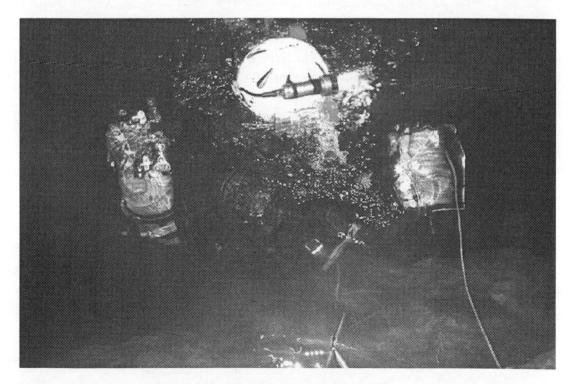

Picture 6. Cave diver immerging with a yellow guide line to sign the path.

Correspondence among time label, day and time of the experimental design, time elapsed (hours) from the beginning to the end of the experiment and the blood drawing location are summarized in Table1. To avoid the confounding effect of food intakes, the cave diver had fasted 8 hours before each blood drawing while food and fluid intakes were selected by himself. Other three blood drawings, as controls, had been performed three days before the performance, at the same resting time envisaged for the day of the experiment, to minimize the specimen processing time influences and any circadian fluctuations. In addition, the cave diver drank and ate at the same time and had the same food expected for spelunking and cave diving performance.

Technique

The blood was collected, after 5 minutes in seated position, from the antecubital vein in vacuum tubes without anticoagulant for serum analysis and with anticoagulant EDTAK3 in powder form for haemocromocytometric test. A whole blood smear was done immediately at each sampling point. The test tubes and the smears were placed in an insulated polystyrene container [Henry 2001] and the blood samples were analysed within 24 hours after being drawn [Banfi 2003; Dos Santos 2007]

GH assay was performed on Liaison (DiaSorin, Saluggia, Italy), while cortisol on DX1800 (Beckmann Coulter, Fullerton, California, 2004). The precision (intra-assay variation) and the reproducibility (inter-assay variation) of each assay are summarized in Table 2.

Total and differential leukocytes count were performed on Coulter LH 750 ANALYZER (Beckman Coulter, Fullerton, CA, USA). Differential counts were also verified by counting leukocyte subsets on whole blood smears stained with May-Grünwald stain (Sigma-Aldrich, St.Louise, MO).

Lymphocytes subsets were analyzed on the flow cytometer Coulter EPICS-XL (Beckman Coulter, Fullerton, CA, USA) set up for two colour detection and controlled with XL system II software.

Cells were prepared from 100 μl whole blood aliquots to which were added 10 μl of appropriate fluorescent-conjugated monoclonal antibodies IgG1-fluorescein isothiocyanate (FITC) and phycoerythrin (PE)). After 30 minutes of incubation at 4 °C, every tube was processed using the ImmunoPrep reagent system (Beckman Coulter) on the Coulter TQ-Prep Workstation (Beckman Coulter) for 35 seconds before the flow cytometric analysis.

Lymphocytes were gated according to their forward and side scatter properties, and 5000 events were recorded. T cells were identified with a cytogramme analysis as CD3+ PE/CD19-FITC, CD3+ PE/CD4+ FITC, CD3+ PE/CD8+ FITC; B cells were identified as CD19+ FITC/ CD3- PE and NK cells as CD16+ FITC/CD3-PE phenotype.

Results were expressed as the percentage of cells yielding a specific fluorescence in a gated region. Absolute subset count was derived by multiplying the percentage of a specific cell-type by the total number of lymphocytes in unit volume of peripheral blood.

Table 1. Correspondence among time label, day and time of the experimental design, time elapsed (hours) from the beginning to the end of the experiment and the blood drawing location

Time label	Day and time	Time elapsed (hours)	Blood drawing location
T0	7.30 am - day 1	0	Laboratory
T1	7.30 pm - day 1	12	Bottom of the cave
T2	9.30 am - day 1	14	After immersion
T3	7.30 am - day 2	24	Exit of the cave
T4	7.30 am - day 3	48	Laboratory

Table 2. The intra-assay variation and the inter-assay variation of growth hormone (GH) and cortisol

ASSAY	SENSITIVITY	MEAN		CV%	
				Intra-assay	Inter-assay
GH	0.003 µg/l	Level 1:	0.33 µg/l	1.5	3.2
		Level 2:	6.40 µg/l	2.5	2.9
		Level 3:	19.50 µg/l	2.1	3.6
CORTISOL	11 nmol/l	Level 1: 165.50 nmol/l		6.7	7.1
		Level 2: 664.90 nmol/l		4.4	5.1
		Level 3:1059.50 nmol/l		4.4	5.0

The % coefficient of variation is expressed as 90% confidence level for the variance.

Statistical Methods

Since a single spelunker was tested, only descriptive statistics was performed. We analysed the detrended data of hormonal values (i.e. after the removal of control values from experimental values) to understand the temporal changes during the days of the performance and to control the confounding effects of circadian baseline [de Vries 2000; Thuma et al.1995]. Moreover, for each blood drawing (T0, T1, T2, T3 and T4), GH and cortisol responses to exercise were also compared with those on control day. For immune response, we analysed the test values with respect to controls at the following time points: T1: bottom of the cave, T2: exit from the siphon, T3: exit from the cave, T4: after 24 hours of repose.

Results

Since our calculated percentage changes in plasma volume cannot account for the observed marked changes in plasma hormone concentration, in lymphocyte absolute number and in lymphocytes subset cells, we did not correct these data for shift in plasma volume.

A marked rise of GH detrended values was found after about 5 hours of descending, on the bottom of the cave (T1 to T2), 700 m under the surface, and between the arrival on the bottom of the cave and the exit from siphon, after about 46 minutes of immersion. On the contrary, a marked drop was measured between the post immersion and the exit of the cave (T2 to T3) and between the exit of the cave and the morning after 24 hours of rest (T3 to T4).

Considering the analysis of the experimental values of GH with respect to control values (Figure 1) a marked increase was measured in all the time points during the performance while no changes were observed the morning before the beginning of the experiment and the day after 24 hours of repose with respect to control values.

Cortisol detrended values showed high initial values, before the beginning of the performance and a marked increase both between the pre-performance values and the bottom of the cave (T1 to T2), before the siphon exploration, and between the pre siphon and post siphon (T2 to T3) time point, while a marked drop was observed between the finish of the immersion and the exit of the cave (T3 to T4) and between the exit of the cave and the day after 24 hours of repose.

The experimental values of cortisol concentration with respect to control values (Figure2) evidenced an increase at the beginning of the exploration (T1), on the bottom of the cave (T2), after the immersion (T3) and at the exit of the cave (T4), while a drop was reached the following day (T5).

A marked drop of the experimental values with respect to control values was observed for total absolute lymphocytes number (Figure3) and lymphocytes subset T cells CD3+ (Figure4), CD4+ (Figure5) and CD8+ (Figure6) at each time point (T1, T2, T3 and T4); in particular, the biggest drop with respect to controls was measured after the immersion (Table 3).

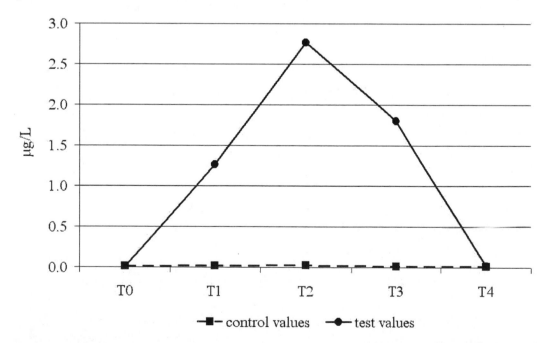

Figure 1. Growth hormone (GH) mean values (control and experimental). Blood drawings were withdrawn at: T0 (before entering of the cave), T1 (bottom of the cave, -700m), T2 (after the immersion), T3 (exit of the cave) and T4 (after 24 h of resting).

CD4:CD8 ratio decreased on the bottom of the cave while out of the siphon and at the exit it increased. No differences were observed the day after repose. A different behaviour was observed for CD16+CD3- (Figure 7); there was a moderate rise on the bottom of the cave while in the following time points a decrease was measured. Also CD16+CD3- cells showed the maximal decrease with respect to control values after the immersion.

Finally, CD19+ (Figure 8) rose with respect to control values on the bottom of the cave and at the exit of the cave, while a drop was measured after the immersion and the day after repose.

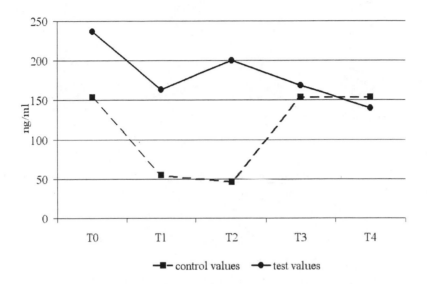

Figure 2. Cortisol mean values (experimental and control). Blood drawings were withdrawn at: T0 (before entering of the cave), T1 (bottom of the cave, -700m), T2 (after the immersion), T3 (exit of the cave) and T4 (after 24 h of resting).

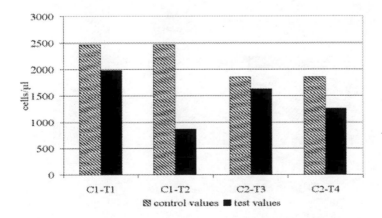

Figure 3. Total absolute number of lymphocytes (control and experimental). C1 – T1: control values – test values measured on the bottom of the cave, C1 – T2: control values – test values reached after the immersion, C2 – T3: control values – test values reached at the exit of the cave, C2 – T4: control values – test values reached the day after 24 hours of repose.

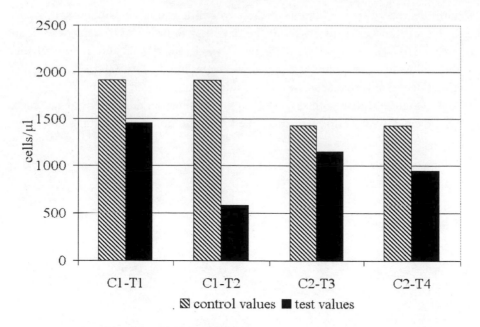

Figure 4. CD3+ cells (control and experimental). C1 – T1: control values – test values measured on the bottom of the cave, C1 – T2: control values – test values reached after the immersion, C2 – T3: control values – test values reached at the exit of the cave, C2 – T4: control values – test values reached the day after 24 hours of repose.

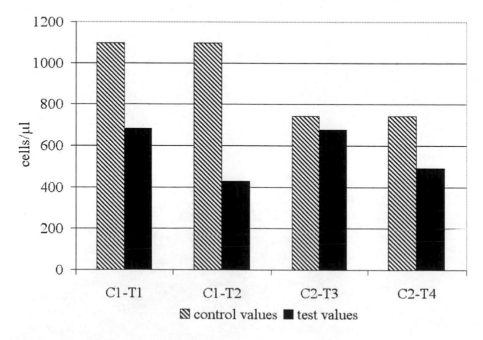

Figure 5. CD4+ cells (control and experimental). C1 – T1: control values – test values measured on the bottom of the cave, C1 – T2: control values – test values reached after the immersion, C2 – T3: control values – test values reached at the exit of the cave, C2 – T4: control values – test values reached the day after 24 hours of repose.

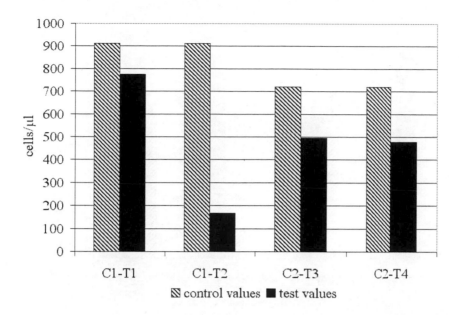

Figure 6. CD8+ cells (control and experimental). C1 – T1: control values – test values measured on the bottom of the cave, C1 – T2: control values – test values reached after the immersion, C2 – T3: control values – test values reached at the exit of the cave, C2 – T4: control values – test values reached the day after 24 hours of repose.

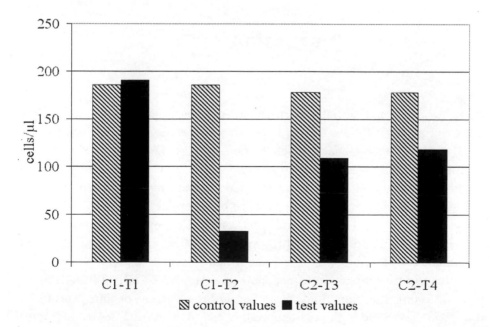

Figure 7. CD16+ cells (control and experimental). C1 – T1: control values – test values measured on the bottom of the cave, C1 – T2: control values – test values reached after the immersion, C2 – T3: control values – test values reached at the exit of the cave, C2 – T4: control values – test values reached the day after 24 hours of repose.

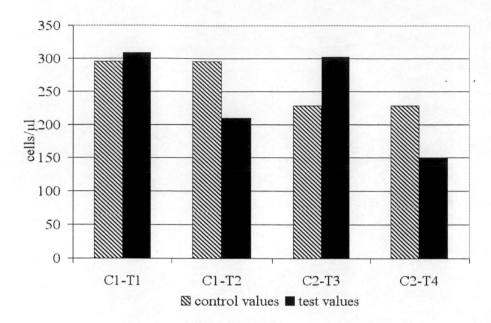

Figure 8. CD19+ cells (control and experimental). C1 – T1: control values – test values measured on the bottom of the cave, C1 – T2: control values – test values reached after the immersion, C2 – T3: control values – test values reached at the exit of the cave, C2 – T4: control values – test values reached the day after 24 hours of repose.

Discussion

Hormonal Responses

It is known that exercise, especially if strenuous, may be a potent stimulus for GH secretion [Godfrey et al. 2003; Pritzlaff et al. 1999; Wideman et al. 2002]. Spelunking is a heavy and long duration aerobic-anaerobic-alternating exercise [Bizzarrini et al. 2002] (usually 15-20 hours) and it is no accident that just on the bottom of the cave, after about 5 hours of descending ropes, carrying heavy sacks, walking and crawling in crouched positions, passing through narrow winding passages, an increase of GH values (detrended data) was reached. Moreover, for spelunkers in general, the compression of the bindings of the climbing sit harness has also to be considered [Stenner et al. 2006]; it could favour, in fact, the regional accumulation of metabolites (i.e lactate) that is one of the earlier processes known to be involved in the stimulation of hypophyseal secretions of GH [Takarada et al. 2000; Reeves et al. 2006]. The poor fluid intake due to the reduction of thirst sensitivity [Vogelaere et al 1993] associated with cold temperature and to the difficulties to find water during the way for the bottom of the cave as well as to the impossibility to take inside enough water for a so long duration exercise, could have influenced exercise-induced GH response too, either enhancing [Saini et al. 1990] or inhibiting [Peyreigne et al. 2001] the secretion.

Focusing on the immersion time interval (T1-T2), the increase of GH values (detrended values) during cave diving is likely due to the great intensity of cave diving effort both to cover the difficult route during the immersion and to pass a lot of restrictions wearing bulky technical equipment with the associated risk of getting stuck. The exposure to cold, instead, is unlikely to have favoured the increase of GH secretion; it is generally accepted, in fact, that cold influences GH response blunting it [Wheldon et al. 2006]. Moreover, the fact that the immersion was performed during the evening reasonably did not affect the magnitude of GH response to exercise, since this is not modified by the time of the day [Kanaley et al. 2001].

Interestingly, the maximum values of GH were detected after the immersion. Actually GH responses are more related to the peak exercise intensity rather than to duration of exercise or total work output [Kjaer and Dela 1996]. This suggests that for the tested cave diver the most strenuous activity was the diving performance. In fact, although the ascending is of very long duration and is a strenuous exercise, we measured a marked drop between the exit from the siphon and the exit from the cave. Lastly, the initial conditions were restored the third day, after 24 hours of resting, underlining that GH changes are transient.

These findings are evident also observing the differences, at each time point, between test results and control data.

No anticipatory response to performance (T0-C0), previously described [Scavo et al. 1991; Vasankari et al. 1993] was found.

The rise of cortisol detrended values reached on the bottom of the cave confirms the well described cortisol response to a long duration and high intensity exercise [Scavo et al.1991; Urhausen et al. 1995]. Moreover, for the spelunkers the enhancing effect of the darkness on cortisol secretion [Pritzlaff et al. 1999] has also to be considered. Interestingly, as it occurred for GH values, the peak of cortisol concentrations was measured after the immersion, pointing out that 46 minutes of immersion have a greater influence on cortisol behaviour than all the rest of the performance. This was, at least in part, an unexpected result because it is known that the plasma concentration of cortisol increases only in relation to exercise of long duration. Thus short term exercise does not increase the cortisol concentration in plasma, and only minor changes in the concentration in plasma cortisol were described in relation to acute time-limited exercise stress of 1h [Galbo1983]. Consequently the marked increase that we measured could be due not only to the intensity of the exercise [Urhausen et al. 1995], but also to the great psychological stress [Steiger 2002]. This athlete, in fact, had to move in darkness with a very low visibility (at the outward going he had about 3 m of visibility while during the return it dropped to 0.5 m) with the awareness that if the guide line broke, it would be very difficult to find the return path. He moved in cold temperatures with an increased risk that the self-contained underwater breathing apparatus would stop to work correctly; since it was a solo exploration of the siphon, he was conscious that if any kind of accident had happened, the situation would become abruptly very critical. Therefore the cortisol levels reached after diving are likely to evidence that the immersion represented the most stressful event during the subterranean exploration. On the contrary, the marked drop reached at the exit, even if after the long and heavy ascent, could represent a positive state that led him to a psychological well being reflected, as previously described, by a reduced cortisol secretion [Lai et al. 2005; Steptoe et al. 2005].

Analyzing the test values with respect to control values, it is evident that there was a marked anticipatory pre-performance elevation in cortisol serum concentrations, a typical stress reaction [Steiger 2002][Vasankari et al. 1993].

The higher test values with respect to control values reached at all the time points, with the exception of the third day, confirm that hypothalamus-pituitary adrenocortical system responds to the heavy and long duration exercise [Scavo et al. 1991][Vaananen et al. 2004][Vaananen et al. 2002][Vasankari et al. 1993] as well as to the aggressive environmental conditions [Castellani et al. 2002][Steiger 2002][VanHelder and Radomski 1989].

In conclusion our data show that the extreme physiological/psychological skills necessary to perform cave diving, especially in deep alpine caves, are stressors that are able to alter the hormonal homeostasis inducing a hypothalamus-pituitary adrenocortical and hypothalamus-pituitary systems response. GH elevation underlines the great intensity and long duration characteristic of this exercise and the cortisol increase evidenced the well known "stress reaction", a prerequisite for the individual survival. The subsequent cortisol drop that took place during spelunking, suggests that an adaptation to both exercise and environment occurred. Finally, the drop of experimental values with respect to control values reached the day after repose demonstrated that this kind of activity needs a long rest period to re-establish the initial physiological conditions.

Immune Responses

It is widely accepted that lymphocyte concentrations increase during exercise, due to the recruitment of all lymphocyte subpopulations to the vascular compartment from other tissue pools [Pedersen and Hoffman-Goetz 2000; Gleeson and Bishop 2005; Pedersen and Toft 2000]. The organs involved include the spleen, the lymph nodes, the gastrointestinal tract and the number of cells that enter the circulation is determined by the intensity of the stimulus [Pedersen and Hoffman-Goetz 2000]. However we measured a marked drop of total absolute number of lymphocytes as well as of CD3+, CD4+ and CD8+ lymphocyte subpopulations, with respect to control values, on the bottom of the cave. This drop appears to be dependant both on the lack of mature cells that can be recruited after some hours of endurance exercise [Pedersen and Hoffman-Goetz 2000] and on the exercise-induced rise in circulating cortisol levels by inhibiting their entry into and facilitating their egress from the circulation to organs [Pedersen and Hoffman-Goetz 2000] The cortisol seems to exert its effect with a time lag of some hours [Pedersen and Hoffman-Goetz 2000; Pedersen and Toft 2000], so that in the most of exercises the immune-suppression effects are reached during the recovery period. On the contrary, in this case the cortisol-induced lymphocytes drop becomes evident even before the exercise has been completed [Pedersen and Hoffman-Goetz 2000; Rowbottom and Green 2000], due to the particularly strenuous and prolonged exercise just during the descending.

Interestingly, we measured the biggest drop with respect to control values of total absolute number of lymphocytes that led to absolute lymphopenia; also lymphocyte subsets CD3+, CD4+ and CD8+ dramatically drop after the immersion, confirming that for this athlete this was the most stressful event during the performance. Cold exposure [Castellani et al. 2002] and such a short period of isolation (5 hours) [Schmitt 1993; Shimamiya 2004] are unlikely to have modulated the lymphocytes and T cells response, as well as darkness since night time physical exercise is able to blunt the nocturnal surge of plasma melatonin and increases the levels of cortisol concentration [Monteleone et al, 1992]. Both these events can blunt the enhancing effect of darkness on cell-mediated and humoral immunity [Pandi-Perumal et al. 2006].

At the exit, the differences of absolute number of total lymphocytes and T cells CD3+, CD4+ and CD8+ with respect to control became lower than out of the siphon; this reflects that there was an increase in the absolute number of cells, maybe due to the influence of the heavy exercise to ascend the cave even if their values were never greater than the control values.

The drop of CD4:CD8 ratio reached on the bottom of the cave evidenced a decrease in CD8+ slower than in CD4+; on the contrary, the marked rise of CD4:CD8 ratio observed both after the immersion and at the exit of the cave, underline a decrease in CD8+ faster than in CD4+.

Exercise of various types, duration and intensities induces also recruitment to the blood of cells expressing characteristic NK cell markers [Rowbottom and Green 2000; Nagatomi 2006]; this effect was observed on the bottom of the cave, while a dramatic drop was found after the immersion. Lastly, the NK cells absolute number was reduced with respect to control values, also at the exit, presumably because of the selective migration from vessels to injured muscles [Shephard et al 1994] to assist the repair process.

B lymphocytes according to the literature [Shek 1996] showed a moderate fluctuation during the performance.

The low absolute number of lymphocytes and all lymphocyte subpopulations reached the third day underlines that the strenuous characteristics of this sport prevent the quick restore of the homeostasis producing a very long duration "open window" (at least 36 hours).

In conclusion, though the importance of the absolute number of lymphocytes and of sub populations is still questioned, even when their changes would be of sufficiently long duration to have major clinical implications, it is possible that a period of frequent subterranean explorations or in a deep cave rescue, during which it can happen to enter the cave twice after poor restoring time, can result in a depression of immunity due to cumulative effects of repeated bouts of intense and long duration exercise.

Considering that in such an extreme sport the perfect physiological and psychological conditions are necessary not only for a good performance but also for survival, the marked immune changes that were observed suggest that a period of total repose between two demanding subterranean performances should be respected to avoid that the immune function becomes impaired, leading to a possible increase of the susceptibility to infections.

Such a field study has some limitations. A critical point is represented by the size of the studied sample, that is due to the high skills required to perform this performance, and to the organizational aspects of the experimental design. Another criticism, considering the short half life of tested hormones, could be the limited number of blood drawings performed during the experiment but, as expected, our priority was given to athlete comfort .

Additional information is needed to confirm our preliminary results.

Authors' Notes

The authors are grateful to the cave diver (Spartaco Savio) and to all the spelunker staff that participated in the experiment both in the cave and at the bivouac. They would also like to express their sincere gratitude to the Commissione Grotte Eugenio Boegan (CGEB), Società Alpina delle Giulie, Trieste, Club Alpino Italiano for giving a part of financial support and technical equipment for this study.

References

Ashford DA, Knutson RS, Sacks JJ. (1999). Injury among cavers results of a preliminary national survey. *J. Sports Med. Phys. Fitness*, 39(1), 71-73.

Axelrod J and Reisine TD. (1984). Stress hormone, their interaction and regulation. *Science*, 224, 452-459.

Banfi G and Dolci A. (2003). Preanalytical phase of sport biochemistry and haematology. *J. Sports Med. Phys. Fitness,* 43(2), 223-30.

Bizzarrini E, Bratina F, Delbello G, Sceusa R, Stenner E, Lamberti V and Princi T. (2002). Sportivi in grotta. *Sport e Medicina*, 4, 33-41.

Castellani JW, Brenner JK and Rhind SG. (2002). Cold exposure: human immune responses and intracellular cytokine expression. *Med. Sci. Sports Ecerc*, 34(12), 2013-2020.

de Vries WR, Bernards Nol TM, de Rooij MH and Koppeschaar Hans PF. (2000). Dynamic exercise discloses different time-related responses in stress hormones. *Psychosom. Med.,* 6, 866-872.

Dos Santos AP, Bertho AL, de Menezes Martins R and Marcovistz R. (2007). The sample processing time interval as an influential factor in flow cytometry analysis of lymphocyte subsets. *Mem .Ins.t Oswaldo Cruz*, 102(1), 117-120.

Frankland JC. (1975). Caving and cave rescue. *Community Health,* 7(2), 108-115.

Galbo H. Hormonal and Metabolic adaption to exercise. New York: Thieme Verlag; 1983.

Gleeson M and Bishop NC. (2005). The T cell and NK cell immune response to exercise. *Annals of transplantation*, 10(4), 44-49.

Godfrey RJ, Madgwick Z and Whyte GP. (2003). The exercise-induced growth hormone response in athletes. *Sports Med.,* 33(8), 599-613.

Heiser P, Dickhaus B and Schreiber W. (2000). White blood cells and cortisol after sleep deprivation and recovery sleep in humans. *Eur. Arch. Psychiatry Clin. Neurosci.,* 250, 16-23.

Henry JB and Kurec AS. Preanalytical testing. In: John Bernard Henry, M.D, editor. Clinical Diagnosis and Management by Laboratory Methods. W.B.Saunders Company; 2001; 27-33.

Kanaley JA, Weltman JY, Pieper KS, Weltman A and Hartman ML. (2001). Cortisol and growth hormone responses to exercise at different times of day. *J. Clin. Endocrinol. Metab.,*.86(6), 2881-2889.

Kjaer M and Dela F. Endocrine responses to exercise. In: Exercise and Immune function. L. Hoffman-Goetz, editor. Boca Raton, FL. CRC; 1996; 1-20.

Lai JC, Evans PD, Ng SH, Chong AM, Siu OT, Chan CL, Ho SM, Ho RT, Chan P and Chan CC. (2005). Optimism, positive affectivity and salivary cortisol. *Br. J. Health Psychol.*, 10(Pt 4), 467-484.

Monteleone P, Fuschino A, Nolfe G and Maj M. (1992). Temporal relationship between melatonin and cortisol responses to nighttime physical stress in humans. Psychoneuroendocrinology, 17(1), 81-86.

Mount T. Student manual and workbook for safer cave diving. First edition. United States of America. Paul Pettenude editor. 1995.

Nagatomi R. The implication of alterations in leukocyte subset counts on immune function. (2006). *Exerc Immunol. Rev.*, 12, 54-71.

Nielsen HB. (2003). Lymphocytes Responses to maximal exercise. *Sports Med.*, 33(11), 853-867.

Pandi-Perumal SR, Srinivasan V, Maestroni GJ, Cardinali DP, Poeggeler B and Hardeland R. (2006). Melatonin: Nature's most versatile biological signal? *FEBS J.*, 273(13), 2813-2828.

Pedersen BK and Hoffman-Goetz L. (2000). Exercise and the immune system: regulation, integration and adaptation. *Physiol. Rev.*, 80(3),1055-1081.

Pedersen BK and Toft AD. (2000). Effects of exercise on lymphocytes and cytokines. *Br. J. Sports Med.* 34, 246-251.

Peyreigne C, Bouix D, Fédou C and Mercier J. (2001). Effect of hydration on exercise-induced growth hormone response. *Eur. J. Endocrinol.*, 145, 445-450.

Pritzlaff CJ, Wideman L, Weltman JY, Abbott RD, Gutgesell ME, Hartman ML, Veldhuis JD and Weltman A. (1999). Impact of acute exercise intensity on pulsatile growth hormone release in men. *J. Appl. Physiol.*, 87, 498-504.

Reeves GU, Kraemer RR, Hollander DB, Clavier J, Thomas C, Francois M and Castracane VD. (2006). Comparison of hormone responses following light resistance exercise with partial vascular occlusion and moderate resistance exercise without occlusion. *J. Appl. Physiol.*, doi 0:00440.2006v1.

Rowbottom DG and Green KJ. (2000). Acute exercise effects on the immune system. *Med. Sci. Sports Exerc,.* 32(7), S396-S405.

Saini J, Bothorel B, Brandenberger G, Candas V and Follenius M. (1990). Growth hormone and prolactin response to rehydration during exercise; effect of water and carbohydrate solution. *Eur. J. Appl. Physio.l*, 61, 61-67.

Scavo D, Barletta C, Vagiri D, and Letizia C. (1991). Adrenocorticotropic hormone, beta-endorphin, cortisol, growth hormone and prolactin circulating levels in nineteen athletes before and after half-marathon and marathon. *J. Sports Med. Phys Fitness*, 31(3), 401-406.

Schmitt DA and Schaffar L. (1993). Isolation and confinement as model for spaceflight immune changes. *J. Leukoc. Biol.*, 54, 209-213.

Shek PN. (1996). Immunologic changes associated with strenuous exercise. *Clin. J. Sport Med.*, 6(4), 277-278.

Shephard RJ, Rhind S and Shek PN. (1994). Exercise and the immune system. *Sports Med.*, 18(5), 340-369

Shimamiya T, Terada N, Hiejima Y, Wakabayashi S, Kasai H and Mohri M. (2004). Effects of 10-day confinement on the immune system and psychological aspects in humans. *J. Appl. Physiol.*, 97, 900-924.

Shimamiya T, Terada N, Wakabayashi S and Mohri M. (2005). Mood change and immune status of human subjects in a 10-day confinement study. *Aviat Space Environ. Med.,* 76, 481-485.

Steiger A. (2002). Sleep and the hypothalamo-pituitary-adrenocortical system. Sl*eep Med. Rev.*, 6(2), 125-138 .

Stenner E, Gianoli E, Biasioli B, Piccinini C, Delbello G and Bussani A. (2006). Muscular damage and intravascular haemolysis during an 18 hours subterranean exploration in a cave of 700 m of depth. *Br. J. Sports Med.*, 40, 235-238.

E. Stenner, C. Piccinini, B. Biasioli, E. Gianoli, A. Bussani, G. Delbello. Red cell and core temperature in spelunking. *Int. J. Sport Med.* 2007;28:1-5. DOI:10.1055/s-2007-964978

Stenner E, Gianoli E, Piccinini C, Biasioli B, Bussani A and Delbello G. Hormonal responses to a long duration exploration in a cave of 700 m depth. *Eur J. Appl. Physiol.* 2007;100(1):71-78; DOI:10.1007/s00421-007-0408-9

Steptoe A, Wardle J and Marmot M. (2005). Positive affect and health-related neuroendocrine, cardiovascular, and inflammatory processes. *Proc. Natl. Acad .Sci. U S A*, 102(18), 6508-6512.

Takarada Y, Nakamura Y, Aruga S, Onda T, Miyazaki S and Ishii S. (2000). Rapid increase in plasma growth hormone after low-intensity resistance exercise with vascular occlusion. *J. Appl .Physiol.*, 88, 61-65.

Thuma JR, Gilders R, Verdun M and Loucks AB. (1995). Circadian rhythm of cortisol confounds cortisol responses to exercise: implications for future research. *J. Appl. Physiol.*, 78, 1657-1664.

Urhausen Axel, Gabriel H and Kindermann W. (1995). Blood hormones as markers of training stress and overtraing. *Sports Med.*, 20(4), 251-276.

Vaananen I, Vasankari T, Mantysaari M and Vihko V. (2002). Hormonal responses to daily strenuous walking during 4 successive days. *Eur. J. Appl. Physiol.*, 88, 122-127.

Vaananen I, Vasankari T, Mantysaari M and Vihko V. (2004). Hormonal responses to 100 km cross-country skiing during 2 days. *J. Sports Med. Phys. Fitness*, 44(3), 309-314.

VanHelder T and Radomski MW. (1989). Sleep deprivation and the effect on exercise performance. *Sports Med.*, 7, 235-247.

Vasankari TJ, Kujala UM, Heinonen OJ and Huhtaniemi IT. (1993). Effects of endurance training on hormonal responses to prolonged physical exercise in males. *Acta Endocrinol. (Copenh)*, 129(2), 109-113.

Vogelaere P, Savourey G, Deklunder G, Lecroart J, Brasseur M, Bekaert S and Bittel J. (1992). Reversal of cold induced haemoconcentration. *Eur. J. Appl. Physiol.*, 64(3), 244-9.

Wheldon A, Savine RL, Sonksen PH and Holt RI. (2006). Exercising in the cold inhibits growth hormone secretion by reducing the rise in core body temperature. *Growth Horm. IGF Res,* 16(2), 125-131.

Wideman L, Weltman JY, Hartman ML, Veldhuis JD and Welman A. (2002). Growth hormone release during acute and chronic aerobic and resistance exercise. *Sports Med*, 32(15), 987-1004.

In: Sport and Exercise Psychology Research Advances   ISBN: 978-1-60456-157-9
Editors: M. P. Simmons, L. A. Foster, pp. 329-343   © 2008 Nova Science Publishers, Inc.

Chapter XV

Sport Status and Physical Activity Perceptions of Youth

Sarah M. Jeffery[17], *Mark A. Eys, Robert J. Schinke, and John Lewko*
School of Human Kinetics, Laurentian University, Canada

Abstract

Despite the benefits of participation in sport and physical activity, there is a clear prevalence of sport dropout behavior beginning in early adolescence (Gould and Petlichkoff, 1988; Petlichkoff, 1996; Tremblay, Katzmaryzk, and Wilms, 2002). A potential influence on youth sport and physical activity participation is sport status (Connelly, 1992; Gruber and Gray, 1982). The purpose of the present investigation was to examine levels of sport and physical activity participation for youth of various sport status (i.e., high status/starting athlete, low status/non-starting athlete, non-athlete) prior to the academic transition from elementary school (Grade Eight) to high school (Grade Nine) and examine this situation within the Theory of Planned Behavior (i.e., attitudes towards physical activity, perceived behavioral control, subjective norms, intentions to be physically active; Ajzen, 1991). Grade Eight students ($n = 79$) were administered a set of questionnaires to assess physical activity participation, sport participation (including starting status), and perceptions of physical activity (i.e., TPB variables). Multivariate analyses of variance revealed significant differences between sport status levels in perceptions of attitudes towards physical activity, $F(2,76) = 8.98$, $p < .001$, $\eta^2 = .19$, intentions to be physically active, $F(2,76) = 3.64$, $p < .05$, $\eta^2 = .09$, perceived behavioral control, $F(2,76) = 3.46$, $p < .05$, $\eta^2 = .08$, and vigorous physical activity levels, $F(2,76) = 5.14$, $p < .01$, $\eta^2 = .12$. Specifically, post-hoc tests indicated significant differences ($p < .05$) between starting athletes and non-athletes with regard to attitudes, intentions, and vigorous physical activity levels. However, youth athletes with lower sport status held

17 Address correspondence to: Sarah Jeffery, c/o Mark Eys, School of Human Kinetics, Laurentian University, Sudbury, ON, Canada, P3E 2C6, Telephone: (705) 675-1151 ext. 1203, Fax: (705) 675-4845, Email: sm_jeffery@laurentian.ca.

similar perceptions of physical activity (i.e., attitudes and intentions) and engaged in similar levels of vigorous physical activity as both higher status athletes and non-athletes.

Keywords: *Youth, Sport Status, Physical Activity, Theory of Planned Behavior*

Physical activity participation is responsible for a number of benefits for youth with regard to both physical and mental health (Baranowski et al., 2000; Donaldson and Ronan, 2006; Fredricks and Eccles, 2006; Statistics Canada, 2005; Taras, 2005; Yin and Moore, 2004). From a physiological perspective, physical activity decreases the prevalence of obesity (Statistics Canada, 2005), promotes fat-free mass (Baranowski et al., 2000), improves general circulation (Taras, 2005), and reduces the risk of developing several diseases including coronary heart disease, diabetes, osteoporosis, and hypertension (United States Department of Health and Human Services; USDHHS, 2000). Psychosocial benefits of youth physical activity include the facilitation of academic development (Donaldson and Ronan, 2006; Fredricks and Eccles, 2006; Marsh and Kleitman, 2003; Yin and Moore, 2004), moral development (e.g., decreased likelihood of participation in negative behaviors such as gang membership, sexual behaviors, delinquency, smoking, alcohol and drug use; Nelson and Gordon-Larsen, 2006; Seefeldt and Ewing, 1997), and social development through peer and social affiliation (Britsch, 2000; McHale et al., 2005; Smith, 2007; Utter, Denny, Robinson, Ameratunga, and Watson, 2006; Weiss, Smith, and Theeboom, 1996).

Despite the multitude of benefits associated with youth sport and physical activity participation, the drop-out rate for organized youth sport in the United States has been estimated at 35% (Gould and Petlichkoff, 1988), and research has consistently demonstrated that youth become less physically active as they get older (Tremblay et al., 2002). In addition, youth overweight and obesity rates between the years of 1978 and 2004 have doubled and tripled respectively (Statistics Canada, 2005). This situation has inevitably led to numerous health risks for this specific population (e.g., high blood pressure, type II diabetes, nonalcoholic fatty liver disease, polycystic ovary disorder, disordered breathing during sleep; Daniels, 2006), as well as economic burdens for the Canadian government (Katzmarzyk and Janssen, 2004).

Given the above information, it is necessary to examine potential contributors to youth physical inactivity. Previous research has indicated that youth are leaving sport environments or becoming less active due to a number of reasons such as failure to learn new skills, lack of fun, lack of affiliation, lack of thrills and excitement, lack of exercise and fitness, no challenges, a change of interest, other things to do (Gould, Feltz, Horn, and Weiss, 1982), deciding to participate in sedentary activities (e.g., television viewing; Hagar, 2006), being of a lower socioeconomic status (Harper, 2006), and having low perceptions of competence (Gould and Petchlikoff, 1988; Robinson and Carron, 1982; Weiss and Chaumeton, 1992).

With regard to the latter reason, perceptions of competence are affected by a number of personal and situational factors including sport status (Connelly, 1992; Gruber and Gray, 1982). An individual's status is reflected in his or her standing within the group that is based on the amount of prestige possessed by or accorded to people through the attributes they possess (Jacob and Carron, 1994). A recent study was conducted by Jacob-Johnson (2004) with Canadian and East Indian athletes to determine what specific status attributes were salient in a sport environment. Four categories were identified as important status attributes: (a) physical attributes (e.g., performance, experience, appearance, role on team, position), (b) psychological attributes (e.g., positive attitude), (c) demographic attributes (e.g., family status), and (d) relationships with external others (e.g., friendships outside the team).

Minimal empirical research exists that examines perceptions and experiences of athletes based on their respective sport status. However, one clear delineation of status within sport teams that has been examined in past research is the starting status of athletes. Generally, there are two categories of starting status. First, an athlete who usually begins competitions on the playing surface and receives regular playing time has been classified as a starting player (i.e., higher status athlete). Second, an athlete who does not begin competition on the playing surface and typically receives little to no playing time has been classified as a non-starter (i.e., lower status athlete; Gruber and Gray, 1982; Robinson and Carron, 1982). While not necessarily the primary purpose of their studies, researchers have examined differences between starters and non-starters. For example, non-starting athletes have indicated less satisfaction with their contribution to the team, valued their membership on the team to a lesser degree, and had lower affiliation desire (Gruber and Gray, 1982). In addition, non-starters have been shown to perceive the group as less cohesive (Granito and Rainey, 1988), have lower interpersonal attractions to the group (Bergeles and Hatziharistos, 2003), and have a lower need for achievement (Teevan and Yalof, 1980). It has also been demonstrated that the relationships between perceptions of coach leadership behaviors and role ambiguity (i.e., a lack of clear information regarding a person's role; Beauchamp, Bray, Eys, and Carron, 2005) differed between starters and non-starters. Finally, it has been suggested that non-starting athletes may encounter additional issues that lead to dropout such as not feeling like a part of the team, and feeling bitter, rejected, isolated, and incompetent (Connelly, 1992).

Taken together, the above review highlights that (a) physical activity is beneficial for youth, (b) the percentage of youth participating in physical activity decreases with age, (c) reasons for discontinuation are numerous, and (d) status, and specifically starting status, can effect perceptions of the sport environment. The abovementioned studies regarding starting status are very much directed to the immediate sport environment (i.e., perceptions of their current team) and hypotheses could be generated about the likelihood of individuals not participating specifically on that team or in that sport (i.e., sport-specific dropouts). However, Gould and Petlichkoff (1988) also noted the importance of considering those who would drop out of sport altogether (i.e., sport-general dropouts). For example, it could be possible that feelings experienced in a specific sport environment (i.e., bitterness, incompetence; Connelly, 1992) might transfer to perceptions of physical activity as a whole. Consequently, the purpose of the present study was to examine the general perceptions of physical activity held by higher and lower status members of youth sport teams. In addition, non-athletes were examined as a third comparison group.

Given the relative focus of the present study on attitudes toward physical activity and perceptions of competence, the Theory of Planned Behavior (TPB; Ajzen, 1991) was utilized as the underlying framework. The TPB highlights that a direct determinant of an individual's behavior is his/her intention to engage in the behavior. In addition, intentions are derived from an individual's (a) attitude (a product of his or her behavioral beliefs), (b) perceptions of the subjective norm (a product of normative beliefs or beliefs about the expectations of others), and perceived behavioral control (a product of control beliefs). Perceived behavioral control can also directly affect behavior without the presence of intention.

The TPB has been utilized successfully as a framework to understand physical activity behavior. Armitage and Conner (2001) reviewed 161 articles with 185 independent tests in a meta-analysis of the TPB. These studies contained both self-reported behavior measures and independently or objectively rated behavior measures. It was found that the TPB accounted for 39% of the variance in intention, and 27% of the variance in behavior. In a meta-analysis of the TPB with exercise behavior, Godin and Kok (1996) concluded that 42% of the variance in intentions and 36% of the variance in behavior was explained by TPB variables. Important for the present study, the utility of the TPB has also been tested within the context of youth exercise behavior. For example, Mummery, Spence, and Hudec (2000) examined exercise behaviors using TPB variables with Canadian youth from Grades 3 to 11. Results indicated that TPB constructs explained 47% of the variance in intention. Similar findings have been found in other exercise (e.g., Rivis and Sheeran, 2003) and sport studies with youth (e.g., Nache, Bar-Eli, Perrin, and Laurencelle, 2005).

The aforementioned status research allows for the development of specific hypotheses regarding how perceptions of each component of the TPB could be different for starting athletes, non-starting athletes, and non-athletes. First, based on research by Gruber and Gray (1982) indicating that low status athletes had lower levels of satisfaction with their contribution to the team and lower affiliation desire, it was expected that their general attitudes towards physical activity would also be lower than those of high status athletes. Second, Connelly's (1992) descriptions of challenges for low status athletes such as feeling incompetent and perceptions that they will never improve provide support for a hypothesis that low status athletes will hold lower perceptions of perceived behavioral control than would high status athletes. Third, given that low status athletes receive limited playing time and may have negative perceptions of their sport experiences (e.g., Gruber and Gray, 1982), it was hypothesized that low status athletes would hold lower perceptions of intentions, and participate in less actual physical activity (i.e., moderate and vigorous physical activity) than would high status athletes. Fourth, due to their lack of experience in organized physical activity environments, non-athletes were hypothesized to hold the lowest perceptions of physical activity (i.e., attitudes, subjective norms, perceived behavioral control, intentions), as well as participate in the lowest amount of actual overall physical activity (i.e., moderate and vigorous physical activity levels). Finally, due to the lack of empirical research, no a priori hypothesis specific to differences between starting and non-starting athletes was generated regarding subjective norm.

Methods

Participants

As part of a larger project, the general target population was students making the academic transition between elementary (Grade Eight) and high school levels (Grade Nine) within a Northern Ontario (Canada) municipality. Specific to the present study, participants of interest were Grade Eight students from six Northern Ontario elementary schools who returned a signed parent/guardian informed consent form. The mean age of participants was 13.51 years ($SD= .57$). Included in the analysis were 42 starting/high status athletes, 16 non-starting/low status athletes, and 21 non-athletes. Of the 58 athletes, the majority (29.63%) listed soccer as their favorite or most important current sport team. This was followed by basketball and volleyball (16.67% each), hockey (12.97%), baseball/softball (7.41%), football (5.55%), track and field (3.70%), and swimming, dance, canoe club, and tae kwon doe (1.85% each). Gender balance was approximately even ($n_{males} = 40$; $n_{females} = 39$).

Measures

Demographic information. Demographic information was obtained from participants regarding age, gender, socioeconomic status, and secondary school (i.e., high school) they planned to attend.

Physical activity information. The 3-Day Physical Activity Recall (3DPAR) is a self-report questionnaire that was utilized to examine physical activity behavior. It is an extension of the Previous Day Physical Activity Recall (PDPAR; Weston, Petosa, and Pate, 1997) and has been utilized in previous research examining youth physical activity (e.g., Trost et al., 2002). The questionnaire was administered on a Wednesday so that information on the previous three days included a weekend day and two weekdays (i.e., Sunday, Monday, and Tuesday). A list of 55 activities grouped into eating, work, after-school/spare time/hobbies, transportation, sleep/bathing, school, and physical activities/sports were displayed in a numbered list. Each day was scheduled into 30 minute timeblocks in which participants recorded the identification number of their predominant activity during that time. In addition, graphics and definitions were provided on this measure for light activities, moderate activities, hard activities, and very hard activities. Consequently, for each 30 minute increment, participants also checked off the corresponding intensity level (i.e., light, moderate, hard, very hard). Utilizing the guidelines of classification of energy costs of human physical activities proposed by Ainsworth et al. (1993), each timeblock's activity and corresponding intensity level were used to derive a metabolic equivalent (MET) value. Average daily moderate physical activity was calculated by counting the total number of timeblocks indicating activity at a level greater than 3 METs but less than 6 METs and dividing by three. Average daily vigorous physical activity was calculated by counting the total number of timeblocks indicating activity at a level greater than 6 METs and dividing by three. Total average physical activity per day was also calculated (i.e., average blocks per day with > 3 METs). This analytical procedure has been utilized in previous studies examining youth physical activity (e.g., Pate et al., 2005; Trost et al., 2002). Overall, this questionnaire has been validated by comparison with accelerometer-derived count variables (Pfeiffer et al., 2006). Furthermore, it has been indicated that the 3DPAR is a suitable measurement tool for monitoring and surveillance of various adolescent groups (e.g., Lee and Trost, 2005).

Theory of Planned Behavior variables. As outlined above, self-reported physical activity behaviors were obtained from the 3DPAR. Attitudes toward physical activity, subjective norms, perceived behavioral control, and intentions to be physically active were measured with items utilized in past exercise research (e.g., Rhodes and Courneya, 2003) that conform to the suggestions of Ajzen (1991). Specifically, six questions were asked related to physical activity attitudes. These were scored on a seven point Likert-type scale ranging from -3 to +3. An example item would be "I feel that my participating in physical activity at the present time is..." with responses ranging from "useless" (-3), to "useful" (+3). One question (i.e., "Most people who are important to me think I should participate in physical activity on a regular basis") was asked that pertained to the subjective norms component of the TPB, and was scored on a seven point Likert-type scale from strongly disagree (1) to strongly agree (7). Four items were adapted from the Lifestyle Education for Activity Programming (LEAP) II survey (2002) that pertained to the perceived behavioral control component of the TPB. These items were scored on a five point Likert-type scale from 1 (very easy) to 5 (very difficult). An example of a question was "For me to be physically active during my free time on most days would be...". Finally, an additional four questions were adapted from the LEAP II Survey (2002) with regard to intentions for future physical activity. These items were scored on a five point Likert-type scale from disagree a lot (1) to agree a lot (5). An example of a question was "I intend to be physically active during my free time on most days."

Sport team participation information. This section contained three questions that asked participants to list (a) the organized sport teams they were currently involved with, as well as their position and starting status (i.e., the degree to which they contribute to team output; starting athlete/high status or non-starting athlete/low status) on these respective teams, listing their most important team first, (b) the organized sport teams they had been involved with in the past 12 months, as well as the position and starting status on these respective teams, and (c) the organized sport teams they planned to participate on in Grade Nine following the transition to high school. It is important to note that classification of starting status was based upon how each participant responded with regard to their starting status on his/her most important current team (i.e., starting athlete/high status or non-starting athlete/low status.)

Procedure

Initial contact was made with principals of each elementary school following ethical approval from both the authors' university's Research Ethics Board and the public school district. Subsequent to obtaining permission from each school's principal, parental consent forms were distributed to Grade Eight students. Approximately three to four weeks prior to Grade Eight graduation, each student who returned a signed parental consent form was given a package containing the previously mentioned questionnaires to complete during class time on a Wednesday (to accommodate the 3DPAR questionnaire). Students took approximately 30 minutes to complete the questionnaires.

Results

Descriptive Statistics

The means and standard deviations for the total sample and subsamples (i.e., high status athletes, low status athletes, and non-athletes) are presented in Table 1. It is evident that scores for the TPB variables (i.e., attitudes, subjective norms, perceived behavioral control, intentions) are relatively high for each group. Specifically, the mean responses for TPB variables of the overall sample, high status athletes, low status athletes, and non-athletes were well above the median for each respective scale. The mean scores for attitude (-3 to +3 scale range) for the different samples ranged from 1.90 to 2.64. Perceptions of the subjective norm ranged from 5.33 to 6.19. Perceived behavioral control ranged from 4.13 to 4.51. Intentions to be physically active ranged from 3.90 to 4.45. As anticipated, high status athletes had the highest mean scores, followed by low status athletes, and non-athletes for each TPB variable with the exception of subjective norms, on which low status athletes scored slightly higher than high status athletes. Mean scores for physical activity variables (i.e., moderate, vigorous, and total) indicated that the overall sample participated in physical activity an average of 7.02 timeblocks per day. High status athletes had the highest mean *total physical activity* per day (M = 7.65), followed by non-athletes (M = 6.69) and non-starters (M = 6.33). Moderate physical activity levels followed a rather different pattern of results with non-athletes engaging in the most amount of activity at this level (M = 4.69) followed by low status (M = 3.69) and high status athletes (M = 3.57). Finally, the opposite pattern occurred for vigorous physical activity, with high status athletes having the highest mean (M = 4.08), followed by low status athletes (M = 2.65) and non-athletes (M = 2.00).

Table 1. Descriptive Statistics for the Total Sample and the Status Levels

Variable	Total Sample	High Status	Low Status	Non-athlete
Attitudes	2.42 ± 0.70	2.64 ± 0.39	2.44 ± 0.74	1.90 ± 0.93
Subjective Norms	5.93 ± 1.24	6.10 ± 1.30	6.19 ± 0.91	5.33 ± 1.32
Perceived Behavioral Control	4.35 ± 0.59	4.51 ± 0.46	4.28 ± 0.58	4.13 ± 0.71
Intentions	4.23 ± 0.81	4.45 ± 0.73	4.17 ± 0.78	3.90 ± 0.84
Moderate Physical Activity	3.87 ± 2.91	3.57 ± 2.66	3.69 ± 2.57	4.70 ± 3.57
Vigorous Physical Activity	3.19 ± 2.71	4.08 ± 2.73	2.65 ± 2.22	2.00 ± 2.47
Total Physical Activity	7.06 ± 3.70	7.65 ± 3.47	6.33 ± 2.83	6.69 ± 4.55

Inter-correlations between study variables are presented in Table 2 for the total sample, and separately for the specific sub-samples (i.e., high status athletes, low status athletes, and non-athletes). Of particular importance to note was that in accordance with the TPB, attitudes, subjective norms, and perceived behavioral control were all significantly correlated ($p < .01$) with intentions to be physically active.

Also, perceived behavioral control and intentions were significantly correlated with vigorous physical activity levels.

Table 2. Correlations for Study Variables

Variable	Attitudes	SN	PBC	Intentions	MPA	VPA	TPA
Attitudes (T)	-	.34**	.56**	.60**	-.11	.38**	.20
HS	-	(.37*)	(.46**)	(.48**)	(-.04)	(.30*)	(.20)
LS	-	(.12)	(.67**)	(.76**)	(.09)	(.39)	(.38)
NA	-	(.34)	(.51*)	(.65**)	(-.09)	(.32)	(.10)
SN (T)		-	.26*	.41**	-.08	.25*	.127
HS		-	(.12)	(.40**)	(-.22)	(.20)	(-.01)
LS		-	(.37)	(.30)	(-.14)	(.24)	(.06)
NA		-	(.32)	(.39)	(.29)	(.21)	(.34)
PBC (T)			-	.64**	.04	.36**	.30**
HS			-	(.48*)	(.09)	(.23)	(.24)
LS			-	(.93**)	(.07)	(.42)	(.39)
NA			-	(.66**)	(.09)	(.37)	(.28)
Intentions (T)				-	.05	.46**	.37**
HS				-	(.16)	(.43**)	(.45**)
LS				-	(.05)	(.47)	(.41)
NA				-	(.05)	(.33)	(.22)
MPA (T)					-	-.13	.70**
HS					-	(-.14)	(.64**)
LS					-	(-.31)	(.67**)
NA					-	(.11)	(.84**)
VPA (T)						-	.63**
HS						-	(.68**)
LS						-	(.50*)
NA						-	(.63**)
TPA (T)							-
HS							-
LS							-
NA							-

Note. SN: subjective norms, PBC: perceived behavioral control, MPA: moderate physical activity, VPA: vigorous physical activity, TPA: total physical activity, T: total sample, HS: high status athlete, LS: low status athlete, NA: non-athlete.
$*p < .05. **p < .01.$

However, neither of these variables was significantly correlated with moderate physical activity levels.

Starting Status and Physical Activity Perceptions

Prior to reporting further results, it should be noted that the data were screened for missing data and the assumptions of normality and homogeneity of variance necessary for MANOVA were satisfied. A multivariate analysis of variance (MANOVA) was performed to identify potential differences among status levels (i.e. high status athlete/low status athlete/non-athlete) with regard to variables in the TPB (i.e., attitudes, subjective norms, perceived behavioral control, intentions), and physical activity levels (i.e., moderate, vigorous, total). The omnibus MANOVA was significant, Wilks' $\lambda = .69$, $F(14,140) = 2.02$, $p < .05$, $\eta^2 = .17$, indicating that significant differences did exist among status levels. Further univariate analyses of variance (ANOVA) were performed with sport status as the independent variable (three levels: high status athlete, low status athlete, and non-athlete) and attitudes, subjective norms, perceived behavioral control, intentions, moderate physical activity per day, vigorous physical activity per day, and total physical activity per day as the dependent variables. No significant differences were found among groups for subjective norms, moderate physical activity, and total physical activity. However, significant differences between groups were found with regard to attitudes, $F(2,76) = 8.98$, $p < .001$, $\eta^2 = .19$, intentions, $F(2,76) = 3.64$, $p < .05$, $\eta^2 = .09$, perceived behavioral control, $F(2,76) = 3.46$, $p < .05$, $\eta^2 = .08$, and vigorous physical activity levels, $F(2,76) = 5.14$, $p < .01$, $\eta^2 = .12$. Further post-hoc tests indicated that the significant differences ($p < .05$) between status levels for the above variables existed between high status athletes and non-athletes for attitudes, intentions, perceived behavioral control, and vigorous physical activity.

Discussion

The primary purpose of the present study was to compare high status athletes, low status athletes, and non-athletes with regard to their perceptions (i.e., TPB variables; attitudes, subjective norms, perceived behavioral control, intentions) and behaviors (i.e., moderate, vigorous, and total physical activity levels) related to physical activity. A number of issues pertaining to the results of the study warrant further discussion.

The first issue was the consistent trend of high status athletes having more positive perceptions of attitudes towards physical activity, perceived behavioral control, and intentions to be physically active followed in turn by low status athletes and then non-athletes. From a statistical standpoint, post-hoc analyses indicated that high status athletes had significantly higher mean values of these variables only in comparison to non-athletes. Non-starting athletes did not differ statistically from either of the other groups. One possible explanation for the lack of significant difference between low status athletes from both high status athletes and non-athletes could be sample size, as there was an under representation of low status athletes in comparison to the other groups. Regardless, the trends in the data and differences found between starting athletes and non-athletes offer partial support for our initial hypotheses.

A second issue that should be discussed is the differences in physical activity levels among the status levels. As was expected, *vigorous* physical levels were highest among high status athletes, followed by low status athletes and non-athletes. Granted, similar to the previous paragraph, significant differences were only found between starting athletes and non-athletes. Interestingly, while not statistically significant, the opposite pattern existed with regard to the calculated moderate physical activity levels, as they were highest for non-athletes, followed by low status athletes, with high status athletes having the lowest levels of moderate physical activity. This potentially indicates that the sport environment is conducive to encouraging physical activity that is vigorous to its participants.

While the results offer some support for our original hypotheses, a third issue pertaining to measurement centers on the relatively high physical activity levels that could be interpreted from responses given to the 3-Day Physical Activity Recall questionnaire. The overall sample indicated an average of 7.02 thirty minute time blocks per day in which they were physically active (i.e., > 3 METs). If taken literally, this potentially indicates that participants would have been physically active an average of 210 minutes per day. This is obviously well above reported physical activity levels for youth in recent years both in general (e.g., only 21% of Canadian youth are accumulating enough daily activity to meet international guidelines; Cameron, Craig, and Paolin, 2005) and in relation to previous results with the 3-day Physical Activity Recall questionnaire (e.g., Trost et al, 2002; overall sample was considered low active with less than four physically active blocks per day). One potential reason for this could be that participants were asked to respond regarding the "main" activity that they were involved in during the thirty minute timeblock. Thus, for example, a participant that had a fifteen minute walk to and from school may have reported walking as their main activity in one thirty minute timeblock and checked off "moderate" or "vigorous" as the corresponding intensity level. Given that they would take the walk to and from school potentially four times per day (including going home at lunch hour), this leaves a complete hour of actual *inactivity* recorded as being physically active (i.e., essentially doubling the actual physical activity participation). Another potential reason for the high levels of physical activity reported could be that participants may have assumed that just because an activity is classified as a sport, that it is continuously physically active. For example, swimming may have been recorded as the dominant activity from 1:00 p.m. to 4:00 p.m. on a Sunday afternoon, with the corresponding intensity level as "vigorous" for the three hour period. Although technically swimming for the three hours, they may have been engaging periodically in a relatively less active behavior (e.g., floating on a raft, standing in shallow water, etc.). A final possibility for the reporting of elevated levels of physical activity is social desirability. Participants were cognizant of the fact that this was a study on sport and physical activity participation and may have reported exaggerated levels of physical activity. However, while the issue of the literal translation of approximately seven 30 minute timeblocks is raised in this section, it should also be noted that this questionnaire has been successfully validated against other behavioral measures (i.e., pedometers; Lee and Trost, 2005).

A fourth issue that should be highlighted is the method by which perceptions housed under the general Theory of Planned Behavior (TPB) were analyzed. Due to the sample size in two of the groups (i.e., non-starters and non-athletes), the statistical decision was to take a between groups approach; in essence, examining mean differences. However, another approach would be to examine the salience of various relationships among variables in the

TPB overall and separately for each of the groups. Essentially, an ideal analysis would be to examine whether sport status *moderates* specific relationships within the conceptual model. At a general level, the present study provided some additional support for the TPB, particularly in terms of the significant correlations of intentions with attitudes, subjective norms, and perceived behavioral control in the total sample. Also within the total sample, intentions were significantly correlated with vigorous physical activity levels and total physical activity levels. More interesting, from a post-hoc perspective, when correlations were compared between the status levels, it appears that there are differences between the groups, particularly with regard to the perceived behavioral control and intention relationship. The correlation between perceived behavioral control and intention in low status athletes was highest ($r = .93$), followed by non-athletes ($r = .68$), and high-status athletes ($r = .32$). This gives the impression that it may be more important to develop perceptions of control among low status athletes in order for them to have greater intentions to engage in physical activity, whereas this occurs to a lesser degree in non-athletes and high status athletes. Again, due to limited sample size, this suggestion is somewhat speculative but could serve as a basis for future research as this pattern is in alignment with previous suggestions that low status athletes have particular struggles with perceived competence (Connelly, 1992).

Recommendations for Practitioners

The practical implications of this study extend to two primary contexts that exist within the daily lives of youth. First, the potential importance of sport status to levels of physical activity in youth can be recognized by the education system through the development of athletic programs that foster participation and encourage all athletes to contribute equally. Intramural programs may be ideal, particularly for lower status athletes, as they would have equal opportunity for vigorous physical activity participation regardless of their skill level and corresponding status.

A second implication is that identification of specific differences in the physical activity perceptions and patterns of low status athletes can be applied to the context of youth competitive sport. Previous researchers have suggested that role-related interventions may have the potential to increase role clarity and role acceptance in low status athletes (e.g., goal-setting programs, Carron, Hausenblas, and Eys, 2005). Perhaps these interventions, and the corresponding potential increase in satisfaction with the sport environment, will allow low status athletes to increase positive perceptions and levels of physical activity.

Recommendations for Researchers

Future research should address several possible limitations and directions. First, the present study had unequal numbers of high status, low status, and non-athletes. Low status athletes may under-report due to the presence of role ambiguity (i.e., the participant is unclear of their sport status), embarrassment, or social desirability. There is a negative stigma associated with being a low status or non-starting athlete and participants may be hesitant to report holding this role. A consideration for future research may be to examine the under-representation of this population by looking into role interventions to increase the role satisfaction and role acceptance levels of low status athletes, particularly for youth athletes. This may provide an opportunity for more pride in the role, and consequently, a higher likelihood that they will report their role as a low status athlete.

A second area for future research would be to consider the timing of data collection. In the present study, the data was collected in elementary schools during the months of May and June. Future research would be well-directed to choose other time periods as many teachers, parents, and students expressed a lack of interest in additional administrative tasks (i.e., signing consent forms) during the final weeks of the academic year, and thus had a direct impact on the sample size of the current study. Related to this issue of timing, the present study did not address changes in physical activity patterns over time. Physical activity participation could potentially change weekly or seasonally. Future researchers could incorporate repeated measures of physical activity over time in order to gain a more precise representation of overall physical activity.

In conclusion, the well-documented elevated level of physical inactivity and sport disengagement for youth (e.g. Petlichkoff, 1996; Tremblay et al., 2002), despite its numerous health benefits (e.g., reduction of heart disease; USDHHS, 2000), necessitates the analysis of potential reasons why this is the case. Sport status was identified as a potential influence on youth physical activity perceptions and patterns and future researchers should continue to measure the effects of status on physical activity, with specific emphasis on interventions to foster satisfaction within the sport environment for low status athletes during this critical time of their development.

Authors' Note

This project was funded through a SSHRC Canada Graduate Scholarship awarded to the first author. The authors are grateful for the program's support.

References

Ainsworth, B. E., Haskell, W. L., Leon, A. S., Jacobs Jr., D.R., Montoye, H. J., Sallis, J. F. et al. (1993). Compendium of physical activities: Classification of energy costs of human physical activities. *Medicine and Science in Sports and Exercise, 25,* 71-80.

Ajzen, I. (1991). The theory of planned behavior. *Organizational Behavior and Planned Decision Processes. Special Issue: Theories of Cognitive Self-Regulation, 50,* 179-211.

Armitage, C. J., and Conner, M. (2001). Efficacy of the theory of planned behavior: A meta-analytic review. *British Journal of Social Psychology, 40,* 471-499.

Baranowski, T., Mendlein, J., Resnicow, K., Frank, E., Cullen, K. W., Baranowski, J. (2000). Physical activity and nutrition in children and youth: An overview of obesity prevention. *Preventive Medicine, 31,* 1-10.

Beauchamp, M. R., Bray, S. R., Eys, M. A., and Carron, A. V. (2005). Leadership behaviors and multidimensional role ambiguity perceptions in team sports. *Small Group Research, 36,* 5-20.

Bergeles, N., and Hatziharistos, D. (2003). Interpersonal attraction as a measure of estimation of cohesiveness in elite volleyball teams. *Perceptual and Motor Skills, 96,* 81-91.

Britsch, B. M. (2000). The effect of sport participation on female adolescents' gender-role identity and self-concept: The role of motivation, ability, persistence, and team membership. *Dissertation Abstracts International, 61,* 560B.

Cameron, C., Craig, C. L., and Paolin, S. (2005). *Local opportunities for physical activity and sport: Trends from 1999 – 2004.* Ottawa, ON: Canadian Fitness and Lifestyle Research Institute.

Carron, A. V., Hausenblas, H. A., and Eys, M. A. (2005). *Group dynamics in sport* (3rd ed.). Morgantown, WV: Fitness Information Technology.

Connelly, D. (1992). The benchwarmer. *Performance Edge. The Letter of Performance Psychology,* 2.

Daniels, S. R. (2006). The consequences of childhood obesity. *The Future of Children, 16,* 47-67.

Donaldson, S. J., and Ronan, K. R. (2006). The effects of sports participation on young adolescents' emotional well-being. *Adolescence, 41,* 369-389.

Fredricks, J. A., and Eccles, J. S. (2006). Is extracurricular participation associated with beneficial outcomes. *Developmental Psychology, 42,* 698-713.

Godin, G., and Kok, G. (1996). The theory of planned behavior: A review of its application to health-related behaviors. *American Journal of Health Promotion, 11,* 87-98.

Gould, D., Feltz, D., Horn, T., and Weiss, M. (1982). Reasons for attrition in competitive youth swimming. *Journal of Sport Behavior, 5,* 155-165.

Gould, D., and Petlichkoff, L. (1988). Participation motivation and attrition in young athletes. In F. Smoll, R. Magill, and M. Ash (Eds.), *Children in sport* (3rd ed., pp. 161-178). Champaign, IL: Human Kinetics.

Granito, V. J., and Rainey, D. W. (1988). Differences in cohesion between high school and college football teams and between starters and nonstarters. *Perceptual and Motor Skills, 66,* 471-477.

Gruber, J. J., and Gray, G. R. (1982). Responses to forces influencing cohesion as a function of player status and level of male varsity basketball competition. *Research Quarterly, 53,* 27-36.

Hagar, R. L. (2006). Television viewing and physical activity in children. *Journal of Adolescent Health, 35,* 656-661.

Harper, M. G. (2006). Childhood obesity: Strategies for prevention. *Family and Community Health, 29,* 288-298.

Jacob, C. S., and Carron, A. V. (1994). Sources of status in intercollegiate sport teams. *Journal of Sport and Exercise Psychology, 16,* S67.

Jacob Johnson, C. S. (2004, Summer). Status in sport teams: Myth or reality? *International Sports Journal,* 55-64.

Katzmarzyk, P. T., and Janssen, I. (2004). The economic costs associated with physical inactivity and obesity in Canada: An update. *Canadian Journal of Applied Physiology, 29,* 90-115.

Lee, K. S., and Trost, S. G. (2005). Validity and reliability of the 3-Day Physical Activity Recall in Singaporean adolescents. *Research Quarterly for Exercise and Sport, 76,* 101-106.

Marsh, H. W., and Kleitman, S. (2003). School athletic participation: Mostly gain with little pain. *Journal of Sport and Exercise Psychology, 25,* 205-228.

McHale, J. P., Vinden, P. G., Bush, L., Richer, D., Shaw, D., and Smith, B. (2005). Patterns of personal and social adjustment of sport-involved and non-involved urban middle-school children. *Sociology of Sport Journal, 22,* 119-136.

Mummery, W. K., Spence, J. C., and Hudec, J. C. (2000). Understanding physical activity intention in Canadian school children and youth: An application of the theory of planned behavior. *Research Quarterly in Exercise and Sport, 71,* 116-124.

Nache, C. M., Bar-Eli, M., Perrin, C., and Laurencelle, L. (2005). Predicting dropout in male youth soccer using the theory of planned behavior. *Scandinavian Journal of Medicine and Science in Sports, 15,* 188-197.

Nelson, M. C., and Gordon-Larsen, P. (2006). Physical activity and sedentary behavior patterns are associated with selected adolescent health risk behaviors. *Pediatrics, 117,* 1281-1290.

Pate, R. R., Ward, D. S., Saunders, R. P., Felton, G., Dishman, R. K., and Dowda, M. (2005). Promotion of physical activity among high-school girls: A randomized controlled trial. *American Journal of Public Health, 95,* 1582-1587.

Petlickhkoff, L. M. (1996). The drop-out dilemma in youth sports. In O. Bar-Or (Ed.), *The child and adolescent athlete* (pp. 418-430). Cambridge, MA: Blackwell Science.

Pfeiffer, K. A., Dowda, M., Dishman, R. K., McIver, K. L, Sirad, J. R., Ward, D. S., et al. (2006). Sport participation and physical activity in adolescent females across a four year period. *Journal of Adolescent Health, 39,* 523-529.

Rhodes, R. E., and Courneya, K. S. (2003). Investigating multiple components of attitude, subjective norm, and perceived control: An examination of the theory of planned behavior in the exercise domain. *British Journal of Social Psychology, 42,* 129-146.

Rivis, A. and Sheeran, P. (2003). Social influences and the theory of planned behavior: Evidence for a direct relationship between prototypes and young people's exercise behavior. *Psychology and Health, 18,* 567-583.

Robinson, T. T., and Carron, A. V. (1982). Personal and situational factors associated with dropping out versus maintaining participation in competitive sport. *Journal of Sport Psychology, 4,* 364-378.

Seefeldt, V. D., and Ewing, M. E. (1997). Youth sports in America: An overview. *President's Council on Physical Fitness and Sports Research Digest, 2*(11).

Smith, A. L. (2007). Youth peer relationships in sport. In S. Jowett and D. Lavallee (Eds.), *Social Psychology in Sport* (pp. 41-54). Champaign, IL: Human Kinetics. Statistics Canada (2005). *Canadian Community Health Survey: Obesity among children and adults.* Ottawa, ON: Author.

Taras, H. (2005). Physical activity and student performance at school. *Journal of School Health, 75,* 214-218.

Teevan, R. C., and Yalof, J. (1980). Need for achievement in "starting" and in "non-starting" varsity athletes. *Perceptual and Motor Skills, 50,* 402.

Tremblay, M. S., Katzmarzyk, P. T., and Wilms, J. D. (2002). Temporal trends in overweight and obesity in Canada, 1981-1996. *International Journal of Obesity and Related Metabolic Disorders: Journal of the International Association for the Study of Obesity, 26,* 538-543.

Trost, S. G., Pate, R. R., Dowda, M., Ward, D. S., Felton, G., and Saunders, R. (2002). Psychosocial correlates of physical activity in White and African-American girls. *Journal of Adolescent Health, 31,* 226-233.

U.S. Department of Health and Human Services (2000). *Healthy people 2010* (Conference edition, in two vols.). Washington, DC: Author.

Utter, J., Denny, S., Robinson, E. M., Ameratunga, S., and Watson, P. (2006). Perceived access to community facilities, social motivation, and physical activity among New Zealand youth. *Journal of Adolescent Health, 39,* 770-773.

Weiss, M. R., and Chaumeton, N. (1992). Motivational orientations in sport. In T. Horn (Ed.), *Advances in sport psychology* (pp.61-99). Champaign, IL: Human Kinetics.

Weiss, M. R., Smith, A. L., and Theeboom, M. (1996). "That's what friends are for": Children's and teenagers' perceptions of peer relationships in the sport domain. *Journal of Sport and Exercise Psychology, 18,* 347-379.

Weston, A. T., Petosa, R., and Pate, R. R. (1997). Validity of an instrument for measurement of physical activity in youth. *Medical Science Sports Exercise, 29,* 138-143.

Yin, Z., and Moore, J. B. (2004). Re-examining the role of interscholastic sport participation in education. *Psychological Reports, 94,* 1447-1454.

In: Sport and Exercise Psychology Research Advances   ISBN: 978-1-60456-157-9
Editors: M. P. Simmons, L. A. Foster, pp. 345-360   © 2008 Nova Science Publishers, Inc.

Chapter XVI

Regular Exercise May Reduce Oxidative Damage Induced by Psychological Stress

M. Rosety-Rodriguez[18], I. Rosety and F.J. Ordonez

School of Sports Medicine. University of Cadiz. Spain
Pza. Fragela s/n 11003 Cadiz. Spain

Abstract

It is generally accepted emotional stress may increase the risk of several diseases such as arrhythmia, myocardial ischemia, cancer, chronic inflammatory diseases, immunodeficiency, etc.. However the mechanisms regarding how emotional stress causes disruption of homeostasis are complex and remain unclear.

Recent studies have reported it may be explained, at least in part, since psychological stress may change the balance between pro-oxidant and antioxidant factors, inducing oxidative damage. Further, "unhealthy" lifestyle factors such as smoking, sedentary, low-fruit consumption, among others, may be pointed out as potential targets by health care professionals since it was reported a significant synergistic influence on the decrease in the antioxidant capacity when combined to emotional stress.

On the contrary, physical activity is recognized as an important component of a healthy life style and consequently is highly recommended by scientists and clinicians. This finding may be explained at least in part, since regular exercise may improve redox metabolism by increasing significantly antioxidant defense system. At the present moment, this field is at an exciting stage. And fortunately, ample evidence of this progress can be found in the literature.

In this line, several studies focused on the management of emotionally stressed animals concluded regular exercise improved their redox metabolism. In humans, long-term aerobic training program at low-moderate intensity increased significantly both enzymatic and non-enzymatic antioxidant systems. Conversely, short-term supramaximal anaerobic exercise increased significantly lipid, protein and DNA oxidation whose evaluation may provide a significant clue to the magnitude of oxidative damage.

18 Tel. +34 956 01 52 01, Fax: +34 956 01 52 54, Email: manuel.rosetyrodriguez@uca.es.

To explain the double role of physical activity, existing data indicated on one hand that, moderate long-term exercise may cause adaptation of the antioxidant and repair systems, which could result in a decreased base level of oxidative damage and increased resistance to oxidative stress. On the other hand, a single bout of vigorous exercise result in oxidative damage as a sign of incomplete adaptation.

Consequently, in order to be effective and healthy, these intervention programs based on physical activity should be adequately designed and supervised during their application by a multidisciplinary team of healthcare professionals, psychologist, bachelor's degree on exercise science, etc.

I. Emotional Stress is Associated with Oxidative Stress

Psychological stress is supposed to be one of the major ailments that undermine individuals in both their professional and private lifes (Christen 2003; Wang et al. 2007).

Accordingly, it has been shown that emotional stress may increase the risk of several diseases. In this respect, it may induce myocardial ischemia and ventricular arrhythmias in patients with coronary artery diseases (Santana et al. 2003). It may also play a critical role in the origin of cancer as was reported by Bultz et al. (2005), mainly if we take into account it modulates immune response (Liu et al. 2005).

Further it may have adverse implications both on health and performance in athletes (Hanton et al. 2005; Ress et al. 2007).

However the mechanisms regarding how emotional stress causes disruption of homeostasis are complex and remain unclear. Recent studies have reported it may be explained, at least in part, since psychological stress may change the balance between pro-oxidant and antioxidant factors, inducing oxidative damage (Boden-Albala and Sacco 2000; Chalmers et al. 2003).

Immobilization is widely employed to provoke psychological stress since it is less harmful than other stressors such as burn shocks or cold-restraint (Retana-Marquez et al. 2003). It has been believed to be stressful because it produces a variety of physiological disturbances such as increases of corticosterone, ACTH and catecholamine levels in serum as well as abnormal behaviours such as aggressiveness, hyperlocomotion and anxiety-like bahaviours (Chakraborti et al. 2007; Gavrilovic and Dronjak 2005; Gregus et al. 2005; Weiss et al. 2004; Wood et al. 2003).

Further, it was also demonstrated that immobilization was associated with oxidative damage in rats. In this respect, it was reported immobilization leads to formation of free radicals such as superoxide radical, hydroxyl radical, and peroxynitrite, among others, ready to attack biomacromolecules. In addition it was also found levels of malondialdehyde (MDA) and carbonyl groups were significantly increased what suggested lipd and protein oxidation after immobilization (Fontella et al. 2005; Rosety-Rodriguez et al. 2006a).

Evidence linking psychological stress to oxidative damage continues to grow not only in animals but also in humans. In fact, emotional stress was the lifestyle factor that was most markedly associated with a decreased antioxidant capacity (Lesgards et al. 2002).

For example, cardiac surgery represents a major mental stress associated with an increased production of reactive oxygen species that may finally hamper post-operative recovery, increasing hospitalisation times and operative mortality. As a consequence Hadj et al. (2006) conducted a quality assurance and feasibility study to evaluate and monitor the safety and efficacy of a new program of combined pre-operative metabolic (enhanced antioxidant), physical and mental therapy to counter psychological stress prior to cardiac surgery obtaining excellent results.

Mental stress in daily life may also contribute to oxidative stress. Accordingly, Eskiocak et al. (2003) and Sivonova et al. (2004) reported that during university examinations students are under increased oxidative stress. Similarly, burnout seems to involve enhanced oxidative stress among workers (Grossi et al. 2003).

Regarding athletes, who are under severe physiological and psychological stress, the delicate balance between pro-oxidants and antioxidants may be altered increasing the risk of infections (Malm 2006) and sport-related injuries (Atalay et al. 2006). Consquently, supplementation of antioxidants may be desirable under certain physiological and psychological conditions by providing a larger protective margin (Clarckson and Thompson 2000). And not only in professional athletes but also in amateur ones (Reichhart et al. 2003).

Although mechanisms underlying psychological stress related oxidant stress remained to be thoroughly investigated, psychological stress may be considered an appropriate target to promote the health of western population. And consequently, future studies are required for assessing the preventive potentiality of healthy tools such as regular exercise against oxidative damage induced by psychological stress.

For the reasons already mentioned the present chapter entitled "Regular exercise may reduce oxidative damage induced by psychological stress" was performed to support these findings.

II. Psychological Stress may be Associated with other Pro-Oxidant Lifestyle Factors

Regarding the maintenance of an adequate antioxidant homeostasis it is possible to define a "healthy" and "unhealthy" lifestyle patterns.

In this line, recent studies have reported that emotional stress was the lifestyle factor most markedly associated with a decreased antioxidant capacity (Bultz and Carlson, 2005; Irie et al. 2002; Wang et al. 2007). Conversely having no stress at work or at home was weak but significantly related to a high antioxidant defense capacity (Lesgards et al. 2002).

According to the literature several factors have also increased oxidative damage such as: smoking, sedentary habit, low fruit consumption, chronic alcohol consumption, sun exposure, among others (Mimura et al. 2007; Ozbay and Dulger 2002). The most striking feature is that these behaviours have been significantly associated to psychologic stress (Lesgards et al. 2002).

Smoking

In a more detailed way, previous studies have reported a lower antioxidant status and higher lipid peroxidation product levels in plasma of smokers when compared to nonsmokers. Furthermore, pro-oxidant compounds such as nicotine has been involved in atherogenesis through oxidative modification of low density lipoproteins and in lung cancer through oxidation and nitrosation of DNA and other cellular components (Ayaori et al. 2001; Dietrich et al. 2003; Irie et al. 2002; Kim et al. 2003). In any case it should be emphasized it was reported not only in active smokers but also in passive ones (Ayaori et al. 2001). Further the negative contributions regarding antioxidant capacity of low fruit consumption, sedentary habits and regular UltraViolet (UV) exposure tended to be higher in smokers than in non-smokers (Lesgards et al. 2002; Irie et al. 2002).

On the other side, nonsmoking was highly positively related to the antioxidant potential. In short, it is conceivable that whereas nonsmoking strengthened the overall antioxidant defense system, smoking impaired this antiradical defense system.

Low Fruit Consumption

Nutritional habits may also play an important role in redox metabolism since the capacity to enhance antioxidant defense, specially in the forms of vitamins C, E and B or even magnesium, depends on the diet (Anlasik et al. 2005; Kiefer et al. 2004).

However whereas low fruit and vegetable consumption is probably linearly related to a decreased individual antioxidant capacity, it was only reported a weak relation between high intake and increased antioxidant potential (Crujeiras et al. 2006). These results suggested that it was easier to reduce antioxidant defense system by reducing antioxidant intake than to strengthen this system by increasing dietary antioxidants. Several authors concluded to enhance antioxidant capacity it would be better to recommend multivitamin supplementation. In any case, it may explain, at least partly, the beneficial effects of antioxidant supplementation in the reduction of the incidence of cancer and cardiovascular diseases (Anlasik et al. 2005; Kiefer et al. 2004; Trichopoulou and Vasilopoulou 2000).

Sedentary

The prevalence of physical inactivity in adults is increasing. In fact, nearly 40% of the adult population subject themselves to <10 minutes of continuous physical activity per week (Bull, 2003; Kimm et al. 2002). Sedentary lifestyle is associated with increased cardiovascular events although the underlying molecular mechanisms are poorly defined.

Recent studies suggested oxidative stress may play an important role in this process. It may be expained, at least in part, since inactivity increases vascular NADPH oxidase expression and activity and enhances vascular ROS production, which contributes to endothelial dysfunction and atherosclerosis lesion formation during sedentary as opposed to physically active lifestyle (Laufs et al. 2005).

On the contrary, moderate, long-term exercise induces adaptive responses that confer protection against oxidative stress. In this respect it was published it may improve redox metabolism by increasing antioxidant defense system both in experimental (Kakarla et al., 2005; Rosety-Rodriguez et al. 2006a,b,c; Rosety-Rodriguez et al. 2007) and human (Elosua et al. 2003; Ordonez et al. 2006; Ordonez et al. 2007a,b,c) studies. In fact it may increase both enzymatic and non-enzymatic.

Abusive Alcohol Consumption

There are several proposals of a triad relationship between abusive alcohol consumption and ROS generation. In this respect chronic alcoholics have elevated hepatic lipid peroxidation where the degree of lipid peroxidation correlates with the severity of the liver disease. It may be explained since alcohol increases the activity of microsomal NADPH oxidase and mitochondrial NADH cytochrome c reductase resulting in increased ROS generation. Further the existence of ethanol derived radicals such as hydroxyethyl free radicals, formed by a direct reaction of ethanol with hydroxyl radicals has also been suggested (Albano 2006; Wu and Cederbaum 2003).

Free radicals increase the oxidative modification of low density lipoprotein (LDL). This is one of the most important mechanisms, which increases cardiovascular risk in chronic alcoholic patients. (Zima et al. 2001). And even ROS derived from alcohol are suggested as possible causative carcinogenic factors (Seitz and Stickel 2006).

Together these observations provide a rationale for the possible clinical application of antioxidants in the therapy for alcoholic liver disease (Albano 2006).

Ultra Violet (UV) Exposure

Sun exposure was also associated with a decreased antioxidant capacity. This finding may explain, at least in part, that solar radiation is one of the major damaging environmental agents for human skin causing premature sking aging and carcinogenesis (Jin et al. 2007; Sauvaigo et al. 2007; Schneider et al. 2006). This is of particular interest for individuals with phototypes I, II and III as defined by Fitzpatrick (1988). In contrast, lack of UV exposure was weakly associated to an increased antioxidant capacity.

For the reasons already mentioned, these lifestyle factors may be pointed out as potential targets by health care professionals since it was reported a significant synergistic influence on the decrease in the antioxidant capacity when combined to emotional stress.

III. Oxidative Stress: An Update on Health Consequences and Assessment Methods

Health consequences

Free radicals are highly reactive species produced under normal biologic conditions, mainly during oxygen consumption in redox reactions required to generate energy and to eliminate xenobiotic and pathogenic organisms.

The organism is naturally protected against these excessive free-radical attack by both enzymatic and non-enzymatic detoxification systems. Thus, under normal physiologic conditions, a balance state is established between free radical production and antiradical defenses.

Nevertheless, various lifestyle, nutritional, environmental and genetic factors may induce an abnormal increase in free radical production and/or decrease in antioxidant defenses that could alter this balance state and conduct to the so called oxidative stress. (Djordjevic 2004; Lehucher-Michel et al. 2001; Young and Woodside 2001).

A century ago, Fenton published his findings on the oxidation of organic molecules by hydrogen peroxide ($H2O2$) in the presence of iron that was considered the beginning of investigations on the phenomena collectively referred to as oxidative stress (Fenton, 1894). In recent years there has been an increasing interest in assessing oxidative stress since it may induce a pronounced impairment of the cellular metabolism and significant damage of tissues. And consequently, it may increase the incidence of several diseases.

There is increasing evidence for links between oxidative stress and a variety of pathological disorders such as cardiovascular diseases, cancer, immune disorders, chronic inflammatory diseases, neurodegeneration, among others (Arranz et al. 2007; Calabrese et al. 2007; Peake and Suzuki, 2004).

Concerning the contribution of sex to the overall antioxidant capacity, several studies have reported women had a significant higher antioxidant capacity than men (Lesgards et al. 2002; Tiidus et al. 2000). This finding is in accordance with clinical studies that have shown women are more protected than men from atherogenic events which are highly associated with oxidative stress (Nordstrom et al. 2001). Further, the largest difference was observed in the oxidant status between sedentary men and women during autumn and winter, which is considered a period of high coronary risk for men (Balog et al. 2006).

Many studies have also demonstrated that intense muscular work generates considerable amounts of reactive oxygen species (ROS) in elite athletes. Accordingly, oxidative stress has been associated with decreased physical performance, muscular fatigue, muscle damage, and overtraining (Konig et al. 2001).

Assessment methods

Because it is rare that physiologic markers can validate high stress levels evaluated by subjective techniques, the determination of antioxidant capacity in whole blood may be of significant use in detecting and assessing potential psychological stress damage. As a consequence, several methods have been developed to assess redox metabolism. In this respect, the importance of blood is increasing since it may reflect the situation in other less accessible tissues (Rosety-Rodriguez et al. 2005).

Antioxidant defense capacity may be assessed by mean of the selective determination of free radical scavenging or reducing activity of plasma or even by the selective analysis of biological antioxidant compounds (vitamin C, E, etc.).

However, since they do not take into account cellular environment and the numerous interactions between biologic antioxidants, the latter assays would not be highly relevant to the determination of the physiologic antioxidant state.

To avoid these problems, recent studies have reported that the assessment of total antioxidant status (TAS) by diagnostic kits may reflect overall individual antioxidant defense. Similarly, free radical–mediated hemolysis may play an important role in this research area. In this respect emotional stress which is known to produce circulating free radicals, significantly shortened free radical-mediated hemolysis when compared to non-smoking controls (Lesgards et al. 2002).

The importance of the assessment of oxidative stress by means of the determination of end products of oxidative damage has been increasing in the last years (Le Bras et al., 2005).

In vitro and in vivo studies have demonstrated oxidative stress can lead to damage or destruction of cellular macromolecules such as lipids, proteins, and nucleic acids (DNA).

In this respect, lipid and protein oxidation results in the formation of malondialdehyde (MDA) and carbonyl groups respectively whose evaluation may provide a significant clue to the magnitude of oxidative stress (Stadtman and Levine, 2000).

It should be pointed out that protein oxidation occurs more quickly than lipid peroxidation since they involve different mechanisms in vivo (Davies and Goldberg, 1987; Senturk et al. 2005).

Reactive species (RS) of various types are capable of damaging not only proteins and lipids but also DNA, which experimental studies in animals and in vitro have suggested is an important factor in aging, carcinogenesis and degenerative diseases (Lodovici et al. 2007; Nilsson et al. 2004; Wen et al. 2007).

In this respect, levels of DNA base oxidation products such as 8OHdG (8-hydroxy-2'-deoxyguanosine) that may serve as non-invasive biomarker of oxidative DNA damage. In contrast to classical determinations of plasmatic levels of MDA and carbonyl groups, 8OHdG may be assessed from urine samples (Haghdoost et al. 2006; Lin et al. 2004; Sabatini et al. 2005).

Since this non-invasive procedure to determine oxidative stress is clearly preferred by patients and participants several studies have been performed to assess lipid and protein oxidation from urine samples. In this respect, as a biomarker of protein oxidation, o,o'-dityrosine was analyzed in urine samples by a recently developed isotope dilution HPLC-atmospheric pressure chemical ionization (APCI)-tandem-mass spectrometry (HPLC-APCI-MS/MS) methodology. And finally, as biomarkers of lipid peroxidation, 7 aldehydes (i.e. propanal, butanal, pentanal, hexanal, heptanal, octanal and nonanal) and acetone were analyzed in urines by gas chromatography with electron capture detection (Orhan et al. 2004).

Thereby, it is widely accepted that the measurement of above mentioned parameters can provide an indicator that is useful as an integrated evaluation to improve lifestyle habits that are to be understood to induce lifestyle-related diseases. Mainly if we take into account oxidative damage has been proposed as a pathogenic mechanism of atherosclerosis, cell aging, neurodegeneration, carcinogenic events, immunological disorders and chronic inflammatory diseases among others.

IV. Regular Exercise as a Healthy Tool to Reduce Oxidative Stress

Regular Exercise Reduced Oxidative Damage by Improving Antioxidant Defense

Physical activity is recognized as an important component of a healthy life style and consequently is highly recommended by scientists and clinicians (Donaldson 2000).

This finding may be explained at least in part, since regular exercise may improve redox metabolism. Based on these observations it was hypothesyzed that moderate exercise may also reduce oxidative damage induced by emotional stress. At the present moment, this field is at an exciting stage. And fortunately, ample evidence of this progress can be found in the literature.

Fortunately, several studies highlight the potential benefit of a moderate training program to attenuate oxidative damage in animals emotionally stressed by immobilization (Kakarla et al., 2005; Radak et al., 2001; Rosety-Rodriguez et al. 2006a; Rosety-Rodriguez et al. 2007). This finding may be explained since regular exercise improved both enzymatic (Rosety-Rodriguez et al. 2007) and non-enzymatic (Rosety-Rodriguez et al. 2006b) antioxidant defense systems in trained specimens.

In this respect, it should be pointed out swimming is frequently preferred as an exercise model for small laboratory animals such as rats since it may be considered as part of their natural environment (Kramer et al., 1993). In addition, aversive stimulation used to promote running are not required (Mattson et al. 2000). This fact is of particular interest since these stimuli have been associated per se with oxidative stress and consequently may interfere with our results leading to mistaken conclusions.

Fortunately, existing data in the literature also indicate regular exercise may reduce oxidative damage in humans (Elosua et al. 2003; Ordonez et al. 2007, Rosety-Rodriguez et al. 2006d; Semaloglu et al. 2000).

In fact, our research group has recently published a 12-week protocol based on regular exercise improved redox metabolism in obese adolescents. This improvement is due to an increase in both plasmatic total antioxidant status (TAS) as well as the activity of erythrocyte antioxidant enzymes such as glutathione peroxidase (GPX) and glucose-6-phosphate-dehydrogenase (G6PDH).

To get this goal we designed a 12 week intervention program based on aerobic, low-moderate intensity exercise. It comprised 3 sessions/week, consisting of warm up (15 min) followed by a main part (20-35 min [increasing 5 minutes each three weeks]) at a work intensity of 60-75% of peak heart rate (increasing 5% each three weeks) and by a cool-down period (10 min).

It should be emphasized all authors agree it is quite important to be progressive in both duration and intensity of each session as was stated previously by expert panel from American College of Sports Medicine (ACSM).

In this line, Semaloglu et al. (2000) reported aerobic training increased in erythrocytes GPx activity with a subsequent decrease in plasma TBARS levels. Similarly, Elosua et al. (2003) reported a 16-week aerobic training program increased endogenous antioxidant activity and low-density-lipoprotein (LDL) resistance to oxidation, and decreased oxidized LDL concentration in 17 healthy young men and women. Regular swimming at low-moderate insensity had also beneficial effects on both enzymatic nd non-enzymatic antioxidant defence systems in healthy children (Gonenc et al. 200).

On the other side, anaerobic training had no effect on the improvement of antioxidant defense (Semaloglu et al. 2000). On the contrary, Merchefer et al. (2004) concluded extreme running competition decreases blood antioxidant defense capacity. And even it may increase oxidative damage as was reported by Groussard et al. (2003) who found short-term supramaximal anaerobic exercise increased significantly plasmatic levels of malondialdehyde (MDA) and decreased both enzymatic an non-enzymatic antioxidant defense system.

To explain the double role of physical activity on redox metabolism, existing data indicated on one hand, that regular exercise may cause adaptation of the antioxidant and repair systems, which could result in a decreased base level of oxidative damage and increased resistance to oxidative stress. On the other hand, a single bout of vigorous exercise result in oxidative damage as a sign of incomplete adaptation.

It has been well demonstrated that the principal factor responsible for oxidative damage during high-intensity exercise is the increase in oxygen consumption. Muscles oxygen utilization during strenuous exercise can increase as much as 100–200 times than at rest. Consequently, increased electron flux through the rapidly respiring mitochondria in the active muscle may lead to an enhancement of electron leakage and consequent reactive oxygen species (ROS) production (Chevion et al. 2003; Palazzetti et al. 2003).

ROS may be generated during and after an acute bout of strenuous exercise not only in working muscles, but also in the tissues that undergo ischemia-reperfusion such as heart, liver, brain, among others (Peake and Suzuki, 2004). Further, leukocyte activation infiltrating the muscle after injury by exercise may also produce ROS (Peake et al. 2005; Sureda et al. 2007).

Further, other theoretical factors (acidosis, catecholamine autoxidation, ischemia-reperfusion syndrome, etc.) that are known to induce, in vitro, oxidative damage may also be operative during short-term supramaximal anaerobic exercise (Groussard et al. 2003).

Fortunately, long-term exercise has the capability to develop an adaptation of the antioxidant and repair systems against the increased level of ROS production, which could result in a decreased base level of oxidative damage and increased resistance to oxidative stress (Niess and Simon, 2007; Radak et al. 2001). On the contrary, a single bout of vigorous exercise result in oxidative damage as a sign of incomplete adaptation.

Recommendations to Design Training Programs

Intervention programs based on regular exercise to improve health in general and redox metabolism in particular, should be designed and supervised during their application by a multidisciplinary team of healthcare professionals, psychologist, bachelor's degree on exercise science, etc. Consequently, by actively participating in their own healthcare, participants would progress at their own pace through a closely monitored and custom-tailored exercise program.

According to these recommendations, our protocol based on exercise will improve participant's health in general and oxidative damage in particular. Further we prevent sport-related injuries that may finally conduct to many participants, not only the injured one, to leave the program.

Pre-participation physical examination (PPE) is highly recommended by experts and required for all participants to detect potential relative or absolute contraindications.

It is also recommended before starting the exercise program to obtain written informed consent signed by all participants since it represent one of the most important legal and ethical principles.

Another observation one can make when reviewing the literature is that the duration of the intervention program may be essential not only to get proposed objectives but also to guarantee participants follow-up the whole protocol without getting lost.

Previous studies have reported longer programs (one-year, six month, etc.) having less sessions per week and although they obtained good results the problem was that many participants left the program before it finished. In this respect Galan et al (2006) reported a 10-month protocol based on regular exercise having good results in elderly

On the contrary, shorter programs reported (10 and 8 weeks) did not reach their objectives regarding oxidative stress (Rahnama et al. 2007). It may be expected they would obtain better results if they increase the number of sessions per week. However, the inconvenience may be that many participants have low physical condition and as a consequence they have many difficulties to follow the training program and high risk of musculoskeletal injuries that may finally lead to leave it.

It is possible to obtain quickest results improving oxidative stress if we design a mixed protocol including regular exercise as well as dietary and intensive lifestyle modifications (vitamin supplementation; no smoking; etc.).

In this respect, a 2-week combination of diet and exercise ameliorated significantly oxidative stress, inflammation, and monocyte-endothelial interaction in adults with diabetes (Roberts et al. 2006) as well as in overweight children (Roberts et al. 2007). It clearly suggested exercise and hypocaloric (low fat content) diet seem to interact positively. And consequently, if sedentary obese individuals start a combined exercise-hypocaloric diet program the risk of coronary heart disease is lower than for exercise or hypocaloric diet alone as was reported previously by Wood (1994).

Similarly the combination of exercise training and antioxidant supplementation (150 µg of selenium, 2000 IU of retinol, 120 mg of ascorbic acid and 30 IU of alpha-tocopherol,) for 4 weeks increased antioxidant enzyme activities (Margaritis et al. 2003).

For the reasons already mentioned, it may be concluded firstly that psychological stress increases significantly oxidative stress that may finally play an important role in several diseases. And finally, that regular exercise should be recommended as a healthy and effective tool to reduce oxidative damage by improving antioxidant defense system. In any case, further studies on this topic are required.

V. References

Albano E. Alcohol, oxidative stress and free radical damage. Proc Nutr Soc. 2006; 65: 278-90

Anlasik T, Sies H, Griffiths HR, Mecocci P, Stahl W, Polidori MC. Dietary habits are major determinants of the plasma antioxidant status in healthy elderly subjects. *Br. J. Nutr.* 2005; 94: 639-42.

Arranz L, Guayerbas N, De la Fuente M. Impairment of several immune functions in anxious women. *J. Psychosom. Res.* 2007; 62: 1-8.

Atalay M, Lappalainen J, Sen CK. Dietary antioxidants for the athlete. *Curr. Sports Med. Rep.* 2006; 5: 182-6.

Ayaori M, Hisada T, Suzukawa M, Yoshida H, Nishiwaki M, Ito T, Nakajima K, Yonemura A, Ishikawa T. Plasma levels and redox status of ascorbic acid and levels of lipid peroxidation products in active and passive smokers. *Environ. Health Perspect.* 2001; 108: 105-108.

Balog T, Sobocanec S, Sverko V, Krolo I, Rocic B, Marotti M, Marotti T. The influence of season on oxidant-antioxidant status in trained and sedentary subjects. *Life Sci.* 2006; 78: 1441-7.

Bull F. Defining physical inactivity. *Lancet.* 2003; 361: 258–259.

Boden-Albala B, Sacco RL. Lifestyle factors and stroke risk: exercise, alcohol, diet, obesity, smoking, drug use, and stress. *Curr. Atheroscler. Rep.* 2000; 2: 160-6

Bultz BD, Carlson LE. Emotional distress: the sixth vital sign in cancer care. J Clin Oncol. 2005; 23: 6440–1.

Calabrese V, Guagliano E, Sapienza M, Panebianco M, Calafato S, Puleo E, Pennisi G, Mancuso C, Butterfield DA, Stella AG. Redox regulation of cellular stress response in aging and neurodegenerative disorders: role of vitagenes.*Neurochem. Res.* 2007; 32: 757-73

Chakraborti A, Gulati K, Banerjee BD, Ray A.Possible involvement of free radicals in the differential neurobehavioral responses to stress in male and female rats. *Behav. Brain Res.* 2007; 179: 321-5.

Chalmers AH, Blake-Mortimer JS, Winefield AH. The prooxidant state and psychologic stress. *Environ. Health Perspect.* 2003; 111: 16

Chevion S, Moran DS, Heled Y, Shani Y, Regev G, Abbou B, Berenshtein E, Stadtman ER, Epstein Y.Plasma antioxidant status and cell injury after severe physical exercise. *Proc. Natl. Acad .Sci. U S A.* 2003; 100: 5119-23.

Christen Y. Environmental factors of longevity. Presse Med. 2003; 32: 370-6.

Clarkson PM, Thompson HS. Antioxidants: what role do they play in physical activity and health?. *Am. J. Clin. Nutr.* 2000; 72: 637-46.

Crujeiras AB, Parra MD, Rodriguez MC, Martinez de Morentin BE, Martinez JA. A role for fruit content in energy-restricted diets in improving antioxidant status in obese women during weight loss. *Nutrition.* 2006; 22: 593-9.

Davies KJ and Goldberg AL. Oxygen radicals stimulate intracellular proteolysis and lipid peroxidation by independent mechanisms in erythrocytes. *J. Biol .Chem.* 1987; 262: 8220–8226

Davies KJ and Goldberg AL. Proteins damaged by oxygen radicals are rapidly degraded in extracts of red blood cells. *J. Biol. Chem.* 1987; 262: 8227–8234.

Dietrich M, Block G, Norkus EP, Hudes M, Traber MG, Cross CE, Packer L. Smoking and exposure to environmental tobacco smoke decrease some plasma antioxidants and increase gamma-tocopherol in vivo after adjustment for dietary antioxidant intakes. *Am. J. Clin. Nutr.* 2003; 77: 160-6.

Djordjevic VB. Free radicals in cell biology. *Int. Rev. Cytol..* 2004; 237: 57-89.

Elosua R, Molina L, Fito M, Arquer A, Sanchez-Quesada JL, Covas MI, Ordonez-Llanos J, Marrugat J. Response of oxidative stress biomarkers to a 16-week aerobic physical activity program, and to acute physical activity, in healthy young men and women. *Atherosclerosis.* 2003; 167: 327-34.

Eskiocak S, Gozen AS, Yapar SB, Tavas F, Kilic AS, Eskiocak M. Glutathione and free sulphydryl content of seminal plasma in healthy medical students during and after exam stress. *Hum. Reprod.* 2005; 20: 2595-600.

Fenton HJH. Oxidation of tartaric acid in presence of iron. J Chem Soc. 1894; 65: 899-910.

Fitzpatrick TB. The validity and practically of sun-re- active skin types I through VI. *Arch. Dermatol.* 1988; 124: 896-871.

Galan AI, Palacios E, Ruiz F, Diez A, Arji M, Almar M, Moreno C, Calvo JI, Munoz ME, Delgado MA, Jimenez R.Exercise, oxidative stress and risk of cardiovascular disease in the elderly. Protective role of antioxidant functional foods. *Biofactors.* 2006; 27: 167-83.

Gavrilovic L, Dronjak S. Activation of rat pituitary-adrenocortical and sympatho-adrenomedullary system in response to different stressors. *Neuro. Endocrinol. Lett.* 2005; 26: 515-20.

Gonenc S, Acikgoz O, Semin I, Ozgonul H. The effect of moderate swimming exercise on antioxidant enzymes and lipid peroxidation levels in children. *Indian J. Physiol. .Pharmacol.* 2000; 44: 340-4.

Gregus A, Wintink AJ, Davis AC, Kalynchuk LE. Effect of repeated corticosterone injections and restraint stress on anxiety and depression-like behavior in male rats. *Behav. Brain Res.* 2005; 156: 105-14.

Grossi G, Perski A, Evengard B, Blomkvist V, Orth-Gomer K. hysiological correlates of burnout among women. *J. Psychosom. Res.* 2003; 55: 309-16.

Groussard C, Rannou-Bekono F, Machefer G, Chevanne M, Vincent S, Sergent O, Cillard J, Gratas-Delamarche A. Changes in blood lipid peroxidation markers and antioxidants after a single sprint anaerobic exercise. *Eur. J. Appl. Physiol.* 2003; 89: 14-20.

Hadj A, Esmore D, Rowland M, Pepe S, Schneider L, Lewin J, Rosenfeldt F. Pre-operative preparation for cardiac surgery utilising a combination of metabolic, physical and mental therapy. *Heart Lung Circ.* 2006; 15: 172-81.

Haghdoost S, Sjolander L, Czene S, Harms-Ringdahl M. The nucleotide pool is a significant target for oxidative stress. *Free Radic. Biol. .Med.* 2006; 41: 620-6.

Hanton S, Fletcher D, Coughlan G. Stress in elite sport performers: a comparative study of competitive and organizational stressors. *J. Sports Sci.* 2005; 23: 1129-41.

Irie M, Asami S, Nagata S, Miyata M, Kasai H. Psychological mediation of a type of oxidative DNA damage, 8-hydroxydeoxyguanosine, in peripheral blood leukocytes of non-smoking and non-drinking workers. *Psychother. Psychosom.* 2002; 71: 90-6.

Jin GH, Liu Y, Jin SZ, Liu XD, Liu SZ. UVB induced oxidative stress in human keratinocytes and protective effect of antioxidant agents. *Radiat Environ. Biophys.* 2007; 46: 61-8.

Kiefer I, Prock P, Lawrence C, Wise J, Bieger W, Bayer P, Rathmanner T, Kunze M, Rieder A.Supplementation with mixed fruit and vegetable juice concentrates increased serum antioxidants and folate in healthy adults. *J. Am. Coll .Nutr.* 2004; 23: 205-11.

Kim SH, Kim JS, Shin HS, Keen CL. Influence of smoking on markers of oxidative stress and serum mineral concentrations in teenage girls in Korea. *Nutrition.* 2003; 19: 240-3.

Kimm SY, Glynn NW, Kriska AM, Barton BA, Kronsberg SS, Daniels SR, Crawford PB, Sabry ZI, Liu K. Decline in physical activity in black girls and white girls during adolescence. *N .Engl. J. Med.* 2002; 347: 709–715.

Konig D, Wagner KH, Elmadfa I, Berg A. Exercise and oxidative stress: significance of antioxidants with reference to inflammatory, muscular, and systemic stress. *Exerc. Immunol. Rev.* 2001; 7: 108-33.

Lehucher-Michel MP, Lesards JF, Delubac O, Stocker P, Durand P, Prost M. Oxidant stress and human disease: crrent knowledge and perspectives for prevention. Press Med. 2001; 30: 1017-1023.

Lesgards JF, Durand P, Lassarre M, Stocker P, Lesgards G, Lanteaume A, Prost M, Lehucher-Michel MP.Assessment of lifestyle effects on the overall antioxidant capacity of healthy subjects. *Environ. Health Perspect.* 2002; 110: 479-86.

Lin HS, Jenner AM, Ong CN, Huang SH, Whiteman M, Halliwell B. A high-throughput and sensitive methodology for the quantification of urinary 8-hydroxy-2'-deoxyguanosine: measurement with gas chromatography-mass spectrometry after single solid-phase extraction. *Biochem. J..* 2004; 380: 541-8.

Liu H, Wang Z. Effects of social isolation stress on immune response and survival time of mouse with liver cancer. *World J. Gastroenterol..* 2005; 11: 5902–4.

Lodovici M, Luceri C, De Filippo C, Romualdi C, Bambi F, Dolara P. Smokers and passive smokers gene expression profiles: correlation with the DNA oxidation damage. *Free Radic. Biol. Med.* 2007; 43: 415-22.

Machefer G, Groussard C, Rannou-Bekono F, Zouhal H, Faure H, Vincent S, Cillard J, Gratas-Delamarche A. Extreme running competition decreases blood antioxidant defense capacity. *J. Am. Coll Nutr.* 2004 ; 23: 358-64.

Malm C. Susceptibility to infections in elite athletes: the S-curve. *Scand. J. Med. Sci. Sports.* 2006; 16: 4-6.

Margaritis I, Palazzetti S, Rousseau AS, Richard MJ, Favier A. Antioxidant supplementation and tapering exercise improve exercise-induced antioxidant response. *J. Am. Coll Nutr.* 2003; 22: 147-56.

Mimura K, Kobayashi T, Mizukoshi S. Study of quantification of oxidative stresses caused by lifestyle habits. Rinsho Byori. 2007; 55: 35-40.

Niess AM, Simon P. Response and adaptation of skeletal muscle to exercise--the role of reactive oxygen species. *Front Biosci.* 2007; 12: 4826-38.

Nilsson R, Nordlinder R, Moen BE, Ovrebo S, Bleie K, Skorve AH, Hollund BE, Tagesson C. Increased urinary excretion of 8-hydroxydeoxyguanosine in engine room personnel exposed to polycyclic aromatic hydrocarbons. *Occup. Environ. Med.* 2004; 61: 692-6.

Nordstrom CK, Dwyer KM, Merz CN, Shircore A, Dwyer JH. Work-related stress and early atherosclerosis. *Epidemiology.* 2001; 12: 180-5.

Ordoñez FJ, Rosety M, Rosety-Rodriguez M. Regular physical activity increases glutathione peroxidase activity in adolescents with Down syndrome. *Clin. J. Sports Med.* 2006; 16: 355-356.

Ordonez FJ, Rosety MA, Rosety-Roriguez M. Exercise may reduce Oxidative Damage in Down Syndrome by Increasing Total Antioxidant Status. *Med. Sci. Sports Exerc.* 2007a; 39: 31

Ordoñez FJ, Bernardi M; Rosety MA, Macias Amat I, Rosety-Rodriguez M. Erythrocyte membrane fatty acid composition remained unchanged after a training program in adolescents with Down syndrome. *Eur. J. Clin. Invest.* 2007b; 37: 8

Ordonez FJ, Rosety-Roriguez M. Regular exercise attenuated lipid peroxidation in adolescents with Down's syndrome. *Clin. Biochem.* 2007c; 40: 141-2.

Orhan H, van Holland B, Krab B, Moeken J, Vermeulen NP, Hollander P, Meerman JH. Evaluation of a multi-parameter biomarker set for oxidative damage in man: increased urinary excretion of lipid, protein and DNA oxidation products after one hour of exercise. *Free Radic. Res.* 2004; 38: 1269-79.

Ozbay B, Dulger H. Lipid peroxidation and antioxidant enzymes in Turkish population: relation to age, gender, exercise, and smoking. *Tohoku J. Exp. Med.* 2002; 197: 119-24.

Palazzetti S, Richard MJ, Favier A, Margaritis I. Overloaded training increases exercise-induced oxidative stress and damage. *Can. J. Appl. Physiol.* 2003; 28: 588-604.

Peake J, Suzuki K. Neutrophil activation, antioxidant supplements and exercise-induced oxidative stress. *Exerc. Immunol. Rev.* 2004; 10: 129-41.

Peake JM, Suzuki K, Wilson G, Hordern M, Nosaka K, Mackinnon L, Coombes JS. Exercise-induced muscle damage, plasma cytokines, and markers of neutrophil activation. *Med. Sci. Sports Exerc.* 2005; 37: 737-45.

Radak Z, Taylor AW, Ohno H, Goto S. Adaptation to exercise-induced oxidative stress: from muscle to brain. *Exerc. Immunol .Rev.* 2001; 7: 90-107.

Rahnama N, Gaeini AA, Hamedinia MR. Oxidative stress responses in physical education students during 8 weeks aerobic training. *J. Sports Med. Phys. Fitness.* 2007; 47:119-23.

Rees T, Hardy L, Freeman P. Stressors, social support, and effects upon performance in golf. *J. Sports Sci.* 2007; 25: 33-42.

Reichhart M, Wagner KH, Konig D, Berg A, Elmadfa I. Oxidative stress and antioxidant status of athletes and untrained persons. *Forum Nutr.* 2003; 56: 303-4.

Roberts CK, Won D, Pruthi S, Lin SS, Barnard RJ. Effect of a diet and exercise intervention on oxidative stress, inflammation and monocyte adhesion in diabetic men. *Diabetes Res. Clin. Pract.* 2006; 73: 249-59.

Roberts CK, Chen AK, Barnard RJ.Effect of a short-term diet and exercise intervention in youth on atherosclerotic risk factors. *Atherosclerosis.* 2007; 191: 98-106.

Rosety-Rodriguez M, Ordonez FJ, Rosey I, Rosety JM, Rosety M. Erythrocyte antioxidant enzymes of gilthead as early-warning bioindicators of oxidative stress induced by malathion. *Haema.* 2005; 8: 237-240.

Rosety Rodríguez M, Ordoñez FJ, Rosety I, Frias L, Rosety MA, Rosety JM, Rosety M. 8 Week Traning program attenuates mitochondrial oxidative stress in the liver of emotional stressed rats. Histol. *Histhopathol.* 2006a; 21: 1167-1170.

Rosety-Rodriguez M, Ordoñez FJ, Rosety M. Eight week moderate exercise training program increases plasmatic total antioxidant status in rats stressed by immobilization. *Haema.* 2006b; 9: 124-126.

Rosety-Rodriguez M, Ordoñez FJ, Rosety MA, Frias L, Rosety I, Rosety M. Combination of exercise and dietary vitamin supplementation protects mitochondrial ultrastructure in the liver of stressed rats. *Eur .J. Clin. Invest.* 2006c; 36: 25-25.

Rosety-Rodriguez M, Ordonez FJ, Rosety M. Influence of regular exercise on erythrocyte catalase activity in adolescents with Down syndrome. *Med. Clin.* 2006d; 127: 533-4.

Rosety-Rodriguez M, Rosety I, Frias L, Rosety MA, Ordoñez FJ. Liver Superoxide Dismutase Activity was increased by Exercise in Emotionally Stressed Rats. *Med .Sci. Sports Exerc.* 2007; 39: 253.

Sabatini L, Barbieri A, Tosi M, Roda A, Violante FS. A method for routine quantitation of urinary 8-hydroxy-2'-deoxyguanosine based on solid-phase extraction and micro-high-performance liquid chromatography/electrospray ionization tandem mass spectrometry. Rapid Commun Mass *Spectrom.* 2005; 19: 147-52.

Santanna ID, de Sousa EB, de Moraes AV, Loures DL, Mesquita ET, da Nobrega AC. Cardiac function during mental stress: cholinergic modulation with pyridostigmine in healthy subjects. *Clin. Sci. (Lond).* 2003; 105: 161–5.

Sauvaigo S, Bonnet-Duquennoy M, Odin F, Hazane-Puch F, Lachmann N, Bonte F, Kurfurst R, Favier A. DNA repair capacities of cutaneous fibroblasts: effect of sun exposure, age and smoking on response to an acute oxidative stress. *Br. J. Dermatol.* 2007; 157: 26-32.

Schneider LA, Bloch W, Kopp K, Hainzl A, Rettberg P, Wlaschek M, Horneck G, Scharffetter-Kochanek K. 8-Isoprostane is a dose-related biomarker for photo-oxidative ultraviolet (UV) B damage in vivo: a pilot study with personal UV dosimetry. *Br. J.Dermatol.* 2006; 154: 1147-54.

Seitz HK, Stickel F. Risk factors and mechanisms of hepatocarcinogenesis with special emphasis on alcohol and oxidative stress. *Biol. Chem.* 2006; 387: 349-60.

Selamoglu S, Turgay F, Kayatekin BM, Gonenc S, Yslegen C. Aerobic and anaerobic training effects on the antioxidant enzymes of the blood. *Acta Physiol. Hung.* 2000; 87: 267-73.

Senturk UK, Gunduz F, Kuru O, Kocer G, Ozkaya YG, Yesilkaya A, Bor-Kucukatay M, Uyuklu M, Yalcin O, Baskurt OK. Exercise-induced oxidative stress leads hemolysis in sedentary but not trained humans. *J. Appl. Physiol.* 2005; 99: 1434-41.

Sivonova M, Zitnanova I, Hlincikova L, Skodacek I, Trebaticka J, Durackova Z. Oxidative stress in university students during examinations. *Stress*. 2004; 7: 183-8.

Sureda A, Ferrer MD, Tauler P, Maestre I, Aguilo A, Cordova A, Tur JA, Roche E, Pons A. Intense physical activity enhances neutrophil antioxidant enzyme gene expression. Immunocytochemistry evidence for catalase secretion. *Free Radic. Res.* 2007; 41: 874-83.

Tiidus PM.Estrogen and gender effects on muscle damage, inflammation, and oxidative stress. *Can. J. Appl. Physiol.* 2000; 25: 274-87.

Trichopoulou A, Vasilopoulou E. Mediteranean diet and longevity. *Br .J. Nutr.* 2000; 84: 205-209.

Valyi-Nagy T, Dermody TS. Role of oxidative damage in the pathogenesis of viral infections of the nervous system. Histol *Histopathol.* 2005; 20: 957-67.

Wang L, Muxin G, Nishida H, Shirakawa C, Sato S, Konishi T. Psychological Stress-Induced Oxidative Stress as a Model of Sub-Healthy Condition and the Effect of TCM. *Evid. Based Complement Alternat. Med.* 2007; 4: 195-202.

Weiss IC, Pryce CR, Jongen-Relo AL, Nanz-Bahr NI, Feldon J. Effect of social isolation on stress-related behavioural and neuroendocrine state in the rat. *Behav. Brain Res..* 2004; 152: 279-95.

Wen WH, Yang J, Gao XF, Cao SQ, Dong HY, Heng ZC.Study on the association between urinary organic arsenic and 8-hydroxydeoxyguanine in workers exposed to arsenic. Zhonghua Yu Fang Yi Xue Za Zhi. 2007; 41: 193-5.

Wood PD. Physical activity, diet and health: independent and interactive effects. *Med. Sci. Sports Exerc.* 1994; 26: 838-843.

Wood GE, Young LT, Reagan LP, McEwen BS. Acute and chronic restraint stress alter the incidence of social conflict in male rats. *Horm. Behav.* 2003; 43: 205-13.

Wu D, Cederbaum AI.Alcohol, oxidative stress, and free radical damage. *Alcohol Res Health.* 2003; 27: 277-84.

Young IS, Woodside JV. Antioxidants in health and disease. *J. Clin. Patjol.* 2001; 54: 76-86.

Zima T, Fialova L, Mestek O, Janebova M, Crkovska J, Malbohan I, Stipek S, Mikulikova L, Popov P.Oxidative stress, metabolism of ethanol and alcohol-related diseases. *J. Biomed. Sci.* 2001; 8: 59-70.

In: Sport and Exercise Psychology Research Advances   ISBN: 978-1-60456-157-9
Editors: M. P. Simmons, L. A. Foster, pp. 361-391   © 2008 Nova Science Publishers, Inc.

Chapter XVII

Analyzing the Measurement of Psychological Need Satisfaction in Exercise Contexts: Evidence, Issues, and Future Directions

Philip M. Wilson[19], Diane E. Mack, Katie Gunnell, Kristin Oster, and J. Paige Gregson

Department of Physical Education and Kinesiology,
Faculty of Applied Health Sciences
Brock University, St Catharines, Ontario, Canada, L2S 3A1

Abstract

Background: Perceived competence, relatedness, and autonomy embody the basic psychological needs subtheory housed within Self-Determination Theory (SDT; Deci and Ryan, 2002). Fulfillment of these basic psychological needs represents an important avenue for the promotion of well-being and the optimization of motivation for health behaviors including exercise. Few attempts, however, have been made to systematically measure the fulfillment of basic psychological needs in exercise contexts using a construct validation approach (Wilson, Rogers, Rodgers, and Wild, 2006).

Purpose: The main purpose of this article is to review the available evidence attesting to the measurement of psychological need satisfaction in exercise contexts using SDT as a guiding framework. The subpurposes of this review were to identify key issues associated with the current measurement of psychological need satisfaction in exercise using a construct validation framework (Messick, 1995), and illustrate salient issues pertinent to the selection and development of instruments designed to measure perceived competence, autonomy, and relatedness specific to exercise contexts for future research.

19 Correspondence concerning this manuscript can be sent to: Philip M. Wilson, PhD, Department of Physical Education and Kinesiology, Faculty of Applied Health Sciences, Brock University, 500 Glenridge Avenue, St Catharines, Ontario, L2S 3A1, Canada. Tel: (905) 688-5550 Ext. 4997. Fax: (905) 688-8364. Email: phwilson@brocku.ca.

Summary: Early work in this area relied on instruments that had not been developed specifically for measuring perceived psychological need satisfaction in exercise contexts. A number of psychometric concerns were evident in the data reported in these studies including reliability issues and a lack of convincing evidence for convergent and nomological validity. More recent construct validation work has produced the Psychological Need Satisfaction in Exercise Scale (Wilson et al., 2006) and the Basic Psychological Needs in Exercise Scale (Vlachopoulos and Michailidou, 2006). Both instruments appear to hold promise for furthering our understanding of the influential role afforded competence, autonomy, and relatedness perceptions in the context of exercise.

"We must believe that even in prehistoric times Og, the cave man, made rudimentary appraisals of his fellows. He saw Zog go by, made some such judgment as "Big, strong, keep out of way," and acted upon it; or he came upon the campfire of Wog, observed "Small, weak, take dinner," and did so forthwith. But for much of recorded history, the appraisals that man has made of his fellows have been of this crude and subjective type." (Thorndike and Hagen, 1955, p.1).

As the foregoing quote suggests, measurement has a long and often controversial history in human development. Measurement is at the heart of any scientific endeavor (Messick, 1995) and refers generally to the process of assigning numbers to variables of interest according to specified rules or conventions (Stevens, 1946). Despite the importance of this process, Kerlinger (1979) noted that "measurement can be the Achilles' Heel of behavioral research" (p. 141) given that scientists often pay insufficient attention to measurement issues. Marsh (1997) has suggested that theory and measurement are "inexorably intertwined" (p. 27) such that neglecting one aspect during the process of scientific research simultaneously undermines the credibility of the other.

The purpose of this paper is to review the current status of research in exercise contexts that has measured psychological need satisfaction from the perspective of Self-Determination Theory (SDT; Deci and Ryan, 2002). To address this purpose, a brief overview of SDT will be offered highlighting key issues essential to the measurement of psychological need fulfillment (a more complete overview of SDT can be found in Deci and Ryan, 2002). Following this introduction, the measurement of perceived competence, autonomy, and relatedness will be chronicled to illustrate the examples of instrument development using SDT as a framework within exercise psychology. The final section of this review highlights challenges evident in the measurement of psychological need satisfaction in exercise settings and offers suggestions for further instrument development and evaluation research.

Self-Determination Theory: A Brief Overview

SDT is an organismic approach to human development and motivation that concerns the ongoing tensions and struggles between organisms and their surrounding environment (Ryan, 1995). The SDT framework is comprised of four mini-theories that collectively inform different aspects of human development, growth, and assimilation of the self with the social world. Causality orientations theory (COT) concerns the influence of personality traits on human functioning and more specifically describes individual differences in the degree to which people are orientated towards self-determined or controlled functioning across life domains (Deci and Ryan, 2002). Cognitive evaluation theory (CET) describes the effects attributable to varying social conditions on intrinsic motivation (Deci and Ryan, 1985). Recognizing that not all behaviors are intrinsically motivated (Ryan, 1995), organismic integration theory (OIT) posits a differentiated approach to understanding extrinsic motivation that is unique to SDT. More specifically, OIT concerns the degree of internalization with the self associated with the source of extrinsic motivation that can vary from controlled psychological processes (namely *external* and *introjected* regulations) to more volitionally endorsed or self-determined processes (*identified* and *integrated* regulations). Basic psychological needs theory (BPN) represents the final subtheory comprising the SDT framework. BPN concerns the active role afforded the basic needs for competence, autonomy, and relatedness in motivational development and the promotion of well-being.

The SDT framework has become a popular approach for examining a broad array of motivational issues in physical activity contexts including exercise (see Hagger and Chatzisarantis, 2007, for a review). This is hardly surprising given that the approach to motivation advocated within SDT specifies the regulatory processes whereby motivational orientations and behavioral regulations shape people's actions (namely OIT and COT), as well as, accounting for the processes through which different motives develop and flourish (namely CET and BPN). According to Deci and Ryan (2002), motivation for a given behavior such as exercise participation varies along a continuum from highly controlled to more volitionally endorsed processes with the latter responsible for enduring behavior and greater well-being. Emerging research in exercise settings has supported many of the propositions set forth by Deci and Ryan (2002) within SDT concerning COT (Rose, Markland, and Parfitt, 2001; Rose, Parfitt, and Williams, 2005), CET (Markland, 1999; Markland and Hardy, 1997), OIT, (Wilson, Rodgers, Fraser, and Murray, 2004), and to a lesser extent BPN (Edmunds, Ntoumanis, and Duda, 2007; Vlachopoulos and Michailidou, 2006; Wilson et al., 2006). Consequently, further consideration of the propositions set forth by Deci and Ryan (2002) within BPN seem worthy of additional research in exercise settings.

One issue that warrants careful research in the exercise psychology literature is the measurement of basic psychological need satisfaction. As advocated by Deci and Ryan (2002), basic psychological needs are innate "nutriments" (p. 7) not merely personal desires or goals that when satisfied authentically promote growth, integration, motivational development, and well-being. In contrast, evidence of ill-being such as maladjustment, fragmentation, and psychological maladies will occur when social contexts fail to fulfill basic psychological needs (Deci and Ryan, 2002). Stated differently, Deci and Ryan (2002) recognize that while the manner in which each psychological need is fulfilled may vary considerably as a function of people, context, or time for example, the net effect of satisfying each need is universal in terms of optimizing motivation and promoting well-being. While this approach is not without controversy (Iyengar and DeVoe, 2003), the BPN subcomponent of SDT is attractive given that it offers a parsimonious account for a broad array of human emotions and behaviors, as well as, delineating targets for intervention to change behavior and thereby improve human functioning (Sheldon, Williams, and Joiner, 2003).

The psychological needs for competence, autonomy, and relatedness have long been advocated by Deci and Ryan (1985) as fundamental for understanding a broad spectrum of motivational and well-being issues. *Competence* stems from the seminal work of White (1959) and refers to the extent to which people feel that they can interact with optimally challenging tasks within one's environment in an effective and capable manner. *Autonomy* draws on the work of deCharms (1968) and involves feeling a sense of personal agency or volition with reference to behavior such that one's actions stem from an internal locus of causality as opposed to feeling like a pawn to external incentives or agenda. *Relatedness* refers to feeling a meaningful sense of connection with others within one's social milieu or more globally within life (Baumeister and Leary, 1995). The satisfaction of these innate psychological needs is proposed to be complimentary such that appeasing one psychological need does not occur at the expense of fulfilling another (Deci and Ryan, 2002).

Basic Psychological Need Satisfaction and Exercise

Several distinct phases of research exploring the importance of basic psychological needs appear evident in the literature as applied to exercise settings. During the *initial phase* an emphasis was placed upon examining the effects of one of the three basic psychological needs that produced mixed evidence with reference to SDT. Research encompassing this phase typically used instruments modified from their original context for the purposes of testing SDT in exercise settings as opposed to context-specific instrument development initiatives seen in later phases of research (e.g., McCready and Long, 1985). A *second phase* of research emerged characterized by two inter-related themes. The first centers around the creation of instruments designed specifically to measure at least one of the key psychological needs comprising the BPN subtheory of SDT (e.g., Markland and Hardy, 1997; Markland, 1999; Rose et al., 2001).[20] The second theme concerned adapting instruments developed in other contexts for the assessment of the three basic psychological needs proposed by Deci and Ryan (2002) in exercise (e.g., Li; 1999; Wilson, Rodgers, and Fraser, 2002a; 2002b; Wilson, Rodgers, Blanchard, and Gessell, 2003).

One important contribution from the research comprising *phase two* concerns the increased attention drawn to the instrumentation used to assess fulfillment of basic psychological needs within the SDT framework in exercise contexts. Towards this end, a *third phase* of research has recently begun with the development of two instruments designed specifically to capture variation in basic psychological need satisfaction in a manner consistent with SDT (Deci and Ryan, 2002). Both instruments were developed by independent research groups and appear to show initial promise for measuring perceived competence, autonomy, and relatedness experienced in exercise. Vlachopoulos and

---

20 Markland and colleagues (Rose et al., 2001; Markland, 1999) recognize that perceived locus of causality does not equate to perceived autonomy or self-determination. The former is concerned largely with the source responsible for initiating the behavior whereas the latter is to a large extent focused on the issue of choice with respect to the target behavior. Notwithstanding this observation, Reeve (2002) indicates that perceptions of volition, choice, and locus of casualty collectively represent the content of perceived autonomy from the SDT perspective.

colleagues (Vlachopoulos, 2007; in press; Vlachopoulos and Michailidou, 2006; Vlachopoulos and Neikou, in press) have developed the Basic Psychological Needs in Exercise Scale (BPNES) using a series of sophisticated structural equation modeling studies with Greek exercisers. Wilson and colleagues (Wilson and Muon, in press; Wilson et al., 2006; Wilson, Mack, and Blanchard, in press; Wilson, Mack, and Lightheart, in press; Wilson, Mack, Muon, and LeBlanc, 2007; Wilson, Rodgers, Murray, Longley, and Muon, 2006) have developed the Psychological Need Satisfaction in Exercise Scale (PNSE) using samples of Canadian exercisers. The BPNES contains 12 items whereas the PNSE contains 18 items equally distributed across one of three subscales per instrument assessing feelings of competence, autonomy, and relatedness experienced in exercise. The initial stages of development for both the BPNES and the PNSE have attended to a number of construct validation steps advocated by measurement experts (Messick, 1995). Consequently, both instruments appear to hold promise for advancing our understanding of the functional role afforded basic psychological need fulfillment in exercise contexts.

Purpose

Despite the popularity of Deci and Ryan's (2002) SDT framework, the lion's share of research in exercise contexts has focused on the nature and assessment of exercise motivation and the motivation-consequence link (see Markland and Ingledew, 2007, for a review). Less evidence is currently available summarizing the measurement issues central to advancing our understanding of arguments set forth by Deci and Ryan (2002) within the BPN subtheory of SDT. The main purpose of this review, therefore, is to examine the measurement of psychological need satisfaction specific to exercise contexts in studies that have used SDT as a guiding framework. The secondary purpose of this paper is to suggest avenues for further research designed to advance our understanding of the measurement of perceived competence, autonomy, and relatedness needs within exercise contexts.

Method

Selection of the Data

Literature searches were completed to identify studies that measured psychological need satisfaction in exercise settings using both computer- and manual-based searches (see Figure 1). Computer-based searches included a comprehensive examination of the following databases: Academic Search Premier, BioMed Central, MEDLINE, Physical Education Index, PsychLIT, PsychInfo, PubMed, Scholars portal e-journal, SPORTDISCUS, and Web of Science. Keywords entered for the computer-based searches were as follows: Competence, autonomy, relatedness, psychological needs, psychological need satisfaction, psychological need fulfillment, basic psychology needs theory, self-determination theory, belongingness, connectedness, relative autonomy, relative autonomy index, and self-determination index. These key words were selected on the basis of their ability to represent the central concepts proposed by Deci and Ryan (2002) within the BPN subtheory of SDT.

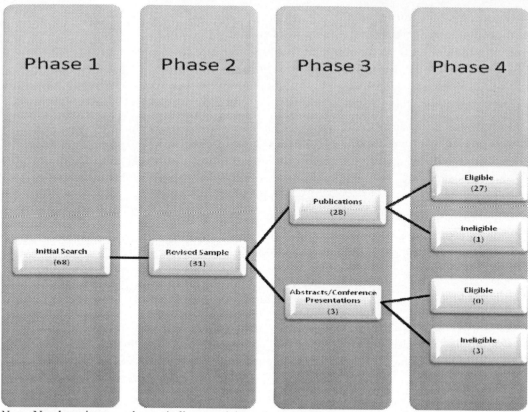

Note. Numbers in parentheses indicate articles selected for retention at each stage of the sampling process. Phase 1 = Number of articles identified based on the initial computer- and manual-based literature searches. Phase 2 = Number of articles retained based on evaluating intitial search results against inclusion/exclusion criteria using study abstracts only. Phase 3 = Catagorization of articles following review of full-text material/article in the revised sample. Phase 4 = The full-text material for each article was examined against the inclusion/exclusion criteria to determine eligibility for retention in the final review.

Figure 1. Flow chart depicting research article selection and retention.

Manual-based searches involved obtaining articles from reference lists contained in relevant empirical studies identified through the computer-based searches. Two authors were contacted to request additional information which was subsequently provided.

Studies identified in the search process were retained if they met the following inclusion/exclusion criteria: (1) The sampling frame was conducted in exercise settings or from populations of current exercisers (this eliminated sport and physical education settings as the major source from which the sample was drawn); (2) The sample was comprised of adults (defined as those 18 years of age and older); (3) The study measured the satisfaction of at least two of the three psychological needs articulated by Deci and Ryan (2002) within the BPN subtheory of SDT; (4) The authors reported sufficient information regarding the assessment of reliability and/or validity of scores derived from the instrumentation used to measure psychological need satisfaction within the study itself (this excluded scientific abstracts presented at academic conferences due to a lack of information for the purposes of this review).

Data Coding

Consideration to developing clear and detailed coding rules was afforded a priori to limit concerns over ambiguity and reliability (Cooper, 1982). Variables coded included (1) sample characteristics (sample size, gender, age, race/ethnicity), (2) study characteristics (method of sampling, sampling frame, presence of manipulation, study design), (3) the measurement of psychological need satisfaction within the study (focus of item content, instrument modifications), and (4) the results reported specific to estimating both reliability and construct validity of psychological need satisfaction scores with reference to SDT's nomological network (Cronbach and Meehl, 1955) which included indices of motivation and behavior (drawn mainly from OIT) alongside proxy markers of well-being (drawn mainly from BPN). Assessment of construct validity evidence in this review was based on select aspects of the framework advocated by Messick's (1995) work in the educational testing literature. In brief, Messick (1995) contended that construct validation concerns the suitability of score interpretations derived from tests as opposed to the instruments themselves and outlined six sources of potential construct validity evidence. Our focus in this investigation concerned four of the six (i.e., content, external, structural, and generalizability-based evidence) sources outlined by Messick (1995) given that substantive and consequential-based validity evidence are more applicable to educational testing than exercise psychology research.

Two coders independently coded all studies selected for inclusion in this review. The primary researcher trained each coder with respect to the substantive nature of the constructs of interest (e.g., competence, autonomy, and relatedness) and the assessment procedures outlined in the coding sheet. Training proceeded in sequential stages. First, each coder was asked to code a random sampling of articles ($n = 3$) that served to familiarize coders with the assessment protocol and the foundation to discuss ambiguities that arose during coding. Second, modifications to the coding sheet were discussed and implemented based on experiential feedback from the coders with the intent of providing greater clarity specific to statistical techniques used to examine the psychometric characteristics of test scores and domain clarity with reference to the item content of instruments used in the coded studies. Any discrepancies that were found between the two coders were brought to the primary investigator for discussion, and a decision was made after deliberation. As a final check, one separate member of the research team with formal training and substantive experience in meta-analytic investigations reviewed all studies coded to ensure consistency of data reporting from each coder.

Results

Study Characteristics

Twenty-seven published (including in press) empirical research articles produced thirty-three studies that met inclusion criteria (see Table 1). One study attempted to experimentally manipulate psychological need satisfaction postulated within SDT using a randomized design with 97.0% ($n = 32$) of the studies classified as non-experimental. Five studies (15.6%)

assessed changes in psychological need satisfactions via exercise over time. The majority of studies 84.8% ($n = 28$) utilized purposive sampling, whereas 15.2% ($n = 5$) used convenience sampling techniques.

Participant Characteristics

Studies retained for inclusion yielded an overall sample size of 10,451 ($R = 26 - 1872$). Age was reported in 97.0% ($n = 32$) of studies included in this review ($M_{age} = 30.64$; $SD = 8.01$). Gender was reported in 90.9% ($n = 30$) of studies, with 83.3% ($n = 25$) of these investigations using mixed gender samples and 16.7% ($n = 5$) using women only. All studies reporting sample ethnicity identified participants were of mixed ethnic origin 27.3% ($n = 9$). Exercise mode was not reported in 9.10% ($n = 3$) studies. When reported, participants engaged in various modes of exercise in 70.0% ($n = 21$) of the studies, with 26.7% ($n = 8$) and 3.3% ($n = 1$) reporting participants engaging in aerobic or resistance training exercise only. Two studies examined exercise-specific feelings of psychological need satisfaction in symptomatic populations (i.e., cancer survivors, exercise on prescription affiliates), whereas conclusions derived from 93.9% ($n = 31$) of the studies were from adult populations recording no symptomatic health conditions.

The Measurement of Psychological Need Satisfaction in Exercise

Various instruments were used to measure psychological need satisfaction in exercise across the 33 studies coded. The majority of studies (90.9%; $n = 30$) used varied instruments containing context-specific item content to measure psychological need satisfaction in exercise. Over one-third of the coded studies used instrumentation developed expressly to examine the fulfillment of basic psychological needs in exercise contexts including the PNSE (24.2%; $n = 8$) and the BPNES (15.2%; $n = 5$). The remaining studies incorporated either proxy instruments to measure psychological need satisfaction in exercise (24.2%; $n = 8$), used single item indicators (18.2%; $n = 6$), employed instruments adapted to exercise from other contexts (15.2%; $n = 5$), or used an unpublished instrument (3.0%; $n = 1$).

Descriptive Statistics

Consideration of descriptive statistics indicated that participants reported moderate-to-high levels of psychological need satisfaction in exercise regardless of the instrument used (see Table 1). Satisfaction of competence and autonomy needs in exercise settings were more strongly endorsed by exercisers than relatedness needs across the majority of coded studies.

Table 1. Evidence informing the interpretation of test scores for instruments measuring perceived psychological need satisfaction in exercise (studies are sorted alphabetically by first author)

Author (Year)	Measure of Psychological Need Satisfaction / Reliability	Descriptive Statistics / Evidence for score validity derived from psychological need satisfaction instruments
Edmunds, Ntoumanis, and Duda (2006a)		Purpose: Examined the relationship between psychological need satisfaction, motivational regulation, and exercise behavior.
	Basic Need Satisfaction at Work (Deci et al., 2001) modified for exercise context. *Reliability*[@] Study 1: α_C = .65; α_A = .65, α_R = .85; Study 2: α_C = .65; α_A = .64, α_R = >.70	*Descriptive Statistics* Study 1: M_C = 5.02; SD_C = .95; M_A = 5.49; SD_A = .82; M_R = 5.10; SD_R = 1.15. Study 2: M_C = 5.07; SD_C = .90; M_A = 5.25; SD_A = .82; M_R = 5.16; SD_R = 1.03. *External Validity* 1. Pattern of relationships between PNS sub-scale scores ($r_{A,R}$ = .37 - $r_{C,R}$ = .52). 2. Study 1: Pattern of relationships between PNS scores and motivational regulation ($r_{C,ER}$ = -.22 – $r_{C,INT}$ = .47; $r_{A,ER}$ = -.33 - $r_{A,INT}$ = .26; $r_{R,ER}$ = -.12 - $r_{R,INT}$ = .34). Study 2: After controlling for gender, age, and perceived autonomy support, INT was predicted by (β_C = .38; β_A = .02; β_R = .02) and IDENT by (β_C = .45). 3. Exercise intensity: trend toward stronger correlations with increased intensity ($r_{C,mild}$ = -.09 – $r_{C,strenuous}$ = .38; $r_{A,mild}$ = .02 – $r_{A,total}$ = .16; $r_{R,moderate}$ = -.01 – $r_{R,strenuous}$ = .17). After controlling for gender and age, total exercise was predicted by (β_C = .22; β_A = .09; β_R = -.04) and strenuous exercise by (β_C = .36; β_A = -.01; β_R = -.06).
Edmunds, Ntoumanis, and Duda (2006b)		Purpose: Examined whether those classified as 'non-dependent-symptomatic' or 'nondependent-asymptomatic' for exercise dependence differed in terms of psychological need satisfaction, self-determined vs. controlling motivation, and exercise behavior.
	Basic Need Satisfaction at Work (Deci et al., 2001) modified for exercise context. *Reliability*[@] α_C = .63; α_A = .66, α_R = .85	*Descriptive Statistics* Symptomatic: M_C = 5.13; SD_C = .90; M_A = 5.49; SD_A = .83; M_R = 5.15; SD_R = 1.14. Asymptomatic: M_C = 4.76; SD_C = .94; M_A = 5.47; SD_A = .82; M_R = 4.97; SD_R = 1.21. *External Validity* 1. Exercise intensity: After controlling for gender and age ($n_{symptomatic}$ = 198), 5% unique variance in total exercise attributed to PNS scores (R^2_{adj} = .09; β_C = .16; β_A = .16; β_R = .01); 8% unique variance in strenuous exercise attributed to PNS scores (R^2_{adj} = .15; β_C = .32; β_A = .01; β_R = -.02). After controlling for gender and age ($n_{asymptomatic}$ = 141), 3% unique variance in strenuous exercise attributed to PNS scores (R^2_{adj} = .14; β_C = .26; β_A = -.03; β_R = -.15). 2. Effect size estimates discriminating between symptomatic and asymptomatic samples (d_C = .40; d_A = .02; d_R = 15).

Table 1. (Continued)

Author (Year)	Measure of Psychological Need Satisfaction Reliability	Descriptive Statistics Evidence for score validity derived from psychological need satisfaction instruments
		Purpose: To examine whether overweight/obese individuals who adhered more to their exercise prescriptions reported greater levels of psychological need satisfaction compared to those who adhered less to their exercise program.
Edmunds, Ntoumanis, and Duda (2007)*	9 – Item instrument developed by Tobin (2003). *Reliability*[@] $\alpha_C = .72 - .83$; $\alpha_A = .55 - .62$; $\alpha_R = .74 - 88$ across three time points.	*Descriptive Statistics* Baseline: $M_C = 3.35$; $SD_C = 1.69$; $M_A = 4.01$; $SD_A = 1.62$; $M_R = 3.50$; $SD_R = 1.69$. One month: $M_C = 3.82$; $SD_C = 1.34$; $M_A = 4.15$; $SD_A = 1.53$; $M_R = 3.73$; $SD_R = 1.45$. 3 months: $M_C = 3.66$; $SD_C = 1.05$; $M_A = 4.05$; $SD_C = 1.58$; $M_R = 3.37$; $SD_R = 1.32$. *External Validity* 1. Pattern of relationships between PNS sub-scale scores averaged across three test administrations ($r_{A,R} = .10 - r_{C,R} = .49$). 2. Pattern of relationships between PNS scores and motivational regulation averaged across three test administrations ($r_{C,INTR} = .26 - r_{C,IDENT} = .66$; $r_{A,ER} = -.29 - r_{A,INT} = .57$; $r_{R,INTRE} = .08 - r_{R,ER} = .48$). Positive β weights associated with self-determined forms of motivation. Positive and negative β weights predictive of more controlling forms. Effect of autonomy on motivational regulations increased over time ($\beta_{INT} = 10$; $\beta_{IDENT} = .15$; $\beta_{INTRE} = .19$) as did perceptions of competence ($\beta_{INTRE} = .18$). 3. Pattern of relationships with indices of well-being ($r_{C,SWL} = -.09 - r_{C,SV} = .34$; $r_{A,NAffect} = -.35 - r_{A,PAffect} = .38$; $r_{R,NAffect} = -.29 - r_{R,SV} = .46$). Autonomy was a positive predictor of satisfaction with life ($\beta = .36$) and increased over time ($\beta = .20$). 4. Women reported greater increases in relatedness across the 3 month period ($\beta = .51$). 5. Exercise adherence: Small correlations with PNS scores averaged over a 3 month period ($r_C = .13 - r_R = .24$). At 3 months, weak negative relationship with autonomy ($r = -.08$) and small positive relationships with competence ($r = .13$) and relatedness ($r = .34$). Adherers demonstrated greater increases in relatedness at 1 and 3 months ($\beta = .21$) with women reporting greater increases over time than men.

Hagger, Chatzisarantis, and Harris (2006)	Purpose: To investigate the influence of global level psychological need satisfaction on exercise behavior.
	Global measure of psychological needs (Sheldon et al., 2001). *Reliability* Composite α = .87	*External Validity* 1. Structural paths between global PNS scores and relative autonomous motives (β = .16). 2. Factor correlations between global PNS scores and exercise (φ = .15). *Structural Validity* Correlations between latent PNS factors (φ$_{Mdn}$ = .54).
Kowal and Fortier (1999)	Purpose: Examined the relationships between situational motivational determinants and flow.
	Adapted versions of the Perceived Competence Scale for Children (Harter, 1982); the Autonomy Perceptions in Life Contexts Scale (Blais and Vallerand, (1992) and; the Perceived Relatedness Scale (Richer and Vallerand, 1998). *Reliability* α$_C$ = .69; α$_A$ = .54, α$_R$ = .81	*Descriptive Statistics* Weighted means based on tertile splits: M_C = 5.24; SD_C = .88; M_A = 4.64; SD_A = 1.37; M_R = 5.55; SD_R = 1.00. *External Validity* 1. Pattern of relationships between PNS scores and motivational determinants ($r_{C:transformationoftime}$ = -.07 - $r_{C:challenge-skillbalance}$ = .63; $r_{A:transformationoftime}$ = -.03 - $r_{A:concentration}$ = .25; $r_{R:transformationoftime}$ = .11 - $r_{R:challenge-skillbalance}$ = .50).
Kowal and Fortier (2000)	Purpose: To test Vallerand's (1997) hierarchical model of intrinsic and extrinsic motivation in a physical activity context.
	Adapted versions of: Competence (Fortier, Vallerand, and Guay, 1995); the Autonomy Perceptions in Life Contexts Scale (Blais and Vallerand, 1992) and; Perceived Relatedness Scale (Richer and Vallerand, 1998). *Reliability:* Situational α$_C$ = .60; α$_A$ = .51; α$_R$ = .82. Contextual: α$_C$ = .83; α$_A$ = .79; α$_R$ = .86	*Descriptive Statistics* Situational: M_C = 5.29; SD_C = .85; M_A = 4.85; SD_A = 1.24; M_R = 5.36; SD_R = .91. Contextual: M_C = 4.89; SD_C = 1.16; M_A = 4.65; SD_A = 1.41; M_R = 5.47; SD_R = .82. *Validity* 1. Pattern of relationships between situational PNS sub-scale scores ($r_{A:R}$ = -.03 - $r_{C:R}$ = .35) and contextual PNS sub-scale scores ($r_{C:A}$ = -.14 - $r_{C:R}$ = .27). 2. Patterns of relationships between situational PNS and situational and contextual motivation ranged from r_A = .27 - r_C = .54 and r_A = .21 - r_C = .36 respectively. Patterns of relationships between contextual PNS and situational and contextual motivation ranged from r_C = .28 - r_R = .31 and r_C = .20 - r_R = .42 respectively. Flow was positively associated with all PNS subscale scores with greatest magnitude associated with situational and contextual relatedness (r_s = .47 and .44 respectively).

Table 1. (Continued)

Author (Year)	Measure of Psychological Need Satisfaction Reliability	Descriptive Statistics Evidence for score validity derived from psychological need satisfaction instruments
Levy and Cardinal (2004)		Purpose: To examine the effect of a mail-mediated intervention based on self-determination theory on adult's exercise behavior.
	Adapted sport competence subscale of the Physical Self-Perception Profile (Fox, 1990); autonomy via the Locus of Causality for Exercise Scale (Markland and Hardy, 1997); relatedness via the Social Support for Exercise Questionnaire (Sallis et al., 1987). *Reliability* Specifics not reported.	*Descriptive Statistics* Competence generally increased over time. Autonomy and relatedness increased Baseline – Time 1 and decreased slightly at Time 2. *Content Validity* 1. Specifics not reported. *External Validity* 1. Females: Reported changes in autonomy across the three test administrations ($\eta^2 = .07$). 2. Exercise behavior: Increased exercise behavior for females ($\eta^2 = .20$) only. Interventions based on SDT did not result in significant behavior change compared to control.
Li (1999)	Purpose: To construct an exercise motivation scale and provide initial evidence of its psychometric properties.	
	Contextual competence: Sport competence subscale of the Physical Self-Perception Profile (Fox, 1990); autonomy: adapted Exercise Objectives Locus of Control Scale (McCready and Long, 1985); relatedness: adapted Social Support Scale for Children (Harter, 1985). *Reliability*[@] $\alpha_C = .87; \alpha_A = .87, \alpha_R = .76$	*External Validity* 1. Competence positively related to exercise motivation ($\gamma_{ER} = .12 - \gamma_{IDENT} .22$); autonomy positively related to self-determined forms (γs ranged from .16 to .32) and negatively related to non-determined forms (γs ranged from -.20 to -.23); relatedness positively related to self-determined forms (γs ranged from .15 to .18) and negatively related to non-determined forms (γs ranged from -.14 to -.17).
Markland (1999)	Purpose: To determine whether self-determination moderates the effects of perceived competence on intrinsic motivation or whether self-determination and perceived competence have independent effects.	
	Contextual competence: IMI – PC (McAuley et al., 1989); Autonomy: Locus of Causality for Exercise Scale (Markland and Hardy, 1997). *Reliability* $\alpha_C = .81; \alpha_A = .87$	*Descriptive Statistics* $M_C = 4.27; SD_C = 1.30; M_A = 4.20; SD_A = 1.33$. *External Validity* 1. Factor correlations ($r_{C,A} = .45$) 2. Effect for competence on enjoyment/interest in physical activity ($R^2 = .24$). When autonomy entered, ($R^2 = .52; R^2_\Delta = .28$).

Markland and Hardy (1997)	Purpose: The development of a perceived locus of causality scale.	
	Contextual competence: modified IMI – PC (McAuley et al., 1989); Contextual autonomy: Locus of Causality for Exercise Scale (Markland and Hardy, 1997).	*Descriptive Statistics*
		M_C 4.15; $SD_C = 1.34$; $M_A = 4.07$; $SD_A = 1.42$.
		External Validity
		1. Factor correlations ($r_{C.A} = .62$).
	Reliability	2. Patterns of interrelationships with $r_{C.pressure} = .55 - r_{C.effort} = .68$ and $r_{A.effort} = .75 - r_{A.pressure} = .78$.
	$\alpha_{C=} .81$; $\alpha_{A=} .82$	
Parfitt, Rose, and Markland (2000)	Purpose: To compare the effects of preferred vs. prescribed intensity exercise on affect and enjoyment.	
	IMI - perceived competence and perceived choice (McAuley et al., 1989) modified to the exercise mode.	*External Validity*
		1. Discriminant validity supported a large effect ($d = 2.03$) with perceived choice and weak effect ($d = .12$) for perceived competence between preferred and prescribed intensity exercise.
	Reliability	
	Specifics not reported.	
Peddle, Plotnikoff, Wild, Au, and Courneya (in press)	Purpose: To evaluate medical, demographic, and psychosocial correlates of exercise in colorectal cancer survivors.	
	PNSE (Wilson et al., 2006).	*External Validity*
	Reliability	1. Pattern of relationships between PNS sub-scale scores ($r_{A.R} = .38 - r_{C.A} = .59$).
	$\alpha_C = .95$; $\alpha_A = .95$, $\alpha_R = .96$	2. Pattern of relationships between PNS scores and motivational regulation ($r_{C.ER} = -.16 - r_{C.INT} = .49$; $r_{A.ER} = -.21 - r_{A.INT} = .35$; $r_{R.ER} = -.07 - r_{R.INT} = .49$).
		3. PNS scores predicted INTRO: ($\beta_A = -.19$; $\beta_R = .15$); INDENT ($\beta_C = .27$; $\beta_R = .13$).
		4. Exercise Intensity: Pattern of relationships with moderate/vigorous exercise ($r_C = .29$; $r_A = .22$; $r_R = .29$).

Table 1. (Continued)

Author (Year)	Measure of Psychological Need Satisfaction Reliability	Descriptive Statistics Evidence for score validity derived from psychological need satisfaction instruments
Thorgersen-Ntoumani, and Ntoumanis (2007)	Purpose: To examine motivational predictors of body image concerns, self-presentation, and self-perceptions.	
	Basic Need Satisfaction in Life Scale (Gagné, 2003) as a global measure. *Reliability*[@] $\alpha_C = .60$; $\alpha_A = .76$, $\alpha_R = .75$	*Descriptive Statistics* $M_C = 5.36$; $SD_C = 0.76$; $M_A = 5.27$; $SD_A = 0.85$; $M_R = 5.65$; $SD_R = 0.77$. *External Validity* 1. Pattern of relationships between PNS sub-scale scores ($r_{A.R} = .48$ - $r_{C.A} = .54$). 2. Pattern of relationships between PNS scores and motivational regulation ($r_{C.INTRO} = -.36$ - $r_{C.INT} = .21$; $r_{A.INTRO} = -.29$ - $r_{A.INT} = .16$; $r_{R.INTRO} = -.26$ - $r_{R.INT} = .29$). 3. Pattern of relationships with self-esteem ($r_{R} = .44$ - $r_A = .58$) and PSW ($r_R = .43$ - $r_A = .60$). 4. Discriminant validity support demonstrated as those not a risk for eating disorders demonstrated higher PNS scores than those at risk ($d_A = 1.01$ - $d_R = .56$).
Wilson, Rodgers, and Fraser (2002a)	Purpose: To examine the pattern of relationships between the motivation for physical activity measure and psychological needs satisfaction.	
	Three single items measures served as contextual measures of PNS. *Reliability* Not applicable given single item indicators.	*Descriptive Statistics* $M_C = 5.60$; $SD_C = 1.05$; $M_A = 5.62$; $SD_A = 1.18$; $M_R = 4.67$; $SD_R = 1.41$. *External Validity* 1. Pattern of relationships between PNS sub-scale scores ($r_{C.R} = .19$ - $r_{C.A} = .47$). 2. Pattern of relationships between PNS scores and exercise motivation ($r_{C.appearance \, and} r_{C.social} = .12$ - $r_{C.enjoyment-interest} = .45$; $r_{A.appearance} = .07$ - $r_{A.enjoyment-interest} = .48$; $r_{R.appearance} = .03$ - $r_{R.social} = .46$).
Wilson, Rodgers, and Fraser (2002b)	Purpose: To examine the pattern of relationships between the BREQ, psychological need satisfaction and exercise behavior.	
	Three single items measures Served as contextual measures of PNS. *Reliability* Not applicable given single item indicators.	*Descriptive Statistics* $M_C = 5.50$; $SD_C = 1.07$; $M_A = 5.56$; $SD_A = 1.19$; $M_R = 4.56$; $SD_R = 1.48$. *External Validity* 1. Pattern of relationships between PNS sub-scale scores ($r_{C.R} = .23$ - $r_{C.A} = .49$). 2. Pattern of relationships between PNS scores and motivational regulation ($r_{C.ER} = -.18$ - $r_{C.INT} = .46$; $r_{A.ER} = -.07$ - $r_{A.INT} = .40$; $r_{R.ER} = .02$ - $r_{R.INT} = .19$).

Wilson, Rodgers, Blanchard, and Gessell (2003)	Purpose: To examine the relationships between psychological need satisfaction, exercise regulations, and motivational consequences.	
	Activity Feeling Scale (Reeve and Sickenius, 1993) served as a contextual measure of PNS. *Reliability*[@] $\alpha_{C.Time1} = .85$; $\alpha_{C.Time2} = .93$; $\alpha_{A.Time1} = .74$; $\alpha_{A.Time2} = .68$; $\alpha_{R.Time1} = .75$; $\alpha_{R.Time2} = .81$	*Descriptive Statistics* $M_C = 5.04$; $SD_C = 1.01$; $M_A = 6.51$; $SD_A = 0.70$; $M_R = 3.55$; $SD_R = 1.31$. *External Validity* 1. Pattern of relationships between PNS sub-scale scores ($r_{A.R} = -.04 - r_{C.R} = .31$). 2. Pattern of relationships between PNS scores and motivational regulation ($r_{C.ER} = -.16 - r_{C.INT} = .53$; $r_{A.ER} = -.18 - r_{A.IDENT} = .33$; $r_{R.ER} = .01 - r_{R.INTRO} = .19$). 3. Changes in PNS scores across the 12 week intervention ($d_C = .69$; $d_A = -1.19$; $d_R = 1.46$).
Wilson, Muon, Rodgers, and Murray (2006)	Purpose: To examine the relationship between psychological need satisfaction and well-being in exercise.	
	Study 1: Three single items measures served as contextual measures of PNS Study 2: PNSE (Wilson et al., 2006). *Reliability* Study 2: $\alpha_C = .89$; $\alpha_A = .94$; $\alpha_R = .91$	*Descriptive Statistics* Study 1; Time 1: $M_C = 5.25$; $SD_C = 1.42$; $M_A = 5.29$; $SD_A = 1.42$; $M_R = 4.35$; $SD_R = 1.65$. Study 1; Time 2: $M_C = 5.86$; $SD_C = 0.80$; $M_A = 5.97$; $SD_A = 0.96$; $M_R = 3.94$; $SD_R = 1.97$. Study 2: $M_C = 5.19$; $SD_C = 0.73$; $M_A = 5.42$; $SD_A = 0.79$; $M_R = 4.49$; $SD_R = 1.20$. *External Validity* 1. Pattern of relationships between PNS sub-scale scores: Study 1; Time 1: $r_{C.R} = .34 - r_{C.A} = .80$; Time 2: $r_{C.R} = .19 - r_{C.A} = .46$; Study 2: $r_{A.R} = .22 - r_{C.A} = .53$. 2. Relationships between PNS sub-scale scores and indices of well-being: Study 1; Time 1: ($r_{R.SV} = .17 - r_{A.SV} = .42$); Study 1; Time 2: ($r_{R.SV} = .15 - r_{C.SV} = .43$); Correlations with residual change scores ($r_{R.SV} = .08 - r_{A.SV} = .29$). Study 2: ($r_{A.PAffect} = .14 - r_{C.PAffect} = .36$) and ($r_{R.NAffect} = -.13 - r_{C.NAffect} = -.34$). 3. Pattern of weak to moderate relationships between PNSE scores and global PNS scores. ($r_{R.BasicPsychologicalNeeds.Popularity} = -.03 - r_{C.BasicPsychologicalNeeds.PhysicalThriving} = .45$). 4. Study 1: Positive changes in the satisfaction of competence and autonomy scores ($d = .33$) and negative change in relatedness ($d = .19$) across the 12 week period. *Structural Validity* Factorial composition and structure of PNSE scores $\chi^2 = 340.29$, $df = 132$, $p < .01$, CFI = .93, IFI = .93, RMSEA = .09; 90% CI = .08 - .11. Interfactor correlations (φ) were moderate to strong.

Table 1. (Continued)

Author (Year)	Measure of Psychological Need Satisfaction Reliability	Descriptive Statistics Evidence for score validity derived from psychological need satisfaction instruments
Wilson, Rodgers, Loitz, and Scime (2006)	Purpose: To examine the pattern of relationships between the BREQ, psychological need satisfaction and exercise behavior.	
	Three single items measures served as contextual measures of PNS *Reliability* Not applicable given single item indicators.	*Descriptive Statistics* $M_C = 5.61$; $SD_C = 1.27$; $M_A = 5.88$; $SD_A = 1.13$; $M_R = 5.61$; $SD_R = 1.25$. *External Validity* 1. Pattern of relationships between PNS sub-scale scores ($r_{A.R} = .31 - r_{C.A} = .75$). 2. Pattern of relationships between PNS scores and motivational regulation ($r_{C.ER} = -.26 - r_{C.INT} = .54$; $r_{A.ER} = -.17 - r_{A.INTE} = .55$; $r_{R.ER} = .00 - r_{R.INTE} = .29$). 3. Stronger effects were noted between PNS and autonomous ($R^2_{adj} = .19 - .31$) vs. controlled ($R^2_{adj} = .06$) motives. Structure coefficients demonstrated that competence predicted less controlling motives and greater intrinsic regulation, autonomy predicted more autonomous motives, and relatedness both autonomous and controlling motives.
Wilson, Rogers, Rodgers, and Wild (2006)	Purpose: To provide construct validity evidence for scores derived from the PNSE. *Reliability* $\alpha_C = .91$; $\alpha_A = .91$; $\alpha_R = .90$ for Study 1 and Study 2.	*Descriptive Statistics* Study 1: $M_C = 5.36$; $SD_C = 0.65$; $M_A = 5.50$; $SD_A = 0.59$; $M_R = 4.57$; $SD_R = 0.99$. Study 2: $M_C = 5.31$; $SD_C = 0.68$; $M_A = 5.54$; $SD_A = 0.60$; $M_R = 4.48$; $SD_R = 1.07$. *Content Validity* Forty experts with diverse but relevant content domain expertise rated each item according to item content relevance and representation. Aiken's item content validity (V) coefficient supported relevance ($M_V = 0.92$; $SD = 0.07$) and representation ($M_V = 0.87$; $SD = 0.05$) of PNSE items. *External Validity* 1. Pattern of relationships between PNS sub-scale scores (Study 1: $r_{A.R} = .09 - r_{C.A} = .46$; Study 2: $r_{A.R} = .10 - r_{C.A} = .46$). 2. Study 2: PNSE scores most highly correlated with proxy measures ($r_{C.IMcompetence} = .65$; $r_{A.IMchoice} = .32$; $r_{R.IMaffiliation} = .48$). *Structural Validity* Study 1: Total variance accounted for 63.3%. Inter-factor correlations ranged from $r_{A.R} = .01 - r_{C.A} = .46$). Study 2: Pattern of factor loadings ranged from .69 - .90 on target factors. Measurement model total sample: goodness of fit statistics: $\chi^2 = 688.03$; $df = 132$; $CFI = .94$; $IFI = .94$; $SRMSR = .07$; $RMSEA = .09$; $90\% CI = .08 - .09$. Comparable fit indices across gender. *Generalizability validity* Invariance tests suggested PNSE score interpretations are relatively robust to gender.

Wilson, Mack, and Blanchard (in press)	Purpose: To examine the role of psychological need satisfaction on affective responses in an exercise context.	
	Study 1: Three single items measures served as contextual measure of PNS. *Study 2*: PNSE (Wilson et al., 2006). *Reliability* *Study 1*: Gloabl PNS α = .62 *Study 2*: α_C = .91; α_A = .94; α_R = .92	*Descriptive Statistics* *Study 1*: M_C = 5.63; SD_C = 0.91; M_A = 5.60; SD_A = 1.05; M_R = 4.68; SD_R = 1.39. *Study 2*: M_C = 4.82; SD_C = 0.91; M_A = 4.96; SD_A = 0.99; M_R = 4.44; SD_R = 1.04. *External Validity* 1. Pattern of relationships between PNS sub-scale scores (*Study 1*: $r_{C.R}$ = .23 - $r_{C.A}$ = .54; *Study 2*: $r_{A.R}$ = .58 - $r_{C.A}$ = .82). 2. Relationships between PNS sub-scale scores and indices of well-being: *Study 1*: ($r_{R.PWB}$ = .20 - $r_{C.PWB}$ = .38); PNS scores negative relationship with PD (φ = .18) and positive relationship with PWB (φ = 2.56). *Study 2*: $r_{R.P.Affect}$ = .52 - $r_{C.P.Affect}$ = .63; Moderate influence of PNSE scores on positive affect (β_C = .54; β_A = .52; β_R = .44) and a small influence on negative affect (β_C = -.20; β_A = -.26; β_R = -.01). *Structural Validity* *Study 2*: Goodness of fit statistics: χ^2 =327.46; df = 132; CFI = .92; IFI = .92; $SRMSR$ = .07; $RMSEA$ = .09; 90% CI = .08 - .11.
Wilson, Mack, and Lightheart (in press)	Purpose: To examine the importance of basic psychological needs to domain specific well-being in female exercisers.	
	Study 1: Three single items measures served as contextual measure of PNS. *Study 2*: PNSE (Wilson et al., 2006). *Reliability* *Study 2*: α_C = .90; α_A = .90; α_R = .87. $\alpha_{females}$ = .88 - .92; α_{males} = .84 - .87	*Descriptive Statistics* *Study 1*: M_C = 5.64; SD_C = 0.94; M_A = 5.68; SD_A = 0.98; M_R = 4.65; SD_R = 1.44. *Study 2*: M_C = 5.21; SD_C = 0.68; M_A = 5.56; SD_A = 0.53; M_R = 4.50; SD_R = 0.92. Similar pattern for males and females. *External Validity* 1. *Study 1*: Pattern of relationships between PNS sub-scale scores ($r_{C.R}$ = .24 - $r_{C.A}$ = .56). *Study 2*: ($r_{A.R}$ = -.01 - $r_{C.A}$ = .42). Females ($r_{A.R}$ = .04 - $r_{C.A}$ = .43); Males ($r_{A.R}$ = -.17 - $r_{C.A}$ = .29). 2. *Study 1*: PNS scores predicted greater physical self-worth (γ = .43; R^2 = .18). *Study 2*: Separate analyses of PNS scores predicted greater physical self-worth with competence accounting for the greatest portion of the variance (R^2_{adj} = .24; β = .47) and relatedness (R^2_{adj} = .08; β = .13) the least. Gender was not a meaningful moderator.

Table 1. (Continued)

Author (Year)	Measure of Psychological Need Satisfaction / Reliability	Descriptive Statistics / Evidence for score validity derived from psychological need satisfaction instruments
Wilson, Mack, Muon, and LeBlanc (2007)	Purpose: To examine whether perceived psychological need satisfaction underpins the endorsement of different motives.	
	PNSE (Wilson et al., 2006)	*Descriptive Statistics*
	Reliability	$M_C = 4.82; SD_C = 0.90; M_A = 4.97; SD_A = 1.00; M_R = 4.44; SD_R = 1.04.$
	$\alpha_C = .91; \alpha_A = .95; \alpha_R = .92$	*External Validity*
		1. Pattern of relationships between PNS sub-scale scores ($r_{A.R} = .59 - r_{C.A} = .82$).
		2. Pattern of relationships between PNS scores and motivational regulation ($r_{C.ER} = -.22 - r_{C.INT} = .67; r_{A.ER} = -.30 - r_{A.INT} = .67; r_{R.ER} = -.06 - r_{R.INT} = .63$). PNSE scores predicted a relative autonomy index of motivation ($R^2_{adj} = .42$) with positive associations between autonomy ($\beta = .53$) and competence ($\beta = .25$) and autonomous motivation and relatedness negatively associated ($\beta = -.12$).
		Structural Validity
		Measurement model: $\chi^2 = 334.36; df = 132; CFI = .92; IFI = .92; RMSEA = .10; 90\% CI = .08 - .11.$
Wilson and Muon (in press)	Purpose: To examine criterion validity of scores derived from the Exercise Identity Scale.	
	PNSE (Wilson et al., 2006).	*Descriptive Statistics*
	Reliability	$M_C = 5.15; SD_C = 0.76; M_A = 5.51; SD_A = 0.70; M_R = 4.60; SD_R = 0.95.$
	$\alpha_C = .91; \alpha_A = .92; \alpha_R = .89$	*External Validity*
		1. Pattern of relationships between PNS sub-scale scores ($r_{A.R} = .15 - r_{C.A} = .50$).
		2. Exercise Intensity: ($r_C = .32; r_A = .11; r_R = .29$).
Vlachopoulos (2007)	Purpose: To provide structural and predictive validity of test scores.	
	BPNES (Vlachopoulos and Michailidou, 2006).	*Descriptive Statistics*
	Reliability	Descriptive not reported.
	$\alpha_C = .86; \alpha_A = .84; \alpha_R = .92$	*External Validity*
		1. Pattern of relationships between PNS sub-scale scores ($r_{A.R} = .63 - r_{C.A} = .74$).
		2. IMI interest-enjoyment ($R^2_{adj} = .56; \beta_C = .31; \beta_A = .34; \beta_R = .17$).
		Structural Validity
		Pattern of factor loadings ranged from .59 - .90; $\chi^2 = 209.87; df = 51; CFI = .98; NNFI = .97; RMSEA = .06; 90\% CI = .05 - .07.$ Three factor model superior fit compared to two and one factor model.
		Generalizability Validity
		Measurement invariance noted between community and private exercise participants. [#]

Vlachopoulos and Michailidou (2006)	Purpose: The development and initial validation of the Basic Psychological Needs in Exercise Scale.	
	BPNES (Vlachopoulos and Michailidou, 2006). *Reliability* $\alpha_C = .81$; $\alpha_A = .84$; $\alpha_R = .92$ *Test-retest Reliability* ICC = .97 for all scores.	*Descriptive Statistics* Time 1: $M_C = 3.80$; $SD_C = 0.57$; $M_A = 3.94$; $SD_A = 0.66$; $M_R = 3.70$; $SD_R = 0.73$. Time 2: $M_C = 3.81$; $SD_C = 0.59$; $M_A = 3.97$; $SD_A = 0.67$; $M_R = 3.74$; $SD_R = 0.75$. *Content Validity:* Item generation resulted in 10, 13, 8 items for competence, autonomy, and relatedness respectively. Items developed examined by 3 judges with expertise in basic psychological needs consistent with SDT. Based on comments 1 item deleted from Competence and Autonomy and two items added to Relatedness. 20 exercise participants evaluated items for writing, clarity, and personal relevance. *External Validity* 1. IMI interest-enjoyment: ($R^2_{adj} = .58$; $\beta_C = .51$; $\beta_A = .25$; $\beta_R = .05$) 2. Exercise Frequency: ($R^2_{adj} = .10$; $\beta_C = .21$; $\beta_A = .14$; $\beta_R = -.03$). *Structural Validity* Sample 1: Pattern of factor loadings ranged from .59 - .91; $\chi^2 = 166.43$; $df = 51$; $CFI = .96$; $NNFI = .96$; $SRMR = .04$; $RMSEA = .06$; 90% $CI = .05 - .07$. Sample 2: Pattern of factor loadings ranged from .60 - .89; $\chi^2 = 122.28$; $df = 51$; $CFI = .97$; $NNFI = .97$; $SRMR = .03$; $RMSEA = .05$; 90% $CI = .04 - .06$.
Vlachopoulos (in press)	Purpose: To examine measurement invariance across gender of scores derived from BPNSE.	
	BPNES (Vlachopoulos and Michailidou, 2006). *Reliability* Females ($\alpha_C = .83$; $\alpha_A = .84$; $\alpha_R = .92$); Males ($\alpha_C = .84$; $\alpha_A = .83$; $\alpha_R = .92$)	*External Validity* 1. Pattern of relationships between PNS sub-scale scores: Females ($r_{C,R} = .53$ - $r_{C,A} = .74$); Males ($r_{A,R} = .56$ - $r_{C,A} = .84$). *Structural Validity#* Females ($n = 1147$): $\chi^2 = 161.75$; $df = 51$; $CFI = .99$; $NNFI = .98$; $RMSEA = .04$; 90% $CI = .04 - .05$. Males ($n = 716$): $\chi^2 = 145.82$; $df = 51$; $CFI = .98$; $NNFI = .98$; $RMSEA = .05$; 90% $CI = .04 - .06$. Items loadings ranged from .67 - .91. *Generalizability Validity* No support for measurement invariance by gender.

Table 1. (Continued)

Author (Year)	Measure of Psychological Need Satisfaction Reliability	Descriptive Statistics
		Evidence for score validity derived from psychological need satisfaction instruments
Vlachopoulos and Neikou (in press)		Purpose: To investigate the relative contribution of each of the three needs to the prediction exercise adherence over 6 months.
	BPNES (Vlachopoulos and Michailidou, 2006). *Reliability* Females: $\alpha_C = .92$; $\alpha_A = .94$; $\alpha_R = .92$; Males: $\alpha_C = .73$; $\alpha_A = .81$; $\alpha_R = .93$	*Descriptive Statistics* Females: $M_C = 3.39$; $SD_C = 0.92$; $M_A = 3.52$; $SD_A = 0.98$; $M_R = 3.07$; $SD_R = 0.90$. *Males*: $M_C = 3.59$; $SD_C = 0.62$; $M_A = 3.71$; $SD_A = 0.73$; $M_R = 3.31$; $SD_R = 0.91$. *External Validity* 1. Pattern of relationships between PNS sub-scale scores: Females ($r_{C,R} = .43 - r_{C,A} = .90$); Males ($r_{A,R} = .55 - r_{C,A} = .67$). 2. Exercise Attendance: Females ($\beta_C = .53$; $\beta_A = -.11$; $\beta_R = -.02$); Males ($\beta_C = .31$; $\beta_A = -.07$; $\beta_R = -.02$). After controlling for age and gender OR predicted adherers ($n = 77$) vs. dropouts ($n = 96$) over six months ($OR_C = .32$; $OR_A = .83$; $OR_R = 1.21$). 3. Estimates of effect size discriminating between males and females ($d_C = .25$; $d_A = .22$; $d_R = .27$). *Structural Validity* Females ($n = 120$): $\chi^2 = 76.90$; $df = 51$; $CFI = .98$; $NNFI = .98$; $RMSEA = .07$; $90\%\ CI = .03 - .09$; Males ($n = 108$): $\chi^2 = 98.74$; $df = 51$; $CFI = .94$; $NNFI = .92$; $RMSEA = .09$; $90\%\ CI = .07 - .12$.

Note: [*] additional analyses provided from first author; @ concerns over reliability expressed and in some cases, items deleted; # = data analyzed on similar participant pool. A = Perceived Autonomy; C = Perceived Competence; R = Perceived Relatedness; ER = External Regulation; INTRO = Introjected regulation; IDENT = Identified Regulation; INTE = Integrated Regulation; INT = Intrinsic Motivation; CFI = Comparative Fit Index; NNFI = Non-Normed Fit Index; IFI = Incremental Fit Index; SRMSR = Standardized Root Mean Square Residual; RMSEA = Root Mean Square Error of Approximation; CI = 90% Confidence Interval for RMSEA; ICC = Intra-class correlation; α = Cronbach alpha (Cronbach, 1951); β = Standardized Beta; d = Cohen's d (Cohen, 1988); η^2 = Eta squared; φ = Phi Coefficient; ψ = Standardized Path Coeffient; IMI = Intrinsic Motivation Inventory; ICC = Intra-class correlation coefficient; OR = odds ratio; PD = SEES Psychological Distress; PWB = SEES Positive Well-being; SWL = Satisfaction with Life; PA_{ffect} = Positive Affect; NA_{ffect} = Negative Affect. The purpose statement accompanying each cited article in Table 1 represents the present author's interpretation of the measurement-related focus of the article for the purposes of this review.

Measurement of Psychological Need Satisfaction – Reliability

Where possible, internal consistency reliability estimates (coefficient α; Cronbach, 1951) were recorded (see Table 1). Examination of the coded studies suggests a trend whereby lower estimates of internal consistency reliability were reported within studies using instrumentation that was either adapted, considered a proxy marker of need fulfillment (e.g., IMI-Perceived Choice subscale), or modified from other contexts (e.g., work) for the purposes of assessing psychological need satisfaction in exercise. More recent studies utilizing instruments developed specifically for exercise settings (i.e., PNSE and BPNES) demonstrated higher reliability coefficients. Three studies using either the PNSE or BPNES reported comparable internal consistency reliability estimates for item scores across gender. Evidence of high score stability in the form of test-retest reliability was documented in one study using the BPNES across a 4 week period.

Measurement of Psychological Need Satisfaction – Validity

Content Validity

Three coded studies (9.1%) reported data suggesting evidence of content validity. Two studies reported information specific to item generation and expert review procedures. One study reported statistical evidence supporting the item content relevance and representation of the initial PNSE items using the procedures advocated by Dunn, Bouffard, and Rogers (1999).

External Validity

Pattern of inter-relationships between psychological need satisfaction scores. Nineteen studies (57.8%) reported inter-factor correlations testing relationships between scores for competence, autonomy, and relatedness in exercise. A consistent pattern of low-to-moderate correlations were observed with the relationship between the fulfillment of autonomy and relatedness needs the weakest in 14 (73.7%) studies and competence and autonomy needs the strongest in 17 (89.5%) studies. The pattern of relationships remained similar across studies using both the BPNES and PNSE; however, considerable overlap (i.e., correlations ≥ 0.80) between scores from subscales of both instruments has been noted particularly for the relationship between competence and autonomy perceptions.

Psychological need satisfaction scores and exercise motivation. Seventeen studies (51.5%) examined relationships between basic psychological need satisfactions in exercise with indices of motivation. Consistent with SDT (Deci and Ryan, 2002), perceived competence, autonomy, and relatedness demonstrated consistently stronger associations with more self-determined motives (i.e., *identified* and *intrinsic* regulations) than controlling motives (i.e., *introjected* and *extrinsic* regulations). Research examining the predictive nature of basic psychological need satisfaction scores on motivation suggested a homogenous pattern of more positive associations with self-determined motives and a heterogeneous pattern of relationships with controlling motives. The need for competence, followed by autonomy and relatedness respectively, predicted the greatest portion of variance in more self-determined motives.

Psychological need satisfaction scores and well-being. Eight studies (24.2%) examined whether the fulfillment of psychological needs via exercise was related to well-being markers. Small-to-moderate positive relationships were reported between psychological need satisfaction in exercise scores and well-being markers (e.g., positive affect, physical self-worth) and negatively associated with markers of ill-being such as negative affect. Relatedness consistently demonstrated the lowest pattern of relationships in terms of magnitude with indices of well-being.

Psychological need satisfaction scores and exercise behavior. Nine studies (27.3%) examined the relationship between psychological need satisfaction and exercise behavior. In all studies, exercise behavior was assessed through self-report questionnaires with the instrumentation chosen to assess behavior reflecting various markers of intensity, frequency, and adherence. The pattern of inter-relationships suggests a small positive relationship between psychological need satisfaction scores and exercise behavior with perceived competence accounting for the greatest portion of exercise behavior variance. Five studies looked at changes over time in exercise-specific feelings of competence, autonomy, and relatedness. Patterns of change were assessed between one and six months. Available data suggests subtle fluctuations in psychological need fulfillment scores over time with a general trend towards increased perceptions of competence, autonomy, and relatedness from baseline as a result of regular exercise. Two studies noted the greatest increases occurred in perceived relatedness over the course of 12 week exercise programs. Perceptions of competence most strongly discriminated between exercise program adherents and non-adherers.

Structural and Generalizability Validity

A total of 9 studies (27.27%) have tested the structural validity of scores derived from either the PNSE (*n* = 5) or BPNES (*n* = 4) using structural equation modeling procedures. Inspection of the results across the 9 studies indicate consistent support for the structural validity of score interpretations for both the PNSE and BPNES, as well as, the reproducibility of each instrument's proposed factor structure across multiple samples of active exercisers. Score interpretations from both instruments have demonstrated evidence of invariance across gender and one study documents support for the invariance of BPNES scores across public versus private exercise settings.

Conclusion

The purpose of this review was to summarize and evaluate the development of instruments designed to measure basic psychological need satisfaction in exercise from the perspective of Deci and Ryan's (2002) SDT. Ongoing attention to measurement principles represents an important (and often overlooked) process in advancing scientific knowledge and refining theory (Kerlinger, 1979; Marsh, 1997; Messick, 1995; Stevens, 1946). Construct validation is at the heart of the measurement process (Marsh, 1997; Messick, 1995) and a move towards systematic programs of construct validation that blend applications of relevant theory (such as the BPN subtheory from SDT) with the mosaic of available evidence to inform score interpretations is now recommended (Messick, 1995). In light of this focus, it appears that instrument development research aimed at assessing basic psychological need fulfillment in accordance with SDT (Deci and Ryan, 2002) is progressing towards systematic programs aligned with Messick's (1995) vision. Overall, the results of the present review suggest that the available evidence informing the interpretation of BPNES and PNSE scores is largely consistent with the theory informing the development of both instruments.

What Does the Evidence Tell us About Measuring Psychological Need Satisfaction in Exercise?

Observations noted in this review suggest that the measurement of psychological need satisfaction in exercise from the perspective of Deci and Ryan's (2002) SDT has followed a familiar route for self-perception instruments (Fox, 1997). Results of this review indicate that initial phases of research in this area were dominated by the use of instrumentation developed in an ad hoc fashion to measure concepts integral to the BPN subtheory of SDT which have recently been supplanted by approaches using context-specific instruments to capture variation in psychological need satisfaction experienced by exercisers. Both the BPNES and PNSE have been developed using the approach to construct validation advocated by Messick (1995) and show initial signs of promise as instruments to measure exercise-specific feelings of competence, autonomy, and relatedness in a manner consistent with SDT (Deci and Ryan, 2002). The data noted in this review imply that scores from both instruments can be interpreted meaningfully given the research offering supporting evidence for structural validity (including gender invariance) and criterion validity with reference to a select portion of SDT's nomological network (Cronbach and Meehl, 1955). Combined with evidence that scores from both instruments exhibit minimal error variance in samples of young adult Greek or Canadian exercisers, the addition of both instruments appears promising and provides an avenue to explore Ryan's (1995) contentions regarding the importance of testing of SDT in applied settings (such as exercise) where contextual nuances alongside relevant theory can inform effective social change.

While the available evidence attesting to the construct validity of scores from both the PNSE and BPNES is favorable, Messick (1995) argued that construct validation requires ongoing attention to the nature and quality of evidence available to inform decisions about test score interpretation. Several issues germane to Messick's (1995) construct validation framework warrant further investigation. A number of anomalies have been noted already in research employing the PNSE and BPNES which do not coalesce easily with propositions set forth by Deci and Ryan (2002). For example, excessively large relationships between scores derived from subscales of both the PNSE (Wilson et al., 2007) and BPNES (Vlachopoulos and Michailidou, 2006) raise questions regarding either instrument's ability to discriminate between relevant constructs embedded within BPN. Further, certain studies report criterion validity coefficients from structural equation modeling analyses with indices of motivation especially for perceived relatedness that appear potentially incongruent with SDT (Vlachopouls and Michailidou, 2006; Wilson et al., 2007). It seems imprudent to suggest at this juncture that the available evidence provides a forum for distinguishing between the BPNES and the PNSE as the instrument of choice without additional research to address anomalous findings and other components of Messick's (1995) construct validation framework.

What Measurement Issues Require Further Attention in Exercise Psychology Research?

Considering the importance of instrument development and evaluation in science (Kerlinger, 1979; Marsh, 1997; Messick, 1995), it appears that a number of issues pertaining to the measurement of basic psychological need satisfaction in exercise warrant further attention. Such continued focus would be consistent with Messick's (1995) contention regarding the nature of construct validation processes in applied sciences such as exercise psychology. On the basis of the present review, it appears that at least two directions would be useful for future research to consider when measuring the satisfaction of basic psychological needs through exercise participation. These directions represent conceptual and empirical issues that arise from joint consideration of previous studies and the underlying theory providing the framework from which to interpret BPNES and PNSE scores.

One direction worthy of additional inquiry concerns an examination of areas within Messick's (1995) construct validation framework that have yet to be sufficiently addressed in applications of the BPN subtheory of SDT to exercise. Content validity issues have yet to be thoroughly tested for items comprising either the BPNES or PNSE using empirical procedures (Dunn et al., 1999) that could highlight domain clarity issues worthy of attention. Moreover, the focus in previous research on adult samples that appear young and asymptomatic using both the PNSE and BPNES restricts the generalizability of score properties for either instrument. Particular attention could be afforded to issues of measurement invariance across subgroups of interest given that a major claim of Deci and Ryan's (2002) BPN subtheory concerns the universal effects of satisfying key psychological needs on well-being irrespective of age, gender, or cultural orientation. Minimal evidence attesting to the invariance of PNSE and BPNES scores is currently available. Future studies should establish this important measurement property across subgroups of interest and meaningful time periods given that analysis of variation in basic psychological needs with time has important implications for optimizing motivation and cultivating well-being (Deci and Ryan, 2002).

A second line of empirical research that seems worthwhile concerns accumulating further evidence of external validity (Messick, 1995). Central to this portion of Messick's (1995) construct validation framework is data supporting the convergence and divergence of scores with relevant constructs articulated within the underlying theory informing an instrument's development. Previous studies have focused largely (albeit not exclusively) on providing convergent validity evidence with less attention given to including constructs that should display patterns of divergence with exercise-induced feelings of psychological need satisfaction. Inclusion of such constructs would be invaluable especially at this early stage of research with both the PNSE and BPNES given that Messick (1995) noted that divergent evidence is important in discounting (or affirming) alternative explanations for the focal constructs of interest. Arguments set forth concerning the nature of perceived autonomy (Ryan and Deci, 2007), for example, could be used to evaluate both PNSE and BPNES subscales assessing this portion of SDT's nomological network by examining relationships with perceived choice, volition, internal/external locus of causality, and coercion to more fully inform the interpretations of scores from both instruments.

Corroborating the empirical avenues for further inquiry, the results observed in this review suggest attention to a number of conceptual issues may also be worthwhile. One important conceptual issue concerns the selection and justification of criterion variables used in predictive studies to evaluate the contributions of psychological need satisfaction in exercise. Pedhazur and Pedhazur Schmlekin (1991) have suggested that a program of prediction is only as good as the quality of the criterion variable. Messick (1995) further noted that consideration of the substantive theory underlying instrument development should be given when selecting constructs to include in criterion-validity studies to prevent obfuscation. While this review indicates that an emerging body of research has examined relationships between satisfying competence, autonomy, and relatedness needs through exercise with markers of well-being, it appears that instruments used to assess well-being have been restrictive in scope. Conceptual distinctions have been made between hedonic and eudaimonic forms of well-being with the former focusing on maximizing pleasure or minimizing pain whereas the latter centers on the overall healthy functioning of the organism (Ryan and Deci, 2001). Deci and Ryan (2002) articulated clear links between the satisfaction of basic needs and eudaimonic well-being. In line with this contention, it seems reasonable to suggest that future research estimating criterion validity of either PNSE or BPNES scores give careful consideration to the selection of instruments capable of capturing eudaimonic rather than hedonic well-being.

A second conceptual challenge evident in this review concerns advancing recommendations for the most appropriate statistical treatment of data derived from instruments such as the BPNES and PNSE. Clearly the development of both the instruments has been based on SDT that suggests a multi-dimensional model comprised of three interrelated constructs, namely perceived competence, autonomy, and relatedness experienced when exercising. The conceptual challenge here centers on analyzing data in an appropriate manner to test SDT such that resultant appraisals of construct validity evidence clarify rather than confound the development of literature in this area. One approach would be to model subscales of instruments like the BPNES and PNSE as a series of first-order factors subordinate to a second-order factor representing global need satisfaction within exercise. An alternative approach concerns modeling an instrument's subscale scores individually to evaluate the unique influence attributable to satisfying each psychological need on motivation and well-being issues within exercise settings. Both approaches have merit and appear justifiable theoretically given Deci and Ryan's (2002) contention regarding the complementary nature of satisfying basic psychological needs. Empirical justifications for the first approach could also be advanced given the high relationships noted in select studies reviewed herein amongst indices of exercise-induced feelings of competence, autonomy, and relatedness. Justifications of this variety suffer greatly from beliefs regarding the merits of data-driven refinements to theory (Pedhazur and Pedhazur Schmelkin, 1991). While this conceptual challenge is hardly novel and is likely to pervade, consideration of substantive theory and relevant arguments rather than blind reliance on the 'in vogue' method of data analysis should be the pivotal factor considered in future work.

Limitations and Summary Reflections

While the results of this review are informative and provide a platform for future research with respect to the measurement of basic psychological need satisfaction in exercise, several limitations should be acknowledged pertaining to the nature of the review. First, the review focused on published (or in press) data that is susceptible to publication bias (Bennett, Latham, Stretton, and Anderson, 2004). Second, the focus of this review was restricted to the context of exercise at the expense of other physical activity settings where instrumentation used to measure the fulfillment of SDT-based psychological needs warrants careful attention (e.g., sport, physical education). Finally, no empirical analysis of the available evidence was undertaken in this review. Future research would do well to consider meta-analytical reviews of research applying the BPN subtheory proposed by Deci and Ryan (2002) to issues of exercise motivation as the wealth of available evidence in this area accumulates.

In summary, the purpose of this review was to examine the status of measurement with respect to basic psychological need satisfaction in exercise using SDT as a guiding theoretical framework. The observations gleaned from this review suggest that the measurement of competence, autonomy, and relatedness needs in exercise has matured rapidly since the *initial phase* of research started in the 1980's. The most contemporary phase of research in this area has produced the BPNES (Vlachopoulos and Michailidou, 2006) and the PNSE (Wilson et al., 2006). Both instruments were developed using an approach to construct-validation advocated by measurement experts (Marsh, 1997; Messick, 1995) and appear to hold promise for advancing our understanding of SDT in health promotion initiatives where exercising regularly is pivotal. It seems reasonable to suggest on the basis of this review that attention to measurement principles is crucial to further advancement of SDT-based knowledge in exercise psychology. Perhaps the current phase of research in this area signals 'the end of the beginning' (Churchill, 1942) with respect to our attempts to measure this important subtheory of SDT.

Authors' Note

The first and second authors were supported by grants from the Social Sciences and Humanities Research Council of Canada during the preparation of this manuscript. The third and fourth authors made equal contributions to this article and as such their names appear in alphabetical order in accordance with convention. The fifth author was completing an undergraduate honors thesis under the supervision of the first author at the time of writing this article.

References

¥ Denotes research articles used in this review.

Baumeister, R. F., and Leary, M. R. (1995). The need to belong: Desire for interpersonal attachments as a fundamental human motivation. *Psychological Bulletin, 117*, 497-529.

Bennett, D. A., Latham, N. K., Stretton, C., and Anderson, C. S. (2004). Capture-recapture is a potentially useful method for assessing publication bias. *Journal of Clinical Epidemiology, 57*, 349-357.

Blais, M. R., and Vallerand, R. J. (1992). *Dèveloppement et validation de l'èchelle des perceptions d'autonomie dans les domains de vie* [Development and validation of the Autonomy Percvpetion in Life OCNtexts Scale]. Unpublished manuscript. Universitè du Quèbec á Montrèal.

Churchill, W. (1942). "The end of the beginning". Retrieved September 9th, 2007, from The Churchill Centre. Web site: http://www.winstronchurchill. org/i4a/pages/ index. cfm? pageid=1.

Cohen, J. (1988). *Statistical power analysis for the behavioral sciences* (2nd ed.). Hillsdale, NJ: Lawrence Earlbaum Associates.

Cooper, H. (1982). Scientific guidelines for conducting integrative research reviews. *Review of Educational Research, 52,* 291-302.

Cronbach, L. J. (1951). Coefficient alpha and the internal structure of tests. *Psychometrika, 16*, 297-334.

Cronbach, L. J., and Meehl, P. E. (1955). Construct validity in psychological tests. *Psychological Bulletin, 52*, 281-302.

deCharms, R. (1968). *Personal causation: The internal affective determinants of behavior*. New York, NY: Academic Press.

Deci, E. L., and Ryan, R. M. (1985). *Intrinsic motivation and self-determination in human behavior*. New York: Plenum Press.

Deci, E. L., and Ryan, R. M. (2002). *Handbook of self-determination research*. Rochester, NY: University of Rochester Press.

Deci, E. L., Ryan, R. M., Gagné, M., Leone, D. R., Usunov, J., and Kornazheva, B. P. (2001). Need satisfaction, motivation, and well-being in the work organizations of a former Eastern Bloc country. *Personality and Social Psychology Bulletin, 27*, 930-942.

Dunn, J. G. H., Bouffard, M., and Rogers, W. T. (1999). Assessing item content relevance in sport psychology scale-construction research: Issues and recommendations. *Measurement in Physical Education and Exercise Science, 3*, 15-36.

¥Edmunds, J. K., Ntoumanis, N., and Duda, J. L. (2006a). A test of self-determination theory in the exercise domain. *Journal of Applied Social Psychology, 36*, 2240-2265.

¥Edmunds, J. K., Ntoumanis, N., and Duda, J. L. (2006b). Examining exercise dependence symptomatology from a self-determination perspective. *Journal of Health Psychology, 11*, 887-903.

¥Edmunds, J. K., Ntoumanis, N., and Duda, J. L. (2007). Adherence and well-being in overweight and obese patients referred to an exercise on prescription scheme: A self-determination theory perspective. *Psychology of Sport and Exercise, 8*, 722 – 740.

Fortier, M. S., Vallerand, R. J., and Guay, F. (1995). Academic motivation and school performance: Toward a structural model. *Contemporary Educational Psychology, 20*, 257-274.

Fox, K. R. (1990). *The Physical Self-perception Profile Manual*. Dekalb, IL: Office for Health Promotion, Northern Illinois University.

Fox, K. R. (1997). *The physical self: From motivation to well-being*. Champaign, IL: Human Kinetics.

Gagné, M. (2003). The role of autonomy support and autonomy orientation in prosocial behavior engagement. *Motivation and Emotion, 27*, 199-223.

Hagger, M. S., and Chatzisarantis, N. L. D. (2007). *Intrinsic motivation and self-determination in exercise and sport*. Champaign, IL: Human Kinetics.

¥Hagger, M. S., Chatzisarantis, N. L. D., and Harris, J. (2006). From psychological need satisfaction to intentional behavior: Testing a motivational sequence in two behavioral contexts. *Personality and Social Psychology Bulletin, 32*, 131 – 148.

Harter, S. (1982). The perceived competence scale for children. *Child Development, 53*, 87–97.

Harter, S. (1985). *Manual of the Self-Perception Profile for Children*. University of Denver, Denver, CO.

Iyengar, S. S., and DeVoe, S. E. (2003). Rethinking the value of choice: Considering cultural mediators of intrinsic motivation. In V. Murphy-Berman and J. Berman (Eds.), *Cross-Cultural Differences in Perspectives on the Self* (pp. 129-174). London: University of Nebraska Press.

Kerlinger, F. N. (1979). *Behavioural research: A conceptual approach*. New York, NY: Holt, Rinehart, and Winston.

¥Kowal, J., and Fortier, M. S. (1999). Motivational determinants of flow: Contributions from self-determination theory. *The Journal of Social Psychology, 139*, 355 – 368.

¥Kowal, J., and Fortier, M. S. (2000). Testing relationships from the hierarchical model of intrinsic and extrinsic motivation using flow as a motivational consequence. *Research Quarterly for Exercise and Sport, 71*, 171 – 181.

¥Levy, S. S., and Cardinal, B. J. (2004). Effects of a self-determination theory based mail-mediated intervention on adults' exercise behaviour. *American Journal of Health Promotion, 18*, 345-349.

¥Li, F. (1999). The exercise motivation scale: It's multifaceted structure and construct validity. *Journal of Applied Sport Psychology, 11,* 97-115.

¥Markland, D. (1999). Self-determination moderates the effects of perceived competence on intrinsic motivation in an exercise setting. *Journal of Sport and Exercise Psychology, 21,* 351-361.

¥Markland, D., and Hardy, L. (1997). On the factorial and construct validity of the intrinsic motivation inventory: Conceptual and operational concerns. *Research Quarterly for Exercise and Sport, 68,* 20-32.

Markland, D., and Ingledew, D. K. (2007). Exercise participation motives: A self-determination theory perspective. In M. Hagger and N. L. D. Chatzisarantis (Eds.), *Intrinsic Motivation and Self-Determination in Exercise and Sport* (pp. 23-34). Champaign, IL: Human Kinetics.

Marsh, H. W. (1997). The measurement of physical self-concept: A construct validation approach. In K. R. Fox (Ed.), *The physical self: From motivation to well-being* (pp. 27-58). Champaign, IL: Human Kinetics.

McAuley, E., Duncan, T., and Tammen, V. V. (1989). Psychometric properties of the Intrinsic Motivation Inventory in a competitive sport setting: A confirmatory factor analysis. *Research Quarterly for Exercise and Sport, 60,* 48-58.

McCready, M. L., and Long, B. C. (1985). Locus of control, attitudes towards physical activity, and exercise adherence. *Journal of Sport Psychology, 7,* 346-359.

Messick, S. (1995). Validity of psychological assessment: Validation of inferences from persons' responses and performances as scientific inquiry into score meaning. *American Psychologist, 50,* 741-749.

Mullan, E., Markland, D., and Ingledew, D. K. (1997). A graded conceptualisation of self-determination in the regulation of exercise behaviour: Development of a measure using confirmatory factor analytic procedures. *Personality and Individual Differences, 23,* 745-752.

¥Parfitt, G., Rose, E., and Markland, D. (2000). The effect of prescribed and preferred intensity exercise on psychological affect and the influence of baseline measures of affect. *Journal of Health Psychology, 5,* 231-240.

¥Peddle, C. J., Plotnikoff, R., Wild, C., Au, H., and Courneya, K. S. (in press). Medical demographic and psychosocial correlates of exercise in colorectal cancer survivors: An application of self- determination theory. *Supportive Care in Cancer.*

Pedhazur, E. J., and Pedhazur Schmlekin, L. (1991). *Measurement, design, and analysis: An integrated approach.* Hillsdale, NJ: Lawrence Erlbaum.

Reeve, J. (2002). Self-determination theory applied to educational settings. In E. L. Deci and R. M. Ryan (Eds.), *Handbook of self-determination research* (pp. 183-204). Rochester, NY: University of Rochester Press.

Reeve, J., and Sickenius, B. (1993). Development and validation of a brief measure of the 3 psychological needs underlying intrinsic motivation: The AFS scales. *Educational and Psychological Measurement, 54,* 506-515.

Richer, S. F., and Vallerand, R. J. (1998). Construction et validation de l'Échelle du sentiment d'appartenance sociale. *Revue européenne de psychologie appliquée, 48,* 129-137.

Rose, E. A., Markland, D., and Parfitt, G. (2001). The development and initial validation of the Exercise Causality Orientations Scale. *Journal of Sports Sciences, 19*, 445-462.

Rose, E. A., Parfitt, G. and Williams, S. (2005). Exercise causality orientations, behavioural regulation for exercise and stage of change for exercise: exploring their relationships. *Psychology of Sport and Exercise, 6*, 399-414.

Ryan, R. M. (1995). Psychological needs and the facilitation of integrative processes. *Journal of Personality, 63,* 397-428.

Ryan, R. M., and Deci, E. L. (2001). On happiness and human potentials: A review of research on hedonic and eudaimonic well-being. In S. Fiske (Ed.), *Annual Review of Psychology* (Vol. 52; pp. 141-166). Palo Alto, CA: Annual Reviews, Inc.

Ryan, R. M., and Deci, E. L. (2007). Self-regulation and the problem of human autonomy: Does psychology need choice, self-determination, and will? *Journal of Personality, 74*, 1557-1586.

Sallis, J. F., Grossman, R. M., Pinski, R. B., Patterson, T. L., and Nadar, P. R. (1987). The development of scales to measure social support for diet and exercise behaviours. *Preventive Medicine, 16*, 825-836.

Sheldon, K. M., Elliot, A. J., Kim, Y., and Kasser, T. (2001). What is satisfying about satisfying events? Testing 10 candidate psychological needs. *Journal of Personality and Social Psychology, 80,* 325-339.

Sheldon, K. M., Williams, G., and Joiner, T. (2003). *Self-determination theory in the clinic.* New Haven, CT: Yale University Press.

Stevens, S. S. (1946). On the theory of scales of measurement. *Science, 103*, 677-680.

[¥]Thørgersen-Ntoumani, C., and Ntoumanis, N. (2007). A self-determination theory approach to the study of body image concerns, self-presentation, and self-perceptions in a sample of aerobic instructors. *Journal of Health Psychology, 12, 301-315.*

Thorndike, R. L., and Hagen, E. (1955). *Measurement and evaluation in psychology and education.* New York, NY: Wiley.

Tobin, V. (2003). *Facilitating exercise behavior change: A self-determination theory and motivational interviewing perspective.* Unpublished doctoral dissertation. University of Wales, Bangor.

White, R. W. (1959). Motivation reconsidered: The concept of competence. *Psychological Review, 66*, 297-333.

[¥]Wilson, P. M., Rodgers, W. M., and Fraser, S. N. (2002a). Cross-validation of the revised motivation for physical activity measure in active women. *Research Quarterly for Exercise and Sport, 73*, 471-477.

[¥]Wilson, P. M., Rodgers, W. M., and Fraser, S. N. (2002b). Examining the psychometric properties of the Behavioral Regulation in Exercise Questionnaire. *Measurement in Physical Education and Exercise Science, 6*, 1-21.

[¥]Wilson, P. M., Rodgers, W. M., Blanchard, C. M., and Gessell, J. (2003). The relationship between psychological needs, self-determined motivation, exercise attitudes, and physical fitness. *Journal of Applied Social Psychology, 33*, 2373-2392.

Wilson, P. M., Rodgers, W. M., Fraser, S. N., and Murray, T. C. (2004). The relationship between exercise regulations and motivational consequences. *Research Quarterly for Exercise and Sport, 75*, 81-91.

¥Wilson, P. M., Rodgers, W. M., Loitz, C. C., and Scime, G. (2006). "It's who I am really!" The importance of integrated regulation in exercise contexts. *Journal of Applied Biobehavioral Research, 11*, 79-104.

¥Wilson, P. M., Longley, K., Muon, S., Rodgers, W. M., and Murray, T. C. (2006). Examining the contributions of perceived psychological need satisfaction to well-being in exercise. *Journal of Applied Biobehavioral Research, 11*, 243 – 264.

¥Wilson, P. M., Rogers, W. T., Rodgers, W. M., and Wild, C. (2006). The Psychological Need Satisfaction in Exercise Scale. *Journal of Sport and Exercise Psychology, 28*, 79-104.

¥Wilson, P. M., Mack, D. E., and Blanchard, C. (in press). The role of perceived psychological need satisfaction in exercise related affect. *Hellenic Journal of Psychology*.

¥Wilson, P. M., Mack, D. E., and Lightheart, V. (in press). How important are basic psychological needs to women's well-being? In J. P Coulter (Ed.), *Progress in Exercise and Women's Health Research*. Hauppauge, NY: Nova Science.

¥Wilson, P. M., Mack, D. E., Muon, S. and LeBlanc, M. (2007). What role does psychological need satisfaction play in motivating exercise participation? In L. A. Chiang (Ed.), *Motivation of Exercise and Physical Activity* (pp.1-18). Hauppauge, NY: Nova Science

¥Wilson, P. M., and Muon, S. (in press). Psychometric properties of the Exercise Identity Scale in a university sample. *International Journal of Sport and Exercise Psychology*.

¥Vlachopoulos, S. P. (2007). Psychometric evaluation of the Basic Psychological Needs in Exercise Scale in Community Exercise Programs: A cross validation approach. *Hellenic Journal of Psychology, 4,* 52-74.

¥Vlachopoulos, S. P., and Michailidou, S. (2006). Development and initial validation of a measure of autonomy, competence, and relatedness in exercise: The Basic Psychological Needs in Exercise Scale. *Measurement in Physical Education and Exercise Sciences, 10*, 179 – 201.

¥Vlachopoulos, S. P. (in press). The Basic Psychological Needs in Exercise Scale: Measurement invariance over gender. *Structural Equation Modeling*.

¥Vlachopoulos, S. P., and Neikou, E. (in press) . A prospective study of the relationships of autonomy, competence, and relatedness with exercise attendance, adherence and dropout. *Journal of Sports Medicine and Physical Fitness*.

Index

F

J

K

L

M

P

S

T

U

V